Toward a New Definition of Health
PSYCHOSOCIAL DIMENSIONS

Current Topics in Mental Health

Series Editors: Paul I. Ahmed
U.S. Office of International Health, H.E.W.
and
Stanley C. Plog
Plog Research, Inc.

STATE MENTAL HOSPITALS: What Happens When They Close
Edited by Paul I. Ahmed and Stanley C. Plog

COPING WITH PHYSICAL ILLNESS
Edited by Rudolf H. Moos

THE PRINCIPLES AND TECHNIQUES OF MENTAL
HEALTH CONSULTATION
Edited by Stanley C. Plog and Paul I. Ahmed

TOWARD A NEW DEFINITION OF HEALTH
Edited by Paul I. Ahmed and George V. Coelho

THE YEAR 2000 AND MENTAL RETARDATION
Edited by Stanley C. Plog and Miles Santamour

Toward a New Definition of Health

PSYCHOSOCIAL DIMENSIONS

Edited by

Paul I. Ahmed

Public Health Advisor
U.S. Office of International Health
Department of Health, Education, and Welfare
Rockville, Maryland
and
Lecturer, Department of Health Education
University College
University of Maryland
College Park, Maryland

and

George V. Coelho

Senior Social Scientist
Office of the Assistant Director
  For Children and Youth
National Institute of Mental Health
Rockville, Maryland

With the Assistance of

Aliza Kolker

Assistant Professor
George Mason University
Fairfax, Virginia

PLENUM PRESS · NEW YORK AND LONDON

Library of Congress Cataloging in Publication Data

Main entry under title:

Toward a new definition of health.

(Current topics in mental health)
Includes index.
1. Medicine and psychology. 2. Health. 3. Social medicine. I. Ahmed, Paul I. II. Coelho, George V. III. Kolker, Aliza.

R726.5.T68   362.1'04'2   79-9066
ISBN-13: 978-1-4613-2993-0   e-ISBN-13: 978-1-4613-2991-6
DOI: 10.1007/ 978-1-4613-2991-6

© 1979 Plenum Press, New York
Softcover reprint of the hardcover 1st edition 1979
A Division of Plenum Publishing Corporation
227 West 17th Street, New York, N.Y. 10011

To the late
Margaret Mead (1901–1978)
a friend
and a master anthropologist

Contributors

Paul I. Ahmed, M.A., L.L.B., Public Health Advisor, Office of International Health, U.S. Department of Health, Education and Welfare, Rockville, Maryland, and Lecturer, Department of Health Education, University College, University of Maryland, College Park, Maryland

Peter G. Bourne, M.D., Coordinator, United Nations Development Program, International Drinking Water and Sanitation Decade, United Nations, New York, New York. Former Special Assistant to the President for Health Issues

Rosalynn Carter, Honorary Chairperson, The President's Commission on Mental Health (1977–1978), The White House, Washington, D.C.

George V. Coelho, Ph.D., Senior Social Scientist, Office of the Assistant Director for Children and Youth, National Institute of Mental Health, Rockville, Maryland

Henry P. David, PhD., Director, Transnational Family Research Institute, Bethesda, Maryland

Robert Davis, Public Health Consultant to the Office of International Health, U.S. Department of Health, Education and Welfare, Rockville, Maryland

S. Paul Ehrlich, Jr., M.D., Deputy Director General, Pan American Health Organization, Washington, D. C.

Horacio Fabrega, Jr., M.D., Professor of Psychiatry and Professor of Anthropology, Western Psychiatric Institute and Clinic, University of Pittsburgh, Pittsburgh, Pennsylvania

Renee White Fraser, Ph. D., Visiting Lecturer, University of Southern California, Los Angeles, California

James S. Gordon, M.D., Research Psychiatrist, Center for Studies of Child and Family Mental Health, National Institute of Mental Health, Rockville, Maryland

Robert J. Havighurst, Ph.D., Emeritus Professor of Education and Human Development, Department of Behavioral Sciences, University of Chicago, Chicago, Illinois

Stephen P. Hersh, M.D., Director, Division of Children and Adolescent Services, St. Elizabeth's Hospital, Washington, D.C.

James S. House, Ph.D., Research Scientist, Institute for Social Research, University of Michigan, Ann Arbor, Michigan

Mark F. Jackman, Research Associate, Department of Sociology, Duke University, Durham, North Carolina

Deidre S. Klassen, Research Associate, The Greater Kansas City Mental Health Foundation, Kansas City, Missouri

Arthur Kleinman, M.D., M.A. Associate Professor and Head, Division of Social and Cross-Cultural Psychiatry, Department of Psychiatry and Behavioral Sciences, School of Medicine, University of Washington, Seattle, Washington

Aliza Kolker, Ph.D., Assistant Professor of Sociology, Department of Sociology, George Mason University, Fairfax, Virginia

Margaret Mead, Ph.D., Late former curator, Museum of Natural History, New York, New York

Rudolf H. Moos, Ph.D., Professor and Director, Social Ecology Laboratory, Department of Psychiatry, Stanford University School of Medicine, Palo Alto, California

Karen S. O'Connor, R.N.S., Director of Education and Research, Rainbow Mental Health Center, Kansas City, Kansas

William A. O'Connor, Ph.D., Associate Professor, Department of Psychiatry, School of Medicine, University of Missouri, Kansas City, Missouri

Jonas Robitscher, J.D., M.D., Henry R. Luce Professor of Law and the Behavioral Sciences, Emory University Schools of Law and Medicine, Atlanta, Georgia

Jerry L. Weaver, Social Science Analyst, Agency for International Development, Washington, D.C.

Allan Young, Ph.D., Associate Professor, Department of Anthropology, Case Western Reserve University, Cleveland, Ohio

Laurie Zivetz, M.P.H., Public Health Researcher, Research Triangle Institute, Office for International Programs, Research Triangle Park, Durham, North Carolina

Foreword

It is generally recognized today that the United States has a need to contribute to the improvement of health throughout the world. The need stems from the interrelationships that exist between the health of Americans and the health status of the rest of the people on "Spaceship Earth." Disease does not respect national boundaries, and the frequency of travel and trade between countries increases each year. It further relates to the opportunities found in international settings to help solve health problems more effectively and efficiently. This includes the unique human resources that are found throughout the world as well as certain natural ecological conditions that cannot be duplicated in the United States.

The United States also has a responsibility to contribute to improved health status. Our tradition of humanitarianism alone supports such a responsibility, but our comparative wealth of technical and financial resources dictates a requirement to participate. Modern political realities define relationships between developed and developing countries that will not allow us to isolate ourselves from the compelling health needs of a majority of the world's population.

The difficult question is not *if* we should be involved in international health but *how* we should participate. Unfortunately, recent history does not provide any positive guidelines to follow. In most cases we have followed a natural instinct to export to other countries what we know best, and what we also think is best. This is the Western model of institutionally centered health care delivery, including all the advanced technology and specialized manpower that accompanies a modern health center.

For most of the countries of the developing world the model does not work. It tends to concentrate extremely limited resources in support of a hospital or similar institution that is accessible to only a small percentage of the population. Further, the technology and manpower associated with the institution have frequently been developed and trained to deal with health problems of only limited importance in developing countries. There are numerous examples of countries that spend 90% of their limited health budgets on maintenance of an institution that at best can serve 10% of the population. Prevalent conditions, such as infant diarrhea and tropical diseases, are all but completely ignored. The majority of rural residents and the urban poor frequently have no access to any form of modern health care.

The international health community has only recently formally recognized this situation. In 1974, the World Health Assembly adopted its first resolution calling for the establishment of basic health services to serve the needs of the estimated one billion people in the world without access to health services. In 1976, Dr. Halfdan Mahler, the director-general of the World Health Organization advanced the goal of "health for all by the year 2000."

This sudden shift in the definition of the world's health problem coincides with the entry of the People's Republic of China on the international scene, and their membership in the WHO. After over 20 years of isolation from the community of nations, stories of their successful conquest of major disease problems began to spread. The barefoot doctor, traditional medicine, and local community development and involvement seemed to be the necessary ingredients for this country of over 700 million people ravaged by poverty and disease.

Their success with health programs represented the antithesis of the Western model. It appeared to offer a possibility to achieve rapid advances in health without major capital or human investments. It relied on the simplest of technologies and reached its objectives by broadly distributing responsibility for health rather than centralizing services and facilities.

The traditional Communist and Socialist countries found the Chinese approach particularly disturbing. Their health model is strongly centralized, with all resources distributed from the top. For many years they had extolled the virtues of their system and found the curiosity and enthusiasm for the concepts surrounding the Chinese model a threat. The resulting sense of competitiveness led to the International Conference on Primary Health Care hosted by the Soviets in Alma Ata to demonstrate the purported advantages of their approach.

Thus, while competing concepts capture the attention of the health community, the methods of establishing basic health services and of reaching the goal set by WHO are still not entirely clear. It goes without saying that the patterns of the past must be discarded. It implies that a country's particular characteristics, including its unique health situation, must be the primary determinant. It also suggests that the donor–recipient relationship that has characterized relationships between developed and developing countries must be changed. This necessarily places more responsibility on the developed country to understand those characteristics that define particular health needs and the possible approaches to meeting those needs. It demands of the developing country a capacity to recognize and deal with its priority problems without the diversion or attraction of advanced technology or other cost-prohibitive methods.

Cooperation and collaboration must now characterize relationships between developed and developing countries. Political realities demand this partnership, but contributions to health improvement cannot be expected without a true sense of mutual respect and participation.

Social and cultural barriers to this partnership must be recognized and dealt with in a forthright manner. The Office of International Health in HEW, the Agency of International Development, and the White House now seem to sense this need. This volume, edited by Drs. Paul Ahmed, of the Office of International Health, and George V. Coelho of the National Institute of Mental Health, can make a major contribution by providing the framework for dealing with these barriers to cooperation and by sensitizing health workers to their existence. It can serve as a most useful guide in understanding the forces that must be considered in working with our colleagues in less fortunate parts of the world.

S. PAUL EHRLICH, JR.

Preface

The need for a new definition of health, going beyond the mere absence of disease, has been recognized for some time. Today, health planning and practice encompass, in addition to the treatment of physiological disease, mechanisms of coping with psychological stress, prevention through environmental and life-style changes, the incorporation of different cultural perspectives, etc. This book presents several important original contributions on these issues, many by well-known authorities.

These contributions are organized into five thematic sections: a reconceptualization of the models of health and illness, specific factors affecting disease and illness, health needs of some special groups in the population, methods for analyzing health needs, and future policy issues and implications of the new definitions of health and illness. It should be noted that because of space limitations, these themes are not treated comprehensively in this volume; rather, the papers illustrate various aspects of the issues.

Part I sets the stage by stating the need to expand the definitions of health and illness to include cultural, psychosocial, and environmental dimensions. The authors contend that future improvements in health care will come primarily through such a reorientation rather than through intensive scientific and technological developments in biomedicine.

Part II focuses on some specific examples of nonbiological factors affecting health. These examples include the contribution of occupational stress to several common diseases, the importance of the socioecological environment of the individual, the sociopsychological problems entailed in cancer, and the professional and cultural biases affecting the diagnosis and treatment of mental illness.

Part III deals with the health needs of some specific groups, particularly age and sex groups. The importance of the family as the central unit for diagnosing, preventing, and treating illness is emphasized, and the health needs of families at different stages in the life cycle are considered. In addition, the special health needs of ethnic minorities in the United States are examined.

Part IV deals with the methodology of health analysis. The articles in this section deal with measuring and assessing some of the factors referred to in the previous sections. In particular, methodologies for assessing the individual's socioecological environment, the sociopsychological climate of family and work, and the needs of the health sectors of the developing countries are presented.

Part V, which opens with a statement by Mrs. Rosalynn Carter and ends with an analysis by Dr. Peter Bourne, presents the policy implications of a broader definition of health. The chapters in this section call for a more humanistic approach to mental health services so as to "strengthen the whole person in his total environment"; for incorporating the cultural perspectives of client populations into the delivery of health services in developing countries; and for restructuring our health concerns to emphasize lifestyle, environmental, and ethical factors.

The authors include specialists in the mental health and the behavioral science field, pragmatic experts who have field experiences in international health projects and researchers who have investigated the impact of contemporary social and urban phenomena on health-related behavior and human development.

They were invited to present their findings and views as forcefully as possible in order to sharpen the issues dramatically and even controversially. The authors and topics selected do not cover all the pertinent issues. It is hoped that this collection of articles will stimulate critical thinking and in-depth studies that will be replicated in different cultures and population groups. It is expected that such systematic research will be planned with the cooperation of different professional, civic, and public policy groups.

We are deeply grateful to the contributors, who showed enviable enthusiasm in preparing their articles and extraordinary patience in cooperating with the editors in completing revisions within deadlines. For the delays in the process of submitting the final manuscript, only the editors are responsible.

Toward a New Definition of Health is intended for a diverse audience. This volume should be useful as a textbook or as a collection of supplementary readings in courses in health sciences or in behavioral sciences offered to students of nursing, medicine, and public health. In particular, students and teachers of health planning, social medicine, family medicine, community health, and sociology of health will find these selections useful. In addition, since most of the selections have been presented in relatively nontechnical language, the book should be of interest to those members of the general public who are interested in broad issues of health and illness.

It would be impossible in this space to acknowledge all the dedicated colleagues and associates who have contributed to this book indirectly, through their influence on the authors. We wish to acknowledge in particular, however, the efforts of Dr. Aliza Kolker, of George Mason University, who shared with us the responsibility for integrating the selections and for writing the introductions to the various parts. She devoted considerable time and skill in the final organization of this volume and brought a broad sociological perspective to the dicussions of major themes and issues presented by the authors.

Special thanks are due to Robert de Caires, Jerry Weaver, Ken Farr, Lynn Beamer, Bob Davis, Chris Rosel, Thomasino Borkman, Tee Guidotti, and others who reviewed various articles in this volume. Thanks are due to Rochelle, Irene, and Paul Jr. of the Ahmed family, for providing support through long hours of work that the editors put into the preparation of this book.

Finally, we appreciate the support services provided by Martha Johnston, Ginnie Cavanaugh, Patti Jacklin, and Jane Montgomery, who carefully prepared various portions of the manuscript for the publisher.

PAUL I. AHMED
GEORGE V. COELHO

Introduction: Toward a Less Agonized Reappraisal

Margaret Mead

At home and abroad, in the industrialized countries and in those countries in the first flush of nationhood, we are going through an agonized reappraisal, a reappraisal that matches, in its intensity and lack of balance, the extravagant hopes with which we entered the postwar era in the late 1940s. There was then a new ethic that included all the peoples of the world as rightful participants in the wonders of technology and insisted that all those who had benefited as custodians had a duty to share the bounty they had experienced. The breadth and extravagance of the vision matched the extraordinary advances of the wartime era that had ushered in the electronic revolution, the capacity to produce nuclear power, synthetic materials of all sorts, instant communication, lightning calculations, and the ability to venture into space and plumb the mysteries of genetics. As this new technology had made us into one intercommunicating world, so also it could solve the age-old problems of hunger and thirst, backbreaking, soul-destroying labor, ignorance and narrowness of understanding, selfishness, and greed. It was also believed that the transformation of the whole world need not be accompanied by the dislocations, the exploitations, and the vast human misery that had marked the industrializing of Europe and America.

We brought to this vision of change our hopes in technology and also our new knowledge of human behavior, of the importance of culture, of the need to take into account the traditional behaviors of the past while preparing to educate children in the necessary behaviors of the future. Faith in the efficacy of heavy industry, urbanization, massive campaigns to eradicate epidemic and endemic diseases was counterbalanced by attempts to tap indigenous strengths—the *madrichim* of Israel and the all-purpose workers of India were the precursors of the much-hailed "barefoot doctors" of modern China. The interest in community organization, reliance on local skills and local forms of political organization was pitted against the reliance on the introduction of types of large-scale industrialization that drew millions to the cities and depopulated the neglected countryside.

And for a period, the thinking world was intoxicated by the apparent success of what the generous perceived as sharing the wealth and skills of the industrialized world and the Western-educated, aspiring young elites of the new nations perceived as taking—with modern cities, airlines, hospitals equipped with X rays, universities dazzling in their architecture—their rightful and long-withheld place in the sun. While the unexpected consequences of the spread of modern medicine and modern technology began to overwhelm an unprepared world, the gap between expectation and fulfillment grew also. Epidemic diseases were brought under control, babies lived but parents died, and the disproportions between those who needed education, medical care, and a place in the productive professions and those who had to manage and develop the new kinds of economies grew. Today, in both the developing and the developed world, we find a comparable disillusionment with our achievements and a comparable movement to repudiate everything that has been accomplished by modern technology and modern medicine. In the United States, as in the deliberations of the parliaments of nations that only yesterday were nonliterate and dependent upon epidemics to maintain a balance between population and food supply, there is a wholesale repudiation of everything connected with the scientific revolution on which our contemporary life-styles have been built.

Those who look at concrete results—the control of epidemic diseases, the growth in literacy and higher education, the enormous increase in access to information, as airplanes have replaced foot travel and beasts of burden and satellites the "bush telegraph"—still feel the surge of excitement or progress that possessed the world in the immediate post-World War II period. In the most remote villages, babies live who would have died, mothers live who would have died, some young people have learned to read, and the impaired sight of the mature can be supplemented by spectacles, even as modern communications bring them something worth reading. The new cities have beauty and style, water piped into the villages replace the hour-long journey to a distant spring, a journey of minutes has replaced the paddling necessary when the wind died. From one point of view, it is as if a giant handkerchief had wiped the runny noses of all the babies in the world.

But from our sharpened perception of contrast, we see the disastrous consequences of many of the policies that were too partial and too ill-conceived, as the newer nations fall into debt, as the poor get poorer, as the number of poor is magnified, even as the proportion of those in need may be reduced. As we focused, in the late 1940s and 1950s, on the gap between the industrialized and subsistence economies of the world, on a gap that could be closed, we have come to focus, with equal one-sidedness, on the way that gap has widened. As the focus in the 1950s led to a too rapid repudiation of traditional culture and indigenous strength, too great a willingness to replace human labor with machines, too great a reliance on sources of power and food imported over great distances, so the present emphasis on the need to rely on traditional cultural skills and indigenous natural resources is going to extremes. We are in serious danger of throwing the baby out with the bath water—a metaphor based on the technology (water collected in tubs and the wanton waste of water used only once).

In the disillusionment of their present assessment of the relative status of rich and poor, developed and undeveloped, privileged and unprivileged, we may be able to introduce answers to the insights that come from the scientific study of human behavior to balance our extraordinary burst of discovery in physics, chemistry, and biology. Where we have filled the environment with danger in our rush to find new artificial forms of agriculture, of the management of disease, or the organization of towns and cities, the study of human behavior, the rereliance on traditional strengths may be presented as a polarized alternative; where reliance on science in the past has produced only trouble, repudiation of the natural sciences and the technology based upon them can be presented with the same blind enthusiasm.

But this is not necessary. The alternative to Western plumbing is a return to carrying water from the well. The alternative to electricity, to light where there was darkness, is not a return to a coconut leaf flare and the dim light of an open fire beside which no one can read, but to new sources of power—local, inexhaustible instead of imported, expensive, and exhaustible from electricity plants. The alternative to reliance on vaccines and new drugs of high specificity is not a return to decimating epidemics every generation and endemic diarrhea from contaminated water. The alternative to single simplistic solutions to population control by pills or IUDs is not the large families of rural and proletarian poor that were intended to compensate for those who died. New respect for the language of one's forefathers, although it may be spoken by a mere handful of people and give little access to the wisdom of the wider world, does not mean a repudiation of languages in which millions can speak easily to each other, by radio and satellite.

We need repudiate nothing that we have learned, as we stress the one-sidedness, the nearsightedness, the narrow self-seeking search for profit and political power that has flourished all over the world. The energy crisis, the disillusionment with the gap between hope and fulfillment gives us a new chance to bring health and knowledgeable participation to all the peoples in the world, the poor within the gates and the poor who before were doomed to always remaining outside. As the energy crisis, the growing pollution crisis, the proliferation of nuclear waste and material, and the appreciation of the gap between the well-being that we might attain for everyone and the misery of two-thirds of the world grow, there is a new chance to use all that has been learned about the advantages of localization of food supply, utilization of traditional skills, health practices that are congruent with the behavior and resources of each people. If we use this new opportunity widely, use all that has been learned in three decades of work with living peoples in the field, with all that has been learned in the laboratory, we can take a genuine step forward rather than prepare for another pendulum swing.

Contents

Chapter 5

Psychosocial Factors and Health: New Program Directions.......... 87

World Health Organization

Chapter 6

The Role of Indigenous Medicine in WHO's Definition of Health. 113

Paul I. Ahmed and Aliza Kolker

Part II: Psychosocial Factors in Disease: Some Specific Examples

Chapter 12

**Toward a Definition of Health Risks for Ethnic Minorities:
The Case of Hypertension and Heart Disease** 255

Jerry L. Weaver

Chapter 13

The Social and Psychological Aspects of Family Planning 269

Laurie Zivetz

Chapter 14

Healthy Family Functioning: Cross-Cultural Perspectives 281

Henry P. David

Chapter 15

**Urban Health Services in Developing Countries:
Culture, Technology, and Politics** 321

Paul I. Ahmed and Robert Davis

Part IV: Methodology for Health Analysis

Chapter 16

Evaluating Family and Work Settings 337

Rudolf H. Moos

Chapter 17

Evaluating Human Service Programs: Psychosocial Methods 361

William A. O'Connor, Deidre S. Klassen, and Karen S. O'Connor

Chapter 18

Health Sector Assessment 389

Paul I. Ahmed and Aliza Kolker

Part V: Implications for Practitioners and Policy Planners

Chapter 19

Toward a More Caring Society

Rosalynn Carter

Chapter 20

Mental Health Services: Alternatives Now and for the Future

James S. Gordon

Chapter 21

International Health Planning: Psychosocial Issues and Implications for Development Assistance

Paul I. Ahmed and Renee White Fraser

Chapter 22

Health Care in the Year 2000 443

Peter G. Bourne

Dimensions of Health and Illness: Toward an Integrated Model

Introduction

The six chapters in this section emphasize the need to incorporate new dimensions into the prevailing definitions of illness and health. Although they employ numerous specific examples, all these articles focus on overall conceptualizations rather than on specific diseases. The different authors show how psychological, social, and cultural factors contribute to all phases of disease—its etiology, its manifestations, its treatment, and its prevention.

The first chapter, by Ahmed, Kolker, and Coelho, reviews the background and limitations of the preponderantly medical definition of health, and the rationale for expanding the definition to include nonmedical dimensions. The authors point out that the medical profession has traditionally defined health as merely the absence of disease, and disease as an observable deviation from a biostatistical norm derived within a given historical experience and language system. They call attention to individual and cultural variations in the perceptions and conceptions of "sickness" and "wellness" held by given population groups. They further contend that both these concepts are more usefully viewed as complex behavioral entities consisting of psychological and sociocultural dimensions in addition to the biological ones.

Contending that the new model provides useful guidelines for preventive action, the authors outline several socioenvironmental and behavioral forces that contribute to disease. They indicate that these forces may be largely controlled through preventive social, educational, and economic policies and through personal changes in life-styles. Thus, the most effective means to *promote* health, they claim, is through nonmedical preventive action, although the role of medical treatment should not be ignored. Echoing other calls for reforming the health care system (see Section V), they reiterate the need to decentralize and "humanize" health care and to place greater emphasis on socioenvironmental prevention.

In the second chapter, Fabrega discusses the complex relationship between biological and cultural factors in the perception of illness and disease. In modern society, he contends, *disease* is a biomedical category, defined in terms of undesirable chemical or physical changes in the body's functioning. The interpretation of the organic changes, however, is culturally determined. The *illness* episode is experienced subjectively by the individual and by those around him.

Fabrega mentions several adaptive functions of illness for individuals and for groups. These functions include calling attention to malfunctioning elements so corrective action (treatment) may be taken, sanctioning nonfulfillment of social roles, contributing to natural selection, and enhancing the functional unity of the group. Symbolically, the phenomenon of illness is linked to questions about the meaning of life and death and about the individual's relation to society.

Furthermore, Fabrega continues, the group's formal body of knowledge about illness (its medical taxonomy), as well as its informal (folk) body of knowledge, are products of the cumulative cultural experience of the group and shape its medical care system. Thus, illness is a category of behavior appropriately studied by behavioral scientists and exhibiting wide cultural variations, although it is delimited by invariable biological structures and processes that are universal among human and nonhuman primates alike.

According to Fabrega, the medical taxonomy of modern society, anchored exclusively in a biomedical frame of reference, deals only with disease as defined by "objective" changes in the organism. It therefore deprives individuals of the means for "interpreting" illness and death, for integrating them into their everyday context, and for coping with them psychologically and socially. Conversely, the fact that people are commonly sensitized only to "illness" (i.e., the presence of behaviorally compelling "symptoms" such as pain or incapacity) but not to "disease" (i.e., the presence or potential onset of certain biological processes) presents additional problems. There is little motivation to seek treatment or prevention in the absence of behavioral "symptoms", and thus the full benefits of the biomedical frame of reference are not achieved. In closing, Fabrega calls for an integration of the behavioral study of illness with the biological study of disease: "Illness constitutes a behavioral alteration that is physiologically and chemically grounded but socially and culturally conditioned."

In the third chapter, Kleinman further explores the sociocultural dimensions of effective care. Reiterating the conceptual distinction between *disease* (the underlying biological or psychological malfunctioning) and *illness* (the culturally determined reaction to disease by the patient and by those around him), Kleinman cites case studies from his previous work in China and in the United States to illustrate variations in subjective meanings assigned to biological symptoms. Thus, for example, in Taiwan both patients and doctors categorize most psychological disorders as medical rather than psychiatric malfunctionings. Consequently, they will ignore psychological symptoms such as depression, and seek medical treatment only for somatic symptoms, although the latter may be psychologically caused.

While the ethnomedical approach typically concentrates on the cultural construction of illness in other societies, Kleinman argues for a similar approach to the study of models of disease in our own society. He reminds us of the discrepancies between the biomedical model espoused by medical practitioners and the popular model held by patients and their families. Since the semantic meaning applied to illness determines the course of action taken by those involved, the failure of the physician to confront the personal and social meaning of disease may seriously undermine effective care.

Kleinman calls for the integration of personally and socially relevant meanings, alongside the biomedical meanings, into both medical science and health care. He offers guidelines for eliciting the patient's and his family's "clinical reality" as a basis for prescribing effective care. However, he realistically notes the political difficulties that will stand in the way of any extensive restructuring of the health professions.

The fourth chapter, by Young, contrasts the drawbacks of the Western medical model with the concrete, although limited, advantages of indigenous medical systems in traditional societies. Young discusses several dimensions of medical rationality. A key dimension is efficacy, i.e., the ability to produce desired results (empirical efficacy), or to organize and manage the circumstances connected with illness (symbolic efficacy). He points out that indigenous medical systems are often nearly as empirically efficacious as Western medicine. He offers several hypotheses to account for this efficacy, including the self-limiting nature of many sicknesses and the common practice of using Western medicine only as a last resort after traditional medical treatment has failed and the case is more or less hopeless. Furthermore, indigenous medical practices are often symbolically efficacious in that they enable people to manage sickness episodes and to orient themselves to threats of illness within the cultural context.

In discussing the limitations of Western medicine, Young points out that while Western medical science is dominated by scientific standards of proof, Western medical practice does not meet the same standards of scientific rationality. This is so because clinical decisions are often constrained by insufficient information and by extraneous considerations such as professional interests. Another drawback of Western medicine is the low productivity inherent in the curative approach—i.e., the fact that it provides adequate medical services primarily for the elite, while contributing little toward optimizing the health of the greatest number of people.

While Young does not propose any concrete alternatives to the Western medical system, he notes the existing juxtaposition in many societies of Western and traditional medicine. He points out that a practical division of labor and an interchange of ideas and practices between them may be advantageous to all the people served.

In the fifth chapter, a paper prepared by the World Health Organization (WHO) for the World Health Assembly in 1977, the writers summarize briefly what is known today about the role of sociological, psychological, and cultural factors in the incidence, the course, and the outcome of disease, and propose guidelines for applying this knowledge to WHO's health programs and policies. For example, we know that low socioeconomic status is correlated with shorter life expectancy; that rapid cultural and social change is correlated with stress and hence with hypertension and cardiovascular disorders; that the severity of mental illness and the probability of recovery depend on the degree of cohesive support forthcoming from the patient's family; and that alcoholism and drug addiction are influenced by psychological, social, and cultural factors.

The authors outline the implications of this knowledge for health policy and practice. They point out the need for training health workers in the behavioral sciences, for incorporating the beliefs and practices of indigenous communities into the health care process, and for coordinating medical efforts with efforts in other sectors in order to achieve maximum benefits for health.

The sixth chapter, by Ahmed and Kolker, asserts that in order to meet WHO's goal for world health, a new approach is needed to health planning in developing countries. This approach, based on Young's thesis presented in the fourth chapter, consists in shifting the emphasis of health delivery to the level of the rural community and in integrating traditional health practitioners into the health delivery system. The WHO's goal, originally set in 1946, asserted the fundamental right of all people to "a state of complete physical, mental and social well-being." While the authors admit that this goal is frankly idealistic, they point out that massive international aid in the past three decades has failed to bring the health level of developing countries to that of industrialized nations.

The reasons for this failure, the authors indicate, include the relatively permanent shortage of trained manpower, the staggering costs of Western technology even when it is nominally free, the variety of new and unanticipated problems created by Western technology, and perhaps most crucially, the cultural incompatibility between the Western medical model and native medical traditions.

The authors discuss the limitations of the Western medical model—in particular its tendency, in its more extreme manifestations, to exclude the cultural, psychological, and social dimensions of health. By contrast, non-Western medical systems view health as a state of harmony between the body, the soul, and the cosmos.

The authors underline some often-overlooked functions of traditional medicine, including convenience, affordability, the relief of anxiety, the involvement of family and community, and mediation between the worlds of tradition and modernity. They call for integrating the resources of traditional medicine into the health delivery system in order to bridge the gap between the goal—optimal health for all people—and the currently available means.

1

Toward a New Definition of Health: An Overview

Paul I. Ahmed, Aliza Kolker, and George V. Coelho

Recent developments in medicine, in mental health, and in the social sciences have called attention to the fact that the concepts "disease" and "health" can no longer be adequately defined in purely medical terms of the presence or absence of "symptoms." We know, for example, that disease may exist in the absence of observed symptoms; that the incidence of disease in human groups is influenced by such demographic characteristics as age, social class, ethnicity, place of residence; and that the very labels "disease" and "health" are culturally determined. Similarly, we know that to promote the health of its people, society must do more than treat known diseases. It must upgrade environmental and social conditions, enable people to live a healthier, less stressful life-style, and focus on promoting the well-being of the "whole person" in the context of his social network.

This book presents several original contributions that address various issues involved in broadening the definitions of health and of disease. The articles, spanning both research reports and theoretical discussions, analyze key social, psychological, environmental, and cultural factors that contribute to health. They emphasize the need to restructure health care to take into account the multidimensionality of illness and of health. In this over-

Paul I. Ahmed • Office of International Health, U.S. Department of Health, Education and Welfare, Rockville, Maryland 20857. Aliza Kolker • Department of Sociology, George Mason University, Fairfax, Virginia 22030. George V. Coelho • Office of the Assistant Director for Children and Youth, National Institute of Mental Health, Rockville, Maryland 20857.

view we will briefly review some of the major contributions of medical sociology and of environmental medicine to the understanding, planning, and delivery of better health care.

The Biomedical Definition: A Brief History

The functions and dysfunctions of the biomedical model of health have been described many times, including in the chapters by Fabrega, by Ahmed and Fraser, and by Ahmed and Kolker in this volume. Here we do not propose to discuss this model in detail but rather to review briefly its development in order to gain a better understanding of its limitations.

The ancient Greek view of health, as formulated by Hippocrates (c. 400 B.C.), stated that human well-being is influenced by the totality of environmental factors: living habits, climate, and the quality of air, water, and food (see Cockerham, 1978). Health results from the equilibrium among the body's four humors (blood, phlegm, black bile, and yellow bile) and from the harmony among the body, the environment, and the person's living habits. Illness results from the disruption of this balance. This "holistic" view has persisted to this day in the folk tradition of many cultures, including the Navajos, for example (see Twaddle & Hessler, 1977). In Europe, however, following the Cartesian revolution in the 17th century, the workings of body and mind came to be separated, with the body viewed as an intricate machine, "disease as the breakdown of the machine, and the doctor's task as the repair of the machine" (Engel, 1977, p. 131).

The positivist view of disease as a deviation from a biochemical norm reached its heyday in 19th-century Europe with the formulation of the germ theory of disease and with the concomitant advances in immunology, pathology, and surgical techniques. These advances in medical technology, coupled with earlier advances in public health, including cleaning up water supplies and providing sanitary living conditions, caused spectacular breakthroughs in health. With the etiology, prevention, and treatment of communicable diseases such as typhoid, cholera, and scarlet fever now understood, morbidity and mortality rates in Europe and North America declined significantly. In fact, so successful did this approach seem that even the functioning and the malfunctioning of the human *mind* came to be viewed positivistically, with the field of psychiatry developing as a subspeciality within medicine.

For all the remarkable successes of the "biomedical" approach, however, many contemporary observers feel that it may be nearing the point of diminishing marginal returns (see Bourne, Chapter 22, this volume; Engel, 1977). For several decades, social scientists as well as health planners and practitioners have perceived the need to return to the premodern conception of disease as a sociocultural phenomenon, and of health as a multidimensional *process* involving the well-being of the whole person in the context of his environment. In the rest of this overview we will consider some social, psychological, and environmental issues in the promotion and preservation of health. We will not attempt an exhaustive, systematic conceptualization, a task beyond the scope of our present work. By highlighting (incompletely though the case may be) what is known about nonmedical dimensions of health, we hope to set the background for the subsequent chapters in this volume.

What Is Health?: Illness and Health as Biosocial Concepts

"A healthy person is someone who has been inadequately studied" (Dr. Alexander Burgess, quoted in Twaddle & Hessler, 1977, p. 96).

To understand the limitations of the biomedical conception of health, we will borrow from sociological theory a distinction among three dimensions of nonhealth: disease, illness, and sickness. Although these terms are often used interchangeably in everyday language, sociologists commonly distinguish among them both logically and empirically (see, for example, Szasz, 1977; Twaddle & Hessler, 1977).

1. *Disease* refers to organic malfunctioning, to objectively measurable disorders. The concept of "disease" underlies the biomedical model mentioned above and is analyzed in detail by Fabrega (1974), Twaddle and Hessler (1977), and others. The study, diagnosis, and treatment of disease has been the traditional focus of modern medicine.

Notwithstanding its incontrovertible usefulness, this concept has serious limitations, notably the lack of objective standards of organic performance against which deviations may be measured and the ambiguity and cultural determination of what constitutes a "disorder." These limitations are particularly glaring in the case of mental illness. Because of the historical accident of psychiatry's development as a subspecialty within medicine, mental illness has come to be conceptualized as analogous to physical illness: an observable deviation from a firmly established "norm." The stigmatizing implications of such a positivistic assumption are only now being fully recognized, as Robitscher (Chapter 10, this volume) elucidates (see also Engel, 1977; Szasz, 1977).

Many writers feel that the overwhelming focus of both medicine and psychiatry on "disease" has resulted in straitjacketing society's approach to the pursuit of health. They claim that cultural variations, environmental factors, and psychosocial dimensions have been excluded from analysis; that the promotion of health through environmental and social preventive measures has been inhibited; and that the integrated treatment of "the whole person" has been neglected. They indicate the need for a new perspective on health, one that takes into account other factors beside the presence or absence of organic disorders.

2. *Illness* refers to subjective feelings of not being well. These feelings include pain, nausea, anxiety, etc., and when reported by the individual may result in others defining him as unhealthy and in his seeking medical care (Twaddle & Hessler, 1977).

It is commonly assumed that illness is caused by disease. Subjective feelings of illness, however, may exist in the absence of observable biological causes, just as organic disorders may exist for long periods without causing pain or discomfort. A growing number of health professionals are now advocating the acceptance of the patient's reported state of feelings as a valid "problem" rather than as a psychosomatic symptom of organic disorder, and view their task as restoring the *feeling* of health, not only the organic "evidence" of health (see, for example, Gordon, Chapter 20, this volume).

3. *Sickness* refers to a social identity, distinguishable from disease, which is a biological concept, and from illness, which is a sociopsychological concept. As social identity, sickness is a label bestowed by others and publicly accepted by the individual. While sickness is usually assumed to reflect disease or illness, it may occur independently of either and must not be confused with them (for more analysis of the process and consequences of *labeling*, see Robitscher, Chapter 10, this volume; Szasz, 1977; Wilson, 1970).

A few examples will help to clarify this. Depending on their personal or cultural constitution, individuals may define themselves as "sick" in response to feelings of illness, e.g., pain, weakness, or nausea; in response to incapacity to perform accustomed tasks; or in response to observed bodily changes, such as unusual lumps. Zborowski (1952), for example, reports that first- and second-generation Italian and Jewish immigrants react overtly and emotionally to pain, whereas "Old Americans" do not.

In addition to individuals, societies also differ in their definitions of sickness, and particularly of mental illness. Some societies define as "sickness" specific forms of political activism, e.g., political dissent in the Soviet Union or the movement for women's suffrage in England in the 1920s. Other societies define as "sickness" some forms of religious expression, e.g., hearing the voice of God, as well as some forms of sexual expression, such as homosexuality or promiscuity. Alternatively, these behaviors may be defined as morally evil or as legally criminal, or they may be accepted as legitimate and "healthy." Indeed, interpretations of specific behaviors have changed in the course of history and vary across societies. In some circles of American society homosexuality and promiscuity are no longer regarded as mental "sickness," i.e., calling for psychiatric treatment, while alcoholism and child abuse have lost their moral and criminal connotations and are often viewed as "sick."

Sociologically speaking, sickness, like crime and sin, is a form of deviant behavior: it refers to a deviation from societal norms. Deviance consists in failure to perform one's role expectations, to fully participate in the social system (see Freidson, 1970; Parsons, 1951). If such failure is perceived as willful, the individual is defined as either a sinner or a criminal, a situation that calls for punishment. If the failure is perceived as involuntary, the individual is defined as sick and thus "entitled" to a reprieve from role obligations (particularly occupational and familial duties), to sympathy, and to treatment. This assumes, of course, that he manifests a desire to "get well"; in fact, he is expected to manifest such desire and to cooperate with the physician in attempting to recover.

Since symptoms are rarely unambiguous, and since individuals differ in their interpretation of the costs and rewards of becoming "sick," the assumption of a "sick" identity involves a process of negotiation between the person, those surrounding him, and the physician. It is with the physician that the ultimate authority to pronounce a person "sick," and hence legitimately excused from role obligations, rests in our society. If there is consensus among the individual, his primary group or social network, and the physician, the "sick" or "well" identity will be unambiguous and the approved course of treatment may begin. Because interpretations vary among individuals and across cultures, however, consensus may be difficult to achieve, a situation that may impede effective treatment. This happens, for example, when a physician refuses to accept as valid the complaints of a patient whom he suspects of being a hypochondriac or a malingerer; or when a Western-trained physician must convince an Indian villager who had always lived with abdominal pain that he is sick and should be treated, or even more radically, that he should routinely boil his drinking water. The problem of reaching a consensus is obviously much more severe in cross-cultural situations than in those where the individual, his family and community, and the health professional share the same cultural model of disease. The presence of conflicting models has been a major obstacle to the wholesale transfer of Western medicine to developing countries, as discussed by Ahmed and Kolker (Chapter 6) in this volume.

Our discussion of the different dimensions of nonhealth—biological, psychological, and sociological—should help to clarify the issues involved in the definition of health. Health may be defined along any of the above dimensions, as the absence of organic disorders, as the absence of subjective feelings of illness, or as a social identity complementary to sickness and continuous with it.

Physicians have traditionally defined health as a by-product of the biomedical definition of disease. Traditionally used to separate out those who can or should be treated by a physician, this definition regards health as merely the absence of disease, an uninteresting residual category (Wilson, 1970).

This definition suffers from all the limitations of the concept of disease, i.e., the fact that symptoms are rarely unambiguous and that cultures and individuals differ on what constitutes biological normality and abnormality. Equally seriously, to define health by default is to displace attention from the analysis and promotion of *well-functioning* to the diagnosis and treatment of *malfunctioning*. "We learn much about what is wrong but little about what is right, and thus we are enfeebled in efforts to prevent illness or to foster superior functioning" (Wilson, 1970, p. 4).

Two approaches to a more positive and more illuminating definition of health involve the notion of "perfect functioning" and the notion of "biologically normal functioning." The first approach conceptualizes health, biologically, as a state in which every cell and every organ is functioning at optimum capacity and in perfect harmony with the rest of the body; psychologically, as a state in which the individual feels a sense of perfect well-being and of mastery over his environment; and socially, as a state in which the individual's capacities for participation in the social system are optimal (Twaddle & Hessler, 1977). It is obvious that the state of perfect health can only exist as an ideal toward which people strive, but which they cannot hope to attain.

The problem with this approach is that if nobody qualifies as healthy, we have created a category of pathology that is both theoretically and practically unmanageable. Furthermore, it will be readily seen that this conception of health—perfect biological, psychological, and social functioning—is irrelevant to everyday demands.

The second approach conceptualizes health not as an ideal state but as a biologically "normal" state—i.e., statistically average. This definition too is of limited usefulness. What is statistically "normal" varies among cultures, social classes, and age groups. The importance of age in establishing criteria, although obvious, should not be overlooked. What is biologically or psychologically "normal" for a 10-year-old is pathological for a 40-year-old.

The salience and interpretation of pathological phenomena may vary cross-culturally as well. In some societies a pathological condition such as yaws or trachoma may be more prevalent than the absence of such a condition, yet we surely would not consider individuals manifesting this condition healthy. Social class is generally considered to be negatively correlated with incidence of some diseases. Yet the *reported* incidence of some diseases may be higher in the upper than in the lower classes, since the rich "can better afford to be sick"—sickness carries the rewards of attention and does not involve the costs of unpaid absence from work or expensive medical care. Thus, in the 17th century such ailments as spleen and vapors were believed to afflict "people of quality" but not "the common run" (Rosen, 1974). Today some forms of neurosis are similarly positively correlated with class. Even such traumatic psychological events as the midlife crisis, which is assumed to be biopsychologically determined, is believed to be a phenomenon of the upper and middle classes (see Sheehy, 1976).

In general, the definition of *normal health* becomes more exacting the higher one goes up the socioeconomic ladder, since the better educated and more affluent people are, the less tolerant they become of any signs of malfunction or discomfort. Similarly, as societies industrialize they generally raise their expectations with respect to both the desirable and the attainable states of health. It is clear, therefore, that defining health in terms of biological or psychological absolutes, i.e., perfect or average conditions, is misleading. The definition must recognize the specific circumstances of the individual and the society.

An approach more useful for our purposes would begin by asking, "Health for what?" as well as "Health for whom?" A mild bronchitis that is inconsequential to an office worker may incapacitate a singer. Low back pain that merely inconveniences an executive may disable a dock worker, while a headache paralyzing to the former may be trivial to the latter. What constitutes normal functioning in a teenager may be both unattainable and undesirable in a middle-aged person. Furthermore, since "normal" functioning is defined culturally rather than psychologically, we must ask, "normal" from whose perspective? Mental patients, for example, often insist on their own sanity, yet it is psychiatrists who are called upon to define behavior as "normal" or "deranged"—with an authority and a finality that may have drastic consequences for the patient's life (see Carter, Chapter 19, this volume).

Our definition of wellness and illness takes into account the specific roles the individual is expected to play in his cultural milieu, as well as the judgments that the individual himself and significant others in his social network make about the adequacy of his performance. In particular, effective functioning in two social roles, the familial and the occupational, tends to be regarded as crucial to the well-being of the individual and of his community. Health, then, must be viewed not merely as a state desirable in itself but as a means toward the fulfillment of strategic role obligations, and illness as an obstacle to such fulfillment. It is important to remember, however, that judgments about role performance may conflict, and that the different perspectives of different actors in the situation must be considered (for more on illness and wellness roles, see Wilson, 1970).

We believe that this approach avoids many of the pitfalls of the earlier ones. It does not assume that role obligations or performance criteria are "fixed," unvarying across cultures and among different members of the same culture. While classical sociological theory tends to view role expectations as "objective," rather like a script for behavior (see Merton, 1968), it is more useful to view social roles as constantly changing task-structures determined by ongoing interaction with "role partners." The "sick role" as well as the various "well roles" are, according to this view, dynamic social identities that must be continuously negotiated between the individual, his immediate social network, and the health professional, with the achievement of eventual consensus by no means guaranteed.

The model of health presented here, which may be called "biosocial," incorporates as objective data the values and expectations of the individual and of those around him. These behavioral and attitudinal data are used to supplement observed biological data in developing an integrated model of health and of disease.

This model need not be completely relativistic, tailored to suit each culture, each individual, and each moment in time. The biological and behavioral regularities that underlie this range of diversity should be spelled out. This can be done, as Fabrega suggests in Chapter 2 in this book and in his earlier work (1974), by specifying the biological underpinnings of behavior and by listing the tasks and activities that make up the grid of everyday life, activities that include walking, talking, sleeping, lifting, and self-grooming. The course of any disease may be charted against the underpinnings and the grid. Disease is thus defined in terms of behavioral disruptions and social costs in addition to biological correlates.

Together with the biomedical analysis of disease, which focuses on diagnosis, etiology, and (usually) chemical corrective action, the sociopsychological and cultural factors may be used to devise an integrated program to treat the illness and to restore health. The integrated biosocial model, then, does not sacrifice the demonstrated advantages of the biomedical model; rather, it seeks to supplement them.

Health and the Environment: The Hazards of Poverty

We have argued for a positive, behaviorally anchored view of health to supplement the default definition of the absence of disease. One advantage of such redefinition is that by shifting the focus from disease to health it enables society and individuals to concentrate on promoting health through prevention rather than primarily through treatment. In the following sections we will examine briefly some social and environmental dimensions of health that are amenable to preventive action.

The leading killers in most of the world today are the communicable diseases—dysentery, tuberculosis, cholera, typhoid, etc.—that used to plague North America and Europe until the late 1800s. In the latter countries, however, chronic and degenerative diseases have long replaced communicable diseases as the major causes of mortality, a fact reflected in drastically lower death rates. The crude death rate in Canada, for example, is 7 per 1,000, compared to 25 per 1,000 in Niger. Since young children are the most common victims of communicable diseases, the differences in the rates of infant mortality are even more glaring: In Niger 200 of every 1,000 babies do not survive their first year, compared to 15 of every 1,000 babies in Canada (UN Statistical Yearbook, 1976).

Since the types and causes of morbidity and mortality differ radically between rich and poor nations, our discussion will be divided into two parts: socioenvironmental factors that affect people in nonindustrialized societies will be discussed here, and those pertinent to industrialized societies will be discussed in the next section. This discussion is intended to be illustrative rather than comprehensive. For a more complete discussion, the reader is referred to Eckholm (1977), Basch (1978), and other works.

Although the causes of death in developing countries are diverse, it is estimated that three categories of disease—infections spread through human wastes, airborne infections, and malnutrition—account for 70–90% of all deaths of children under age 5 in these countries (Eckholm, 1977). These three categories of disease—to which we may add a fourth, uncontrolled reproduction—constitute what the World Bank has termed "the basic disease pattern of poverty."

Researchers have pointed out that most major illness in developing countries is socioenvironmental in nature, or more accurately, results from the interaction of biological causes with the ecological and social environment of poverty (see Martin, 1975). Neither the harmful microorganisms alone nor environmental conditions alone are enough to induce the disease; the combination of the two is lethal. Thus, for example, where sanitary facilities are nonexistent or poor and where water is contaminated, people's contact with disease-causing parasites, viruses, and bacteria is a major hazard to health. Untreated sewage, unsafe water supplies, inadequate amounts of safe water, and the lack of motivation to use safe water when available are responsible for a variety of infectious diseases from diarrhea and schistosomiasis to typhoid. Yet in the developing countries over three-fifths of the population lack adequate supplies of safe water and about two-thirds have no access to safe sewage facilities (see Eckholm, 1977).

Another major link in the vicious cycle of poverty and disease is chronic malnutrition. Chronic calorie–protein deficiency, as well as deficiencies of specific vitamins and minerals, are frequently believed to be more debilitating than actual starvation, a relatively rare occurrence (see Eckholm, 1977). The actual scope and severity of the problem are difficult to establish, both because of poor data collection and because of the difficulty of scientifically determining nutritional requirements for health. Nevertheless, it has been variously estimated that from one-sixth to one-half of the people of the world are undernourished (Eckholm, 1977, p. 41). While the largest proportion of the undernourished live in the teeming countries of Asia, large "pockets" of undernutrition exist in the midst of the world's most affluent societies. In the United States undernutrition continues to endanger the health of the rural poor, migrant workers, the aged, and Indians living on reservations.

The most serious outcomes of malnutrition are not direct starvation, but increased susceptibility to many diseases as well as damage to the physical and intellectual development of children. Infants, children, and pregnant women are most vulnerable to malnutrition, and it is among these people that the interaction effects of malnutrition with gastrointestinal and other infections are most debilitating. Not only initial susceptibility to the disease, but the severity and duration of the disease after its onset, are abetted by preexisting nutritional deficiencies. Diseases such as diarrhea, measles, and chicken pox, considered minor in developed countries, are often lethal to children already weakened by undernourishment.

One of the most widely documented, and most tragic, ironies of "modernization" has resulted from the abandonment of breast-feeding. In countries where parents have no access to sanitary food preparation or to adequate nutritional supplies, bottle-feeding has resulted in sharply increased incidences of malnutrition and infections. One physician even reports that in certain countries "bottle-feeding is the cause of more deaths than cancer" (Eckholm, 1977, p. 61).

The third link in the cycle of misery is uncontrolled reproduction. It is commonly known that effective planning for public health, for adequate nutrition, and for economic growth is all but impossible as long as the population's growth outstrips the most heroic governmental efforts. It is less well known, however, that numerous and frequent births, teenage births, and midlife births take a heavy toll on the lives and health of mothers and babies, as well as those of other members of the family. Not only do women who give birth very early or very late in their childbearing years stand a much higher chance of complications and possible death, but the probability of underweight babies, of birth defects, and of infant mortality also rises sharply in these cases. Again, the risks are exacerbated by the general conditions of illness and malnutrition. Furthermore, with each successive birth the decrease in the amount of food and other resources available to the rest of the family aggravates their condition additionally (see Zivetz, Chapter 13, this volume).

These, then, are the major links in the cycle of poverty—unsanitary environmental conditions (particularly contaminated water supplies and untreated sewage), undernutrition, and uncontrolled reproduction. These conditions, primarily social and economic rather than "medical" in nature, abet the growth and spreading of disease-causing microorganisms and increase people's vulnerability to them. Health planners are becoming increasingly aware that if health conditions in developing countries are to be improved, environmental and social measures are no less important than strictly medical ones.

Most communicable diseases, of course, may be treated with drugs, and the list of "miracle drugs" of modern medicine is long and impressive. Yet the World Bank now believes that public health measures, not scientific and technological measures, are needed to improve the health conditions of the developing countries, just as advances in public health were responsible for the striking improvements in health in industrialized societies. The history of tuberculosis in the West provides a remarkable example. The use of antibiotics to treat tuberculosis became widespread in the 1950s. Yet by that time tuberculosis had all but disappeared as a significant menace to public health, as a result of improved living conditions.

Prevention through ecological and socioeconomic measures is safer than the pharmacological treatment of disease, in view of the known harmful side effects of many drugs. Thus, hycanthone and miridazole, two drugs used to control the debilitating gastrointestinal disorder schistosomiasis, have shown signs of possible carcinogenic or mutagenic effects. Yet many countries have eliminated the disease by reducing human contact with contaminated water that contains the snails that harbor the disease-causing parasite (Eckholm, 1977). Not only is prevention through ecological measures safer, it is also cheaper and more effective, since no medical cures can significantly reduce the incidence of disease so long as the responsible microorganisms are allowed to grow and spread uninhibitedly.

Similar principles must be applied to combating malnutrition. Although malnutrition has severe consequences for health, it is primarily an economic and social problem rather than a medical one, and the ultimate solution must come through economic development. Nevertheless, overall economic development is neither a necessary precondition to alleviating malnutrition nor the most effective means toward it. Independently of economic measures to combat poverty, governments can significantly improve the health of the people by providing direct food supplements to infants and to pregnant women, by adding nutrients to commonly consumed foods (a routine practice in the United States, where bread, milk, and salt are fortified), and by persuading mothers to return to breast-feeding. The latter, according to WHO and other sources, could be the single most significant nutritional intervention (Eckholm, 1977).

It is also clear that family planning, for all its medical significance, is a social rather than a medical intervention. Yet an effective program to promote family planning must be a part of any societal strategy to improve the conditions of health.

In this section we discussed some socioenvironmental factors that interact with disease-causing microorganisms to produce the unacceptably high rates of morbidity and mortality in developing countries. We have argued that the only effective approach to improving the conditions of health in these countries is a socioenvironmental one, including ecological, nutritional, economic, and educational measures to break the vicious cycle of disease and poverty. We now turn our attention to the picture of health in developed countries.

Health and the Environment: The Hazards of Affluence

In the industrialized countries infectious diseases, although by no means extinct, have ceased to claim the major toll that they used to exact at least until the last century. The major medical causes of death in the West are cancer and cardiovascular diseases, which together account for two-thirds of all deaths (Eckholm, 1977).

Although cancer and cardiovascular disease have been labeled "degenerative" diseases, since their incidence seems to rise with age, this label is now viewed as misleading. It has become increasingly clear that cancer, stroke, and heart disease are responsible for many premature deaths and that they are induced by many factors other than the inevitable onslaughts of age. Extensive epidemiological studies have shown that the incidence of cancer varies among different countries and geographic areas, and that the incidence of heart disease varies among cultural and ethnic groups. The data suggest, although in most cases inconclusively, that both environmental and life-style factors may be associated with a higher incidence of various diseases. These factors may include industrial and automobile pollution, dietary habits, smoking, drug use, and psychological stress, factors that vary among geographic areas and subcultural groups.

As in the case of socioenvironmental conditions in developing countries, most socioenvironmental factors in developed countries do not directly "cause" disease but rather appear to increase the chances of the disease through their interaction with pathogenic microorganisms and processes. The same appears true for hereditary factors: they tend to predispose individuals to disease, although the presence of external pathogens such as environmental toxins is usually needed to induce it.

Many of the connections between life-style factors and diseases are poorly understood; yet the statistical correlations are significant. In particular, the link between cigarette smoking and lung cancer has been definitively established. Other suspected relationships involve the harmful effects on health of "the affluent diet"—a diet rich in saturated fats and sugar and poor in natural fiber and in several vitamins; the consequences of the sedentary life-style; the effects of prolonged exposure to solar and nuclear radiation; the effects of excessive consumption of alcohol and of other drugs; and the long-term results of stress. These factors have been linked, with varying degrees of certainty, to the probability of coronary heart disease, of cancer of the bowels, breast, prostate, and esophagus, and of hypertension, diabetes, and a variety of other ailments. As indicated above, many of these relationships appear to be indirect and interactive. Thus, smoking may increase the carcinogenic effects of alcohol and other drugs, while air pollutants such as photochemical oxidants exacerbate existing respiratory problems rather than induce new ones (see House & Jackman, Chapter 7, and Weaver, Chapter 12, this volume).

As in the case of developing countries, it is becoming increasingly clear that major future advances in health will come through environmental, social, and educational efforts rather than through strictly medical ones (see also Bourne, Chapter 22, this volume). Although the findings are not conclusive, there is some indication that if air pollution is controlled, smoking and drinking curtailed, and dietary habits altered, the incidence of cancer, cardiovascular disease, and respiratory disease will decline. This prospect appears particularly promising when it is recognized that medical efforts have yielded diminishing returns in health conditions. It must be remembered that decades of expensive research into the medical causes and cures of cancer have not reduced substantially its death toll, that heroic lifesaving technologies have little relevance to the lives of the majority of the people, and that rapidly growing investments in physicians and in hospitals have yielded relatively few gains in longevity and in freedom from disease.

The obstacles to socioenvironmental measures and to life-style changes are political and educational rather than scientific. These obstacles are formidable. Social scientists are becoming increasingly aware of the extraordinary difficulty of changing human behavior by persuasion (see Kolker, 1978). Similarly, while we know how to reduce automobile and industrial pollution and how to screen synthetic chemicals for possible long-term risks, the social, political, and economic costs of these decisions may be higher than we are prepared to pay. These costs may include higher rates of unemployment, slower economic growth, and increasing governmental interference in private lives (for example, by expanding the prohibitions against smoking in public places). Furthermore, as the environmental problems of industrialized countries spread to the developing countries, the latter will have to face the same agonizing choices of better health versus economic growth, or better health versus individual freedom. Their costs will be even higher, since their initial level of well-being is lower. Yet these choices must be confronted.

In the previous pages we explored some ramifications of broadening the definition of health to emphasize sociocultural and environmental concerns. We reviewed briefly several such factors and considered their effect on health in industrialized and in nonindustrialized nations. We pointed out that prevention through nonmedical action may be a cheaper, more humane, and in the long run more effective way to promote health than is the medical treatment of existing diseases. In the concluding pages we will turn our attention to the implications for the medical system itself of the new definition of health.

Promoting Better Health through Medicine

Since disease and illness will always be a part of the human experience, medical treatment will continue to play a major role in the promotion of health even in a society where prevention has raised the collective level of health to its optimal level.

It is widely recognized that the medical system must change in order to accommodate the new definition of health. There is little consensus, however, on the specific direction of such change. In the last section of this book we will discuss some proposed reforms, which are briefly outlined below. No attempt will be made to explore systematically or comprehensively the ramifications of restructuring the medical care system; that would be the subject of another book.

Broadly speaking, the medical care system must be reoriented to address the spectrum of human needs. Indeed, the trend toward integrated or "holistic" care, which has been growing in many professions, has gained increasing acceptance within medicine. This is indicated by several contributors to this book, including Kleinman (Chapter 3), Hersh (Chapter 9), and Gordon (Chapter 20). At the same time, medical care must be humanized and democratized.

Among the specific reforms recommended by students of the medical profession are the following:

1. Physicians should refocus their training and professional orientation to incorporate social, psychological, and cultural factors into both the diagnosis and the treatment of patients. Instead of becoming ever more specialized, medical care should become more integrated, addressing the whole person within the context of his family and his social network. The growing prestige of family practice as a subspecialty attests to the increasing recognition of this need within the medical profession.

2. Access to health resources should be made available to all people, including the rural and urban poor in developed countries and the traditional populations of developing countries. It is often asserted that auxiliary or paraprofessional health workers and neighborhood- and village-based health centers have helped to reduce the gap between the people and the

medical care system, particularly in the developing nations but also in American ghettoes. Not only is the emphasis on primary health care viewed as more humane than the emphasis on hospital-based, technology-intensive care, but it is believed to be more efficient in raising the level of health in many societies (see, for example, Djukanovic & Mach, 1975).

3. People everywhere should be helped to assume more responsibility for their own health. Instead of being passive recipients of treatment (the traditional patient role), individuals are encouraged to become aware of their own biological and psychological processes, to modify their life-styles for healthier living, and even to partake in their own therapy through self-help groups. Such groups, initially modeled after Alcoholics Anonymous and now covering a broad range of problems from diabetes to infertility, are believed to be successful in fulfilling needs unmet by professional medical care (see Stokes, 1978).

Changes in medical care, as envisioned by reformers, must accompany the policy changes discussed earlier—the promotion of a cleaner environment, of better nutrition, and of healthier living conditions.

The promotion of better health concerns all of us—individuals, whose lives are affected; the medical profession, which has traditionally been charged with the task; and governments, which can effect far-reaching improvements through wise policies. It is a joint endeavor; we must all participate. We hope this book will contribute to such an endeavor.

References

Basch, P. F. International health. New York: Oxford University Press, 1978.

Cockerham, W. C. Medical sociology. Englewood Cliffs, N. J.: Prentice-Hall, 1978.

Djukanovic, V., & Mach, E. P. Alternative approaches to meeting basic health needs in developing countries. Geneva: World Health Organization, 1975.

Eckholm, E. P. The picture of health: Environmental causes of disease. New York: W. W. Norton, 1977.

Engel, G. E. The need for a new medical model: A challenge for biomedicine. Science, 1977, 196, 129–136.

Fabrega, H. Disease and social behavior: An interdisciplinary perspective. Cambridge, Mass.: M.I.T. Press, 1974.

Freidson, E. Profession of medicine: A study of the sociology of applied knowledge. New York: Dodd, Mead, 1970.

Kolker, A. Change without tears. Paper presented at the Conference of the Office of International Health, San Diego, 1978.

Martin, J. F. International health planning: Socioenvironmental dimensions and community participation. American Journal of Public Health, 1975, 65, 175–177.

Merton, R. K. Social theory and social structure. New York: Free Press, 1968.

Parsons, T. The social system. New York: Free Press, 1951.

Rosen, G. From medical police to social medicine: Essays in the history of health care. New York: Science History Publications, 1974.

Sheehy, G. *Passages: Predictable crises of adult life.* New York: Bantam, 1976.

Stokes, B. *Local responses to global problems: A key to meeting basic human needs.* Washington: Worldwatch Institute, 1978.

Szasz, T. *The theology of medicine.* New York: Harper & Row, 1977.

Twaddle, A. C., & Hessler, R. M. *A sociology of health.* St. Louis: C. V. Mosby, 1977.

United Nations Statistical Yearbook. New York, 1976.

Wilson, R. N. *The sociology of health: An introduction.* New York: Random House, 1970.

Zborowski, M. Cultural components in responses to pain. *Journal of Social Issues,* 1952, *8,* 16–30.

2

Disease and Illness from a Biocultural Standpoint

Horacio Fabrega, Jr.

Introduction

A physican or public health official in a nation state is strongly motivated to interpret an individual's reports of illness and disease in terms of specific physiologic systems that may be affected and also in terms of etiology, since these parameters usually dictate the mode of treatment or prevention. In orienting to medical information in this way, he or she runs the risk of losing sight of "atypical" manifestations of illness, and indeed of what the illness means to the individual. The health worker's biomedical model of disease, taken ultimately from textbooks and clinical learning experiences heavily influenced by related frameworks, can be expected to exercise a powerful influence on what he or she looks for and finds during the analysis of a problem. In this sense, medical education or public health training can be seen as the progressive forging of a picture of how a "typical person" functions physiologically and chemically and also how that person is likely to be affected by disease processes that themselves are also "organically" constituted. At the very least, this approach to medical problems progressively deemphasizes the logic and rationale of illness given the patient's perspective.

Horacio Fabrega, Jr. • Western Psychiatric Institute and Clinic, University of Pittsburgh, Pittsburgh, Pennsylvania 15261.

Whereas in Western societies disease stands for physical-chemical changes in bodily functioning, among peoples of simpler societies, terms analogous to *disease* seem to stand for an alteration in the social and moral well-being of an individual. The area of study dealing with the differing approaches of people toward illness and disease is termed *ethnomedicine*. Fundamentals of this field will be touched on presently. Regardless of what kind of ontology members of a social group ascribe to disease, in a compelling way one can say that it is in behavioral disruptions that disease is realized. A review of the literature in anthropology (Fabrega, 1971) supports the relevance of this intuition, for it shows that the degree and persistence of a behavioral interference influences importantly what significance is given to an occurrence of disease. If one recalls the obvious fact that the biomedical frame of reference is a relatively new human invention, then the relative importance of behavioral aspects of disease becomes even more compelling. This, essentially, is the medium in which disease has a "natural" meaning and it behooves one to study it critically.

Ethnomedicine: The Comparative Study of Approaches toward Medical Problems

The boundaries of ethnomedicine can be delimited by the pair of terms *social adaptation* and *social maladaptation*. These terms can refer to activities of persons and/or human aggregates and involve their putative functioning within a specified context or setting. The study of the adaptation of human aggregates or groups is a proper domain of ethnomedical science. The analysis and explanation of how social groups adapt and function from a medical standpoint necessarily brings ethnomedicine into the orbit of population biology, sociology, and history. This particular domain of ethnomedical science will not be discussed in this chapter though elements of it are mentioned later in this section.

It is the reference of social adaptation and maladaptation to persons that needs to be grasped and dealt with at present. In this context, the terms *adaptation–maladaptation* will be given meanings that will embrace the following pairs of notions: ability–disability, social competence–social incompetence, social function–social dysfunction, and nondeviant behavior–deviant behavior. All groups, it would seem, provide their members with distinctions such as these, and it is axiomatic here that indicators of these terms involve aspects of behavior. These behavioral distinctions are used by individuals to characterize their own condition and that of their co-members. Groups also differ in terms of the criteria on which they base these distinctions and the explanations they use to render the distinctions meaningful. Principal attention will be given here to the "negative" or "undesirable" pole of the distinctions captured by the above pair of terms.

On the basis of accumulated knowledge—in the Western nations, scientific knowledge—groups invariably partition the negative pole of the continua described above. For our purposes, this partition may be held to yield two categories, both embracing deviant behavior, which will be denoted by the terms *illness* and *nonillness*. Illness thus refers to a subclass of negative behavioral changes in individuals that in the group are referred to by terms analogous to our *sickness, disease,* etc. The individual and group view the illness as requiring corrective action and to accomplish this they have established procedures and medicines. Their way of dealing with illness is different from their way of dealing with other disvalued behavioral changes of persons (i.e., nonillness). For a more elaborate definition of illness and disease, the reader is referred elsewhere (Fabrega, 1974; Field, 1973; Kelman, 1976; Young, 1976).

Groups differ in regard to criteria and mode of explaining the basic distinction between illness and nonillness. Because the assumptions about and modes of explaining illness vary across groups, persons showing illness will orient differently to it and they will also deal with it differently. Nonetheless, because illness involves a disruption or interference in behavior and gives rise to a need for corrective action, the social matrix of illness may be viewed as invariant across cultures. This, plus the fact that illness can be associated with changes in the chemical-physiologic states of the person—again, a matrix more or less common to man—means that episodes of illness everywhere probably share essential characteristics. For this reason one can assume that there exists a finite set of indicators of illness as well as social types or "forms" of illness. An additional assumption that is made here—an assumption that seems warranted in the light of accumulated findings in ethnomedicine—is that in any one group across time the boundary that separates illness from nonillness is fluid and changing. Behavioral changes that in a particular group are viewed as illness at one particular time may, at a later time, be viewed as nonillness and vice versa.

The accumulated experiences that groups have with illness and with its treatment yield a *formal body of knowledge* that is more or less codified in the group as their (medical) theory of illness. This is an outgrowth of the processes of group adaptation and cultural evolution. This theory of illness and its implied set of directives for treatment provides group members with formal (socially sanctioned) explanations of why and how illness occurs and how it may be eliminated. Groups also possess classifications of and names for the illnesses that are deemed likely or possible. This complex and formal body of knowledge that the group has about illness may be termed its *medical taxonomy*. Rather than constituting a frozen and static scheme, a group's medical taxonomy should be viewed as dynamic, evolving, and furnishing group members with *explanations* of actual occurrences of illness as well as names and a system of classification of illness types. In the modern nation states, the existing medical taxonomy that prevails may be termed *biomedicine*. Biomedicine thus constitutes the formal scientific knowledge that exists about illness in the nation states. The units of this Western medical taxonomy will be termed *disease entities*. The expressions of these in bahavior changes constitute illness and it is these that are of special interest to the ethnomedical scientist.

The medical taxonomy of a group may thus be viewed from two vantage points. On the one hand, it constitutes a cultural trait in the sense that it embodies a formal body of knowledge of the group as a whole. However, this body of knowledge is also used by the medical practitioners of the group as a basis for medical practice and care. The taxonomy here serves as their basis for action embodying principles of diagnosis and methods for treatment; the latter include procedures, medicines, and regimens that are deemed efficacious for dealing with the illnesses of the group. The behaviors of medical practitioners and of their clients are partially patterned and regulated by directives that devolve from the group's medical taxonomy.

The accumulated experiences that groups have with illness and with its treatment also yield what may be termed an *informal* (hereafter, *folk*) body of knowledge of illness. Such knowledge, which also constitutes a cultural trait of the group, serves as the lay (i.e., nonprofessional) basis of orientation and action toward illness. It includes names of illness, lay beliefs about causation, standard remedies and routines for home treatment, and a body of rules and expectations that serve to pattern the behaviors of lay persons who are ill and of those who come into contact with those persons. Many terms and principles of this folk knowledge are drawn from the group's medical taxonomy, but the uses and significance that they have in each system of signification (i.e., folk knowledge versus medical taxonomy) should be viewed as different. Nonetheless, it is assumed here that there is a partial equilibrium between the (formal) medical taxonomy and the (informal) folk knowledge of a group. By this one means that formal knowledge, with time, diffuses and becomes standard and traditional (i.e., "informal") in the lay populace. Conversely, some of the informal, lay-accumulated wisdom about illness that some group members derive contains insights and clues about diagnosis and treatment that the medical professionals use and test out. When this knowledge is "proven" useful, it then becomes systematized and comes to be used by the medical professionals. In this sense, folk knowledge has entered the medical taxonomy of the group as a whole; i.e., it has been "formalized."

The medical taxonomy and folk knowledge of illness of a group, together, give a distinctive ideological cast to what can be termed the group's medical care system (MCS). The MCS constitutes what can be viewed as the group's social approach to disease and illness. It embraces the knowledge, tradition, guidelines, and values that groups have vis-à-vis illness and disease. It also includes their way of handling disease and illness, embracing social institutions, health behavior practices, and rules, and identified personnel and structures involved in the delivery of medical care. The MCS of a group has a functional relation with other social systems of the group. Characteristics of MCS and of its relationship to these other systems, in the light of the many contextual factors of the group (i.e., its size, level of development, habitat, etc.), are what contribute to the level of illness in the group as well as to its "style" and approach to nonillness.

The material discussed so far concerns social medical activities and patterns within a hypothetical group at a specified interval of time. Ethnomedical science also embraces relations, theoretical or empirical, that may exist between groups and/or between time periods. This merges the field of ethnomedicine with historical analyses and the field of social cultural evolution. In this instance, an ethnomedical scientist might be interested in analyzing how definitions of illness and disease change across time in a particular group, as well as the related changes in medical care practices and approaches to nonillness. Alternatively, he may wish to explain the sequence of changes that take place when groups endorsing different medical taxonomies come into contact with each other. Here, then, ethnomedical science deals with activities and processes (of a social medical nature) that take place *between* groups and *across* time periods. Figure 1 illustrates and summarizes diagrammatically the material presented in this section.

A basic distinction that ethnomedical science provides is that between illness and disease. In our system of medicine a disease constitutes a physical-chemical change that takes place in an individual's bodily systems. We define disease in terms of what can be called a biomedical language and our MCS is predicated on it. Lay individuals, especially if they endorse other systems of medicine, have little knowledge or awareness of this language. Medical problems are thus conceptualized quite differently. Research has documented that the presence of physiologic and associated behavioral symptoms constitutes their medical "realities." The latter can be termed illness episodes and are realized in behavioral changes. Because illness involves behavior, and behavior (in humans and mammalian forms) is social, communicative, and somehow "cultural," illness bears the stamp of culture. Illness, behavior, and culture are thus somehow related and all three bear a problematical relationship to underlying physical-chemical events and processes (i.e., a *disease*). A purpose of this chapter is to explicate these relationships and provide a perspective about them.

Culture, Behavior, and the Nervous System

Illness involves disruptions in behavior that are associated with neural processes and that are shaped by cultural influences. In this and the following section, the basic raw materials of illness—namely, culture, behavior,

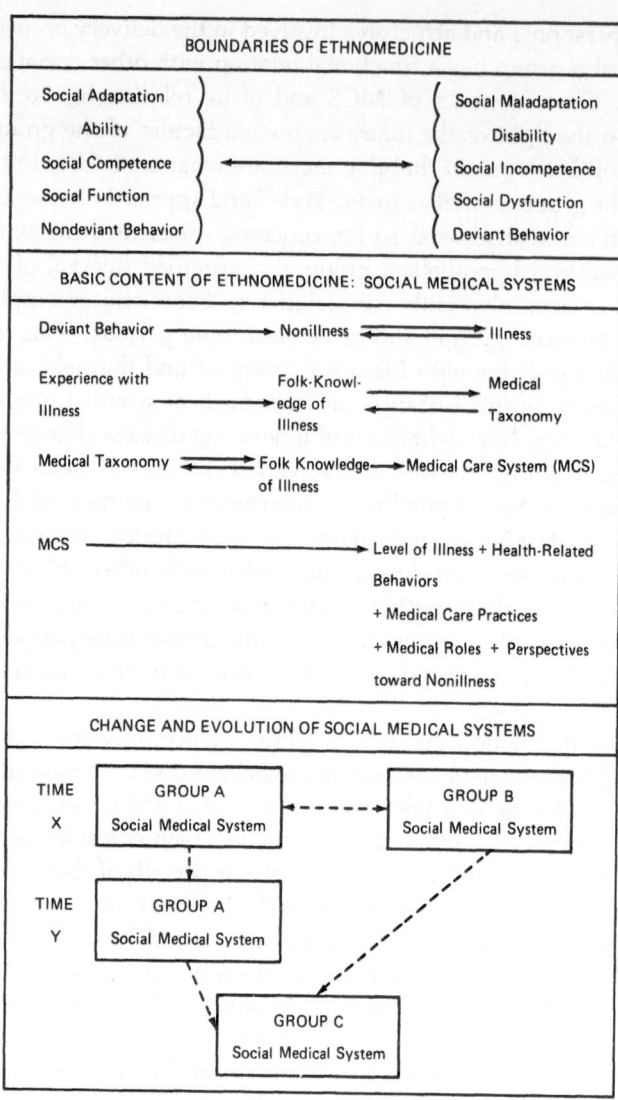

Figure 1. Basic concepts and principles of ethnomedical science.

and the nervous system—are briefly discussed with the aim of assigning a role to each in ethnomedical science.

In order to explicate influences attributed to "culture," it seems appropriate to explicitly restrict the meaning of this term. The reasons for this are obvious: cultural influences, as ordinarily interpreted, are simply too encompassing and embrace phenomena that can effect behavior and nervous system functioning in many different ways. Moreover, if one adopts a historical and populational frame of reference, there is a direct connection between the cultural and the genetic-organic. This is so because a group's way of life encompasses mating rules, dietary habits and practices, activity cycles and patterns, and modification of microclimate—all of which are classically thought to have physiologic or "organic" effects.

Having argued that there exists a need for limiting the rather broad meaning that "culture" can be given, it is necessary to specify precisely how this term is construed here. In this presentation "culture" refers to the symbolic systems of a people. Such symbols are observed and reflected in the style of their social and cognitive behavior. Culture, then, is something one infers or abstracts from the distinctive mode of life of a group. This requires a consideration of the meanings that one can give to behavior.

Behavior is an obviously broad category and needs to be broken down. In this chapter, the following terms will be used. By (1) *social behaviors* we will refer to activities such as gestures, demeanor, facial displays, and simple or coordinated actions, including the social (i.e., performance) aspects of language and speech, which are viewed from an interpersonal and situational standpoint. The appropriate performance of social roles belongs in this category of behavior, as does the "natural" participation in activities that are imbued with shared meanings and that *reflect* norms in the group. The actual norms, together with the accumulated knowledge, guiding themes, and values of a people (derivable from the study of myth and ritual), are somehow "behind" social behavior, although they cannot be included as involving behavior itself. The stylistic patterns of behavior that are observed to take place among co-members can, however. It is very clear that "cultural" groups differ in this type of behavior. It is, in fact, that existence of obvious differences in social behavior among peoples that led to the formulation of the concept culture.

Social behaviors as described above are learned and in many respects may be viewed as "symbolic" insofar as one can point to distinctive stylistic themes and rationales that give them meaning. For analytic purposes it seems useful to single out the individual-centered correlates of the observable social behaviors of a people and term them (2) *cognitive*. This implies that learning has somehow led to the internalization of symbols that members share, it being clearly understood that each category of behavior (i.e., social and cognitive) logically implies the other. Cognitive behaviors embrace phenomena such as thinking, planning, perceiving, remembering, and problem solving. An individual's capacity for and creative use of language will be viewed as a component of this type of behavior. Cognitive behaviors, then, embrace the plans, rules, and means–ends strategems that the individual internalizes during the socialization process. The special categories and processes involved in this type of behavior (e.g., perception, cognition, recall, recognition) are what allow the individual to take in, process, and retrieve information in a "culturally" meaningful way and are thus necessarily implicated in social behavior.

A third category of behavior will be singled out analytically and will be termed (3) *motor behavior.* This category is held to embrace responses viewed purely as sequences of more or less coordinated muscular contractions. The knee jerk, the pupillary contraction to light stimuli, and the salivation produced by the odor of food constitute visible motor "behaviors" that are reflexive. The elementary constituents of overlearned, highly "complex," and social activities (hunting, piano playing, etiquette, etc.) involve the maintenance of posture, muscular tone, the coordination of finely graded muscular contractions, etc., which in their totality constitute motor behaviors. In addition, of course, much motor behavior cannot be directly observed—for example, the relaxation or contractions of viscera when stimulated and the constrictions of blood vessels when the surrounding temperature decreases. This means that "internal" bodily responses can follow motor changes (e.g., hormonal alterations, blood pressure changes, changes in pulse rate). On logical grounds such vegetative changes are placed at this level of "behavior." Motor behaviors, then, constitute overt or covert ("hidden") bodily responses viewed purely as *physical* phenomena. Such behaviors underlie those discussed above and are correlated with them.

In biomedical science, physical-chemical changes of many types ("motor behaviors") importantly influence and subserve social and cognitive behaviors. Moreover, the set of physical, chemical, and physiologic changes is where a biomedical scientist "places" a disease process. Conversely, a social-behavioral scientist whose focus is illness, an entity logically different from diseases, will give principal attention to the categories of behavior termed *social* and *cognitive.*

All the preceding types of behaviors are under the control of the nervous system. For the purposes of this chapter, "nervous system" will refer to phenomena pertaining to that special apparatus or bodily part that is studied by neuroscientists; it encompasses chemical reactions, electrical impulses, and also the actual anatomical parts wherein and between which these neural processes take place. One can distinguish among levels of the nervous system, and three can be delineated based on the following neuroanatomic distinctions. The higher level involves the cortex (outer zones) of the cerebral hemispheres (including its various lobes, frontal, parietal, temporal, and occipital). Certain segments of these hemispheres are called primary sensory areas, to denote the fact that neural impulses generated in the periphery of the body are first registered there. Primary receptive zones are held to be surrounded by secondary and tertiary receptive zones, or analyzers, where impulses are further integrated, transformed, and related to information registered in other sensory zones. More "special" areas of the cortex will be described in later portions of this chapter. The second level will be termed intermediate, and will include the base of the forebrain (the "limbic system"), subcortical structures (e.g., hypothalamus, thalamus), the brainstem (its parts being midbrain, pons, and medulla), and the cerebellum. This "level" is set apart as such purely for analytic convention. It embraces portions of the nervous system importantly implicated in "complex" behaviors—for example, mood, memory, and visceral functioning—as well as in "simpler," more reflexive, behaviors such as the maintenance of posture, coordinated movements of the eyes during fixation on and/or pursuit of objects, and blood pressure. The third and lowest level will include the spinal cord, the autonomic ganglia, the peripheral nerves, and the various nerve endings and receptors in the viscera, muscles, tendons, and body surface.

In juxtaposing categories of behavior and levels of the nervous system we do not mean to draw a strict correspondence between the two. First of all, neither categories of behavior nor levels of the nervous system are mutually exclusive or independent. Moreover, each category of behavior cannot, in a strict way, be equated with a specific level of the nervous system. Distinctions between categories of behavior and levels of the nervous system are thus purely analytic. Behavior as a whole is subserved by an integrated and connected nervous system. Despite the underlying unity of the individual, it is a well-established fact that the nervous system is composed of parts and that its functioning can usefully be conceptualized as involving levels and/or centers, each of which subserves (or contributes to) unique functions and bears a special relation to certain categories of behavior.

Evolutionary Constraints on Cultural Differences

Any "behavioral scientist," even one who is strongly neurologically oriented, can't help but view human social and cognitive behaviors with an intuitive appreciation of its uniqueness when compared to that of the other primates. Moreover, even a casual acquaintance with descriptions of behavior in the anthropological literature is likely to impress one with the striking differences that have been noted among people in both social and cognitive spheres. Nonetheless, when these classes of behavior are viewed abstractly and emphasis is given to well-defined areas of behavior assessed formally and by means of comparable procedures of testing, it is their similarity across peoples and indeed their continuity with the behaviors of the nonhuman primates, especially the apes, that is striking. In recent decades, the field of study of primate behavior has grown enormously, and there now exist a number of reviews of it. In this section, some of the principles and generalizations in this field will be discussed briefly, for they need to be heeded in any explication of the basis of illness and disease.

Studies in ethology and in comparative psychology have amply documented the communicative richness of the social behaviors of nonhuman primates. Indeed, a theme and continuing aim in the field of behavioral biology is to work out the patterns of evolution of the various displays (and their meanings) in mammalian animal forms (Chevalier-Skolnikoff, 1973). In this body of research, a vexing problem is the development of useful categories of behaviors and the assignment of meaning to them. Most biologists would acknowledge that such displays and communicative behavior patterns are the outcome of genetic programs that unfold in (and require sensitization to) social situations. Because of this, the behaviors may be said to be both genetic and learned. The dramatic consequences of socially isolating newborn and infant monkeys are testimony to the importance of rearing influences in higher mammalian forms (Harlow, 1971). Observations of rhesus monkey isolates indicate that a variety of social behaviors among them are thwarted and grossly altered, if not pathologically disturbed. More controlled research has shown that rhesus monkey isolates perform poorly when constrained to send or receive facial displays to other isolates as well as normal conspecifics (Miller, 1974; Miller, Caul, & Mirsky, 1967). Thus, although able to learn ("cognitive") discriminations in an instrumental conditioning situation, in the process responding appropriately in a physiological sense (showing "motor behaviors"), as did normal monkeys, it was the ability to communicate socially through facial displays that was impaired. Such experiments, in verifying the criticalness of social learning for the development of communicative ability in nonhuman primates, support the appropriateness of handling behavior in terms of the three separate (analytic) categories and suggest that relatively independent neurological systems are correlated with them. This body of research is similar in rationale and aims to that involving the communication of emotion. As is well known, facial expressions in certain emotions are currently viewed as universally characteristic of the human species (Ekman, 1972, 1973). These, moreover, are judged as similar (in a structural and contextual sense) to those of nonhuman primates (Eibl-Eibesfeldt, 1972). Elicitors of human facial expressions vary across human groupings, as do the display rules by means of which an individual can mask the expressions, simulate them, and otherwise emblematically use them in discourse (Argyle, 1972). Here, then, one notes universal human patterns (felt to be involuntary, subcortical), which humans can (voluntarily, cortically) use in order to render social behavior creative and symbolically relevant.

Experiments on free-ranging monkeys have underlined the important contributions that the frontal systems of the brain (the cortex of the tip of the temporal lobe and the prefrontal-orbitofrontal cortex) subserve in social behaviors and affect. Bilateral destruction of this system was associated with decreased frequencies and critical alterations of a number of behavior sequences classically termed *social;* for example, allogrooming, facial expressions, and maternal and sexual behavior (Franzen & Myers, 1973a). In another experiment, similar procedures were found to inhibit the sociality of monkeys, these failing to rejoin their social group on release and remaining solitary until death. Increased levels of what was viewed as aimless pacing were also documented (Myers, Swett, & Miller, 1973). Interestingly, these deficits were not observed after prolonged observations of yearling and infant rhesus monkeys whose frontal systems were destroyed. The behavioral deficits appeared with increasing severity among 2- and 3-year-old juveniles. It thus appears that a certain degree of maturation is required for the social effects of destruction of this system to be expressed (Franzen & Myers, 1973b).

Related to these experiments are the findings to the effect that this same neural system appears to regulate the social preferences of monkeys (Suomi, Harlow, & Lewis, 1973). Thus, differences in gender-related social preference patterns were noted between (frontal system) operated and control monkeys. The experimenters were unable to detect gross differences in behavior that might underlie the social discriminations of the monkeys. Insofar as discriminations are involved, one must acknowledge that cognitive behaviors were also affected. Observations noted by these researchers on 11 monkeys with bilateral lesions of the frontal system paralleled those reported above, with operates being more withdrawn and showing less proximity and contact with stimulus animals (Deets, Harlow, Singh, & Blanquist, 1970). Many other behavioral alterations that were noted can easily be brought under the rubric "social." At the same time, these animals also showed distress, "disturbance" behaviors, and differences in aggression, which (see also above) implicate the functioning of the amygdaloid system, with which this frontal system is known to be connected.

Despite the presence of disturbances in various neural and behavioral spheres, one can view the above animal studies as also affirming the value of the analytic category "social behavior." Though operates show some cognitive impairments—which, to be sure, require special methods of procedure for their documentation—many other cognitive capacities are not affected. It is the relative asociality of the operatives that is compelling. A similar relative preservation of cognitive abilities, but with deficiencies in the social sphere (perhaps in the ability to judiciously apply such abilities to real-life social situations), characterizes humans with the frontal lobe syndrome. Such persons can reason "logically," can remember appropriately, and can use language competently. Elementary sensory functions are likewise "normal." Despite their normality in these spheres, they are in certain ways socially compromised. These observations thus suggest that an important component of social behavior is subserved by the frontal systems of the cerebral cortex.

Regarding the evolutionary aspects of behaviors, social and cognitive, the unique functions and consequences of human language are acknowledged though the exact specificities of these, and their differences from that of apes is controversial. There seems to be a consensus that with regard to sensory processes alone, especially audition and vision (including threshold, color, acuity, and movement), few differences exist between man and the higher primates (Mason, 1976). Evidence for other sensory modalities is less substantial and in many instances anecdotal and provocative. For example, it is claimed that chimpanzees may be less sensitive to pain. Nonetheless, the strong commonalities between man and higher primates suggest that their "nervous systems" retrieve comparable amounts, levels, and units of information from the ambient physical energy of the environment. The apes have also been shown to be able to respond to the *relations* among sensory units and to discriminate stimulus arrays on the basis of various "cognitive" criteria (e.g., sameness–difference), which suggests a capability to order sensory phenomena by imposing patterns or creating structures. Rudimentary forms of classification and sorting have been shown to exist among primates, and in some species, actual instances of intermodal integration. All this suggests some capacity for "abstraction" and "concept formation." Similarly, although the data here seem less controlled and more informally derived, it seems to be the case that apes can remember selectively; can anticipate the consequence of their actions; and can show instances of insight, planning, and foresight in the solution of problems, in the process constructively applying information about their immediate environment. The apes have been shown to possess the capacity for a concept of self, a qualitative difference that (together with man) apparently sets them apart from other primates. The spatial memory organization of apes (their ability to remember the location of objects hidden in a spatial territory) is such that it has drawn emphasis to the importance of considering representational processes in any assessment of their memory and learning abilities. Such a representational ability may thus be independent (in an evolutionary sense) from verbal language abilities. It is when projecting action into the more distant future or recalling long past "creative" efforts that their cognitive abilities show a clear discontinuity from those of man. Nonetheless, the existence of such cognitive behaviors among the higher primates, the obvious preadaptations for a form of language and communication, and indeed the stylistic attributes of their group behavior is what has led to the claim of their possessing "culture."

A clear-cut neural-behavior difference between man and the higher primates appears to be the degree of cerebral lateralization in man, that is, asymmetries in function between the left and right sides of the brain. Thus, as recently reported, few primate species show such clear-cut preferences for the use of the same hand or differential behavioral deficits when segments of only one side of the brain are injured (Passingham & Ettlinger, 1974). Indeed, although there are some exceptions (Dimond & Blizard, 1977), the left and right hemispheres among nonhuman primates appear on the whole to be functionally similar. In man, then, unilateral cerebral lesions suffice to produce highly specific and differential behavior defects, whereas in nonhuman primates bilateral lesions seem to be required (Passingham & Ettlinger, 1974). Among nonprimates a normal rate and level of learning seems to require two interconnected hemispheres, whereas man and apparently nonhuman primates can learn a particular ability with only one hemisphere even if the neural system subserving the ability functions optimally with both hemispheres.

The special language capacities of man are held by many to be the principal sources of and bases for cerebral asymmetries of function and brain organization. Language functioning also presents the best evidence of the operation of the principle of mass action in the human brain: Despite the structural differentiation between left and right temporal areas, either hemisphere can subserve language capacities, both seem to be required for optimal language and cognitive development, and a deficiency of cerebral tissue in the corresponding areas during development (in either hemisphere) is associated with cognitive behavior deficits (in language and in other abilities) in adult life. The acquisition and mastery of language may have a priority in the development of adult neural organization and function and the capacity in question appears quite specific in its neuronal requirements. Interestingly, there is evidence to suggest that the right posterior temporal lobe in man, besides subserving spatial orientation, seems to be uniquely involved in the recognition of faces, and in this regard this capacity is also specific in its neuronal requirements. Lateralization of function of this degree is not at present known to be a feature of the brains of other higher primates, though instances of functional asymmetries have been reported (Dimond & Blizard, 1977). Development of the cognitive capacity of apes to somehow "remove" themselves from the here and now (the immediately given), to represent a spatiotemporal model of the world, and to creatively plan, look ahead, and use previous experience as a basis for action is felt to be associated with the trend toward lateralization of cerebral functions, the full realization of which involves the special verbal and visual spatial abilities of man (Levy, 1977).

The reasons for giving attention to nonhuman primate material here seem obvious enough. Similarities in primate (human and nonhuman) modes of neural functioning provide the anchoring points of any physicalistic view of "higher" nervous system function and of behaviors thereby regulated. As pertains to the theme of this chapter, common properties of the behavior and neural functioning of man and the higher primates provide two important guidelines for the comparative study of disease and illness. First of all, since disease processes (which through "motor behaviors" alter the way the nervous system functions) are expressed as "symptoms" or components of illness episodes (i.e., changes in motor *and* social and cognitive behaviors), commonalities between man and other mammalian forms in nervous system functioning imply commonalities in illness and disease. In short, continuities in the way the neural systems of man and primates function necessarily mean continuities in disease and illness since the latter somehow reflect nervous system and behavioral dysfunction. This theme is developed further in this chapter.

At the same time, commonalities in the way the nervous systems of higher mammalian forms function constitute possible boundaries in any examination of cultural differences in disease and illness. In other words, the nervous system properties that man shares with primates are common to all humans, and the form of the behaviors that these properties subserve have to be viewed as constituting some of the human universals of illness and disease. Conversely, man–primate differences in nervous system organization function and behaviors that result from this delimit a class of behavior wherein one might expect to find human ("cultural") differences in illness and disease. More specifically, if the primates, including man, are shown to have identical sensory thresholds to X modality of stimulation, to show identical functional effects when homologous brain areas Y are injured, or demonstrate similar behavioral stereotypies when toxic amounts of pharmacologic agent Z are administered, then primate brain-behavior functions subserving X modality, attributable to areas Y, or underlying stereotypies produced by Z are obviously similar. Given this state of affairs, it is unlikely that one will find human cultural differences when similar means of evaluation are employed. Conversely, if man differs from the rest of the primates and especially from the apes in brain-behavior feature M, then the functioning of this area, center, or circuit does not possess the same degree of phylogenetic fixity (e.g., genetic canalization). It is thus more likely that one *might* find human cultural differences when behaviors (e.g., illness manifestations) subserved by such a neural substrate are evaluated. Quite obviously, the word *might* in the preceding sentence needs to be stressed since there is no guarantee that cultural differences will be found either in behavior or brain organization.

The assumptions lying behind these generalizations are well known and indeed axiomatic in general biology. At different points in the evolutionary time scale, prevailing social conditions served as factors that helped select anatomical and physiologic changes; these, in turn, modified the social conditions of man yielding, as it were, a necessary "feedback" loop between the social and the genetic-organic. This feedback is the reason why there are shared patterns of social and cognitive behaviors between man and other primates and also why the precise origins and "beginnings" of culture are unprecise and blurred. Since the process of evolution is, by definition, cumulative, this means that any gains in adaptation produced by specific changes in the organization of the nervous system and mirrored in "cultural" developments were incorporated in the evolving genome of the hominid line. It also means that specifically human brain-behavior traits are built out of a genetic structure that is shared with the nonhuman primates.

In examining the question of cultural differences in brain organization, behavior, illness, and disease, then, one necessarily probes into the defining properties of species. There is the obvious fact that verbal language and other cultural traits have been and continue to be all-important in the way brain organization in the human species is realized or expressed in behavior. Developments in brain organization conditioned by culture become part of the human species as a whole. It is thus most unlikely that highly unique modes of brain organization and function will depend on specialized attributes of a group's language, culture, or any other social attribute. Rather, since it is a set of general properties of culture, language, etc., which the organization of the human brain necessarily requires for its expression, the properties making up the "average expectable environment," human brain organization will show profound commonalities among cultures. Nonetheless, all anatomists, physiologists, and psychologists acknowledge human variations in their domain of interest; in this light, one asks if these might offer clues that group differences might exist.

The preceding generalizations can be rephrased by stating that evolution equips a member of the human species with *the capacity for* thought, visuospatial orientation, verbal language competence, linear codification of time, musical skills, facial recognition, problem solving, etc., and the capacity to develop disease and illness. Any group differences in the way these capacities are realized neurologically are best interpreted as quantitative and not qualitative. In short, symbolic systems, cultures viewed in the abstract, are more likely to preferentially enhance or deemphasize brain-behavior capacities rather than to generate entirely novel ones, and it is thus highly unlikely that different forms of brain organization will be found across human groups. Any existing group differences will involve areas of functioning that distinguish man unambiguously from the higher primates. When one inquires about how a group's prevailing culture might come to affect disease, illness, brain organization, and behavior, then, one is inquiring about different regions of a general human continuum. On the one hand, the continuum itself is dependent on the basic sociality of man. On the other, different regions of the continuum of human functioning need to be seen as wrought out of a species-wide capability that varies continuously.

Biocultural Implications of Illness

Disease and illness, then, reflect different facets of neural systems malfunctioning. Brain-behavior uniformities provide the conditions for the forms that illness and disease can take in higher mammalian forms and especially man. Here we would like to concentrate on selected features of illness that stem from the special properties of human social and cognitive behavior.

In a formal sense, one can say that illness constitutes an undesirable condition or state that signals that the individual is not able to function adaptively in his group. Since individuals are social beings, illness by implication reflects a setback and poses a dilemma to the group as a whole. In this sense, illness has both a personal and a collective dimension. The view that illness constitutes a maladaptation of an individual that also reflects the group's character of adjustment is ecologic since it takes into consideration social, cultural, and physicalistic aspects of the environments.

There are two interrelated ways in which illness may be said to have a social and cultural meaning. On the one hand, the group's patterns, values, and orientations lead members to assign significance to illness—they value it in a certain way, they describe it in a certain way, they see it as standing for something, and they orient to deal with it in certain ways. In this sense, illnesses are also like cultural traits or complexes, that is, patterns having a significance that is framed in terms of cultural conventions. In a word, illness is a symbolic entity, the meaning of which is given by the medical taxonomy of the group. Illness also has an evolutionary significance since it is (and has been) ubiquitous in human groups and has played an important role in natural selection. Furthermore, since human evolution is a biocultural process, this suggests that in some way illness may have a social "function." Given these considerations, one is led to conjecture that there may be a pattern to the way illness is expressed. In other words, rather than having no meaning or showing no form, one can assume that illness takes on an *organized* form and of such a character that its potential social implications may be apprehended by group members.

Naturalistic observation of nonhuman primates are more and more revealing the social organization that exists in these communities. Matters of vital concern to the individual and group are "noticed," responded to, and communicated about, and when these social activities are carefully analyzed they are seen to possess a biological rationale for the group. Certainly, given the centrality of illness, one can assume that within these groups something similar to illness occurrences are reflected in the social exchanges that occur among co-members—that illness may alter or change the status of social relations among members in patterned ways and this would be mediated in orderly (i.e., meaningful) displays and signals. All this suggests that in altering behavior meaningfully illness may be serving a *communicational function.* If this is so, illness could be described as a ritualized form that is partially encoded in the genome. An important ethnographic task becomes the delineation of the morphology of this ritualized form. This task may be pursued ethologically and with different species that are close to man.

The idea that one must begin to look at illness as a cultural and social form that serves a communicational function and that may thus have an evolutionary significance raises several points. First of all, although it is unquestionably true that nonhuman primates may show well-specified changes in behavior that one can stipulate as illness, it nevertheless is the case that "illness" in this context can only to a limited extent be said to have a "cultural" significance. As far as is currently known it is mainly the observer, on the basis of his culturally derived standards regarding the functioning of living systems, who is able to point to behavioral alterations and classify these as illness. In population biology disease is viewed in genetic and physiological terms and the expression of this as illness involves diminished capabilities, limited success in foraging for food, blunted competitive strivings, withdrawal from sexuality, etc. The "machine" of the living organism is viewed as slowed or its performance less efficient. Naturalistic field studies among the nonhuman primates would allow verifying whether such "mechanical" changes constitute the principal behavioral aspects of illness. It may well be the case that in such communities group members demonstrate additional social alterations in the event of "illness." Perhaps certain selected members are protected when sick, that what we could term *altruistic* sorts of behaviors take place, that dominance positions are not necessarily challenged, that special forms of food giving or borrowing do take place, and that on the whole the behaviors and communications shown by the organism elicit a variety of social readjustments in contrast or in addition to those pure survival constraints that a strict reading of evolutionary principles would suggest. In this latter instance, illness might very well then be said to have a discernible social form and a cultural significance as well.

With regard to human social groups, however, the literature in anthropology amply supports the notion that illness does operate as an organizing and constructive social form. As already implied, all groups have nomenclatural systems by means of which they conduct dialogue about illness. All sorts of "altruistic" social alterations can be said to take place in the context of the sick person's immediate group. The readjustments of group members to accommodate the needs of the sick person and the sanctioned suspension of his or her role obligations attest to the fact that communicationally significant exchanges are taking place. It is precisely because of such obvious socially organized and "constructive" changes in behavior that are implicated in the curing ceremonies and medical practices of all peoples that one is allowed to claim that illness is first of all a *social form*—a creation, of human social groups—and secondly, that it must be seen to have a biologic significance—to reflect and express a common "language" that has proven of great value to the human species.

The social behavioral forms of illness serve several adaptive functions.

On the one hand, their "reading" proves beneficial to the person who is sick —he communicates his disability and thereby elicits concern, sympathy, help, and support. At the same time, such a reading can aid the group to which the individual makes contributions. More specifically, many of the interpersonal weaknesses, maladaptive practices, or socioecologic vulnerabilities that are implicit in the way the group is linked to its habitat are systematically probed in the attempt to undo illness. In the long run, the group arrives at a (medical care) system whose operation protects the group from illness. Groups, of course, develop different types of medical care systems and in each one illness is viewed differently. How well such a system functions depends on which meaning of illness one wishes to concentrate (Fabrega, 1976a).

Disease as a Culturally Ordered Behavioral Form

Thus far, attention has been given principally to social and evolutionary aspects of illness. In this section theoretical aspects of the patternings inherent in the way illness unfolds in the individual will be discussed. In other words, emphasis is given to the logic, rationale, and meaning of illness, given the fact that an individual who becomes ill is a member of a social group.

One can begin by considering the truism that during development man internalizes a representation of his "culture" and that somehow this influences what he thinks and feels and how he behaves. This fact must be held to be reflected during an occurrence of illness, and in this instance the features of culture termed *folk knowledge* and *medical taxonomy* come into play. It is instructive to consider the factors that follow from these rather elementary assumptions. One posits that in illness the individual develops a set of organismic changes (O_i), for example, certain chemical and physiologic changes. Such changes may or may not be directly apprehended, but certainly if pronounced and sustained are reflected in how the individual comes to feel, judge himself, and orient to his social and physical environment. Such changes involving an individual's state of awareness and orientation, in a broad sense, signal his or her sense of disconnectedness and maladaptation. Such changes may add up to experiences similar to those that we have come to call pain, malaise, nausea, altered bodily functioning of various sorts (e.g., respiratory distress, diarrhea), an altered sense of personal identity or awareness, weakness, feelings of helplessness and disarticulation, and the like.

To varying degrees, the individual interprets the altered states of self associated with O_i in terms of the meanings provided him by his culture. Such meanings play a role in and contribute to the final form of the illness.

As an example, if an O_i involves gastrointestinal changes that are reflected in altered abdominal sensations of some sort, they will be perceived and given expression in terms of the relevant cognitive categories that the individual has at his disposal. In the last analysis, such categories derive from the individual's culture and ecological placement. The O_i may be articulated, felt, and reported either as insects in the abdomen, as a cooling of the parts of the abdomen, as a pounding by the spirits, as a common physical object that has been introduced, as the rotting of the inside, or as a fullness and hardening that suggests a "growth" or "tumor," etc. In short, cultural beliefs about self, group, habitat, and illness—which render comprehensible the phenomena of nature—obviously come into play in the interpretation of symptoms.

A basic assumption that has been made is that illness is associated with a set of altered experiences about the self and body that in only a limited sense can be regarded as universal or culture-free. The psychobiologic unity of man necessarily implies that cultural influences color the elemental changes of illness, which, after all, involve complex patterns of nervous-system impulses. Some organismic changes, of course, *necessarily* involve coordinated alterations linked through the structural, chemical, and physiologic systems of the organism. However, for heuristic purposes, it makes sense to judge system structures and their changes as only partially determining specific types of awareness and self-definition. The "segments" of the person that we call mind and body thus become fused and form a unitary whole during illness. This means that whatever sets of symbolic categories are brought to bear in the effort to articulate and make intelligible the altered bodily changes underlying illness, these categories will more than likely have linkages with and/or entail (in a logical sense) other symbolizations that meet in and help define what it is to be a person in this group. Such symbolic connections may reflect structural or functional connections. For example, dreams might be fashioned in line with the symbolic loadings given to the perceptions of insects or spiritual poundings referred to earlier, whichever happen to hold sway. These dreams, in turn, may signal a variety of social judgments that involve the person and his immediate family. As a result of the various changes, the social reality of the individual may be judged as altered; what the individual will be willing to do and tolerate may change, as may also what he is likely to eat and the meanings that he places on physiologic processes such as defecation. In fact, any O_j tied to the original O_i "naturally" (in terms of the apparatus of the person) and culturally (in terms of how the individual is believed constituted) should be seen as interconnected in an "intelligible" manner. The final result of these changes is a network of symbolically related O_i. What is thus "produced" is an ordered psychobiologic whole, which is expressed behaviorally in a socially meaningful way.

If organismic changes underlying an occurrence of illness are read as minor and temporary, they may involve no major modification in the way the individual orients to his immediate social situation and the way co-members relate to him. They may, on the other hand, be correlated with or underlie a degree of withdrawal on the part of the individual, in which case he could be said to be conserving his energy or to be using it more judiciously. In this instance, selected duties and functions might be circumvented or fulfilled cursorily. In either instance, fundamental sensorimotor regularities such as attention, perception, and coordination may be slowed or changed, and the person's efficiency in processing and integrating information cognitively may be interfered with as well. The compellingness of basic biologic drives such as hunger, thirst, sexuality, and sleep may be subtly altered. All these changes, of course, may signal a degree of helplessness and need, marking a state of dependence, and the changes will elicit organized responses from co-members. Conversely, a network of physiologic changes may be "read" as ominous signs that the individual has been maligned, that he has failed, or that he is a liability to his group. In this instance, altogether different social responses will follow. In brief, the social meanings of any organismic changes will vary culturally. They may elicit assistance and support or ostracism and neglect, and distinctive cultural rules will determine this as well as the prescriptions by means of which these are carried out.

To put this matter differently, a characteristic quality of self-awareness, felt wholeness, and psychobiologic competence characterizes any individual. Departures from this state are necessarily calibrated in terms of his or her definition of self and body. What are read as negative departures from a person's normative state are states of awareness that constrain his or her established mode of meeting the requirements and plans of living. Yet, as discussed earlier, such states of illness have social and evolutionary roots. All this suggests that the cultural patterning of illness, which is private to the individual, also has its public side. One must hold that people who are ill show this in subtle but intelligible ways—in their faces, gestures, general demeanor, mode of involvement, level of activity, psychomotor functioning—as well as through gross bodily dysfunctions and in their reports about internal states. Furthermore, to an indeterminate extent, different groups of people probably can "read" the communications and signals of illness of others since this language of illness has (as stated) phylogenetic roots.

Analysis of the beliefs about illness of different groups of people—i.e., of their medical taxonomies, explanations, and curative practices—discloses that three broad domains of reference are implicated. These have been termed the prenatural, the worldly, and the personalistic. A tripartite division of types of symbols included in medical taxonomies has been outlined, though an underlying continuity between them is acknowledged (Fabrega, 1976b). Groups vary in terms of which of the three types of domains of reference are emphasized in the taxonomy and the way in which this is accomplished. Occurrences of illness and treatments that follow, when viewed from a social standpoint, bring into focus matters pertaining to each of these three domains. In light of the present discussion, this means that one can assume that rationalizations of the person about the *experience* of illness reflect (or are isomorphic with) its social significance, which in turn is a product of the group's medical taxonomy. In other words, the *formula* that explains the illness as a social occurrence also orders and punctuates how the individual views himself and his world while sick, and, too, how others view him. Since cultural groups differ in terms of which categories enter into their explanations of illness, so must the individual's conceptions, orientations, and behaviors be expected to differ while ill and in ways consistent with the meaning that the illness is given. For this reason, the representation given to the organismic changes underlying illness (and associated correlates) can be said to show a texture or fabric that is partially dictated by the group's medical taxonomy. In this sense, medical taxonomies also may be judged to structure the feelings, motivations, suppositions, intentions, and behaviors of persons who are diseased. In this light, it makes little sense to judge a moribund person in a particular group as showing the debility, wasting, and emaciation of a parasitic infestation or of cancer. One should, instead, view him and indeed interpret his behavior, actions, and verbalizations as conforming to that of a person showing the extended consequences of what it means to be maligned or punished in ways and through instrumentalities that the group's medical taxonomy articulates. What the individual feels and reports, what he thinks and plans, what he complains about and assuages, and how he behaves and is related to in the group will certainly reflect in an extended sense his medical taxonomy and not that of an observer socialized to believe in the biomedical one.

Illness, Medical Taxonomies, and the Question of Mortality

Perhaps it is appropriate to summarize briefly the logic of the argument that is being developed. The capacity to use social symbols creatively gives a distinctive coloration to human behavior. Such symbols must be held to give significance and make understandable the negative alterations that are signified by the term *illness*. These symbols are part of the group's medical taxonomy and their meanings are drawn from and/or are logically consistent with the inherited myths, knowledge, and basic ideology of the group. An individual interalizes this medical taxonomy and because of this it gives coherence to the organismic changes of illness and to socially relevant behaviors that follow. All this is influenced and conditioned by factors both biologic and cultural. Cultural anthropologists assert that in evolution phenomena glossed by terms such as *consciousness, culture, mind,* and *brain* are fused together and contribute to the experience of self and identity. This holism is implicit here in the attempt to give psychobiologic significance to the universal phenomenon of illness. One has only to add that the changes of illness also reflect what is expected about how the illness may be resolved and about the meaning or purpose that is culturally granted to an individual's existence. This point requires some elaboration.

In all social groups, and particularly so in simpler ones, the phenomenon of illness is strongly linked to the idea of individual finitude—that is, to the set of questions surrounding life and death and of necessity the question of the purposes surrounding human existence. By disrupting the path of personal awareness that sustains the individual in his group, an occurrence of illness necessarily raises the matter of his continuity. The socially connected nature of self and identity is revealed dramatically when human dependency is forced. At the same time, when illness affects significant others, the question of *their* permanence and, by extension, *their* contribution to and influence on the individual's identity is brought into focus. The fragile structure and ultimately social basis of the individual's own world is likewise underscored during such occurrences. Under conditions of human illness, then, the individual is made to question the basis of his placement in the scheme of things.

Now, among other things, medical taxonomies reflect, however indirectly, the existential basis and moral substance of self and personhood. In other words, they constitute a rationale that members use to give meaning to self during illness, and with this they pursue a course of medical treatment. In explaining the basis for an individual's potentially dangerous departure from personal wholeness during an occurrence of illness, the taxonomy confers meaning on how and where that departure may end. In effect, then, explanations for an occurrence of illness with which the individual is provided through his taxonomy also establish why the individual is sick and how his life is to be interpreted. The meaning that illness has and, by implication, the meaning that an individual's life is to be given are both highlighted in the explanations that are drawn from the prevailing medical taxonomy.

One is here simply emphasizing something that has always been evident whenever one is forced to deal with the phenomena of illness and death, phenomena that so often come together. Stated simply, the frame of reference that a person draws on to explain illness (and organismic integrity) is the one that he will ultimately draw on when he is made aware of the possibility of death. This occurs when the person himself is ill, or when those around him on whom he depends are ill. In either case, in explaining the occurrence of illness in a particular manner, that is, in the language of his medical taxonomy, he is in effect forcibly made to imprint a particular meaning upon the life in jeopardy. If a medical taxonomy is anchored in the existential categories that connect meaningfully with the everyday social reality of the person, that illness—and by extension, the purpose of the individual's life—is socially rationalized and made morally coherent. The social processes and personal experiences surrounding illness and death, and those that follow for those who remain, are thereby articulated and made socially comprehensible and purposeful. However, if the prevailing frame of reference vice-à-vis illness is seen to be devoid of a social rationale —in a word, if a group's medical taxonomy is logically uncoupled from social and moral concerns (as indeed is the case with ours)—the individual is deprived of a means of "socializing" illness (and by extension, death) in a coherent and integrated manner. Perhaps it is because of the apparent social insensivity and social inappropriateness of our medical taxonomy that we are confronted so often with those dilemmas (such as the "denial of illness," the "denial of death," and the "lack of compliance with medical regimens") that constantly plague the efforts of our medical practitioners to deal with illness in the narrowly construed manner that is logically dictated by their taxonomy. The ontology given illness in biomedicine must certainly also be held to promote the awkward exchanges across our various helping professions (i.e., medical, religious, etc.) in the context of terminality.

It follows, then, that medical taxonomies not only prescribe meaning and a tangible way of coping with occurrences of illness; they also, it would seem, are linked to more basic matters. A general function of medical taxonomies is that of regularizing and making socially coherent those problems generated by the question of man's mortality and eventual termination. Since the changes tied to an occurrence of illness have the effect of sharpening the fragile and temporary quality of human life, it follows that all medical taxonomies tend to be used to resolve questions and problems of this nature. Among so-called simpler people, this general function continues to be important and is served well, and this is a reason why the taxonomy and MCS of such people can be judged as socially adaptive. In biomedicine, existential questions have been excluded and this in turn has created special problems (Fabrega, 1976a).

Summary and Implications

It is very clear that humans share characteristics or traits with higher mammalian forms. Thus, they live in groups possessing determinate social organizations; they communicate, show emotions, sense physical stimuli of various types, and can solve problems, thereby overcoming obstacles posed by the environment. Such behavioral similarities obviously reflect similar neural systems and, to some extent, constitute evolutionary constraints on human differences. It is also very clear that the human mode of adaptation differs from that of the nonhuman primates. For example, by means of his system of language man is able to speak and develop a more elaborate creative and abstract (removed from the here and now) representation of himself and his condition. He can develop other (more abstract) systems of symbols (e.g., mathematics). He can also create music and use it for the expression of his view of the world, in the process mobilizing bodily motions, as in dance. These differences are somehow tied to the expansion of the brain (the whole process termed *neocorticalization*), though the exact structural and functional features are far from being understood clearly. Arguments will develop about the nature of these human–nonhuman differences: Are they quantitative or are they qualitative? Explanations of these differences in neural terms are likely to draw on concepts of hierarchy, populations of neurons, and emergent functions. Finally, in any examination of the more human modes of adaptation, one can point to seemingly compelling "cultural" differences. Thus, members of human groups speak *different* languages and internalize *different* systems of symbols by means of which they make sense of the world, communicate meaningfully with one another, and relate to the external (whether natural or prenatural) world. More specifically, musical and dance systems appear to differ, as do the modes of using facial expressions and body motion-posture in communication. The way time and space are (conceptually) organized; smells, colors, tastes, and humor interpreted; and sexuality, love, or aggression implemented can in many ways also be shown to be somehow "different." Again, arguments will develop about the nature of these human differences: Are they merely "surface" characteristics or do they reflect differences in "deep" structures? How are such differences accounted for in neural terms? It is clear that explanation of these issues in neural terms raise the question of holism versus locationism.

The above considerations constitute problems and questions that many behavioral and neural scientists ponder at one time or another. The literature in neurobiology does not offer compelling resolution of the problem of how human differences are to be accounted for neurologically. Many of the questions raised in an inquiry about the neural sources of illness and disease no doubt do not lend themselves to an "answer." Most scientists working in areas related to the problems mentioned here believe that many traits (e.g., the perception of color, recognition and expression of emotion, the threshold for pain) are in certain ways universal, but that even the way these are realized in social life is also in certain ways culture-specific. Many scientists would probably agree that most rubrics of human behavior are mixes of universal and cultural-specific (i.e., learned) influences. The social and cognitive behaviors of man involve cortical mediation of some sort; neural centers, analyzer zones, functional systems, and actual pathways subserving the various functions can in many instances be delimited. No scientist, it seems, is in the position to state whether and if so how human social and cognitive behavior differences are physicochemically and cyto-architecturally organized. Rather, it would appear that the nervous system would be judged as containing differentiated neural properties that cultures can draw on, and emphasize or deemphasize, thereby realizing the behaviors in question.

A fundamental assumption of this chapter is that illness constitutes a behavioral alteration that is physiologically and chemically grounded but socially and culturally conditioned. Although social and cultural influences of illness have been emphasized, so has the significance of illness in an evolutionary sense. The social and cultural character of illness is built on the accumulated wisdom that animals have acquired in evolution. In the event of disturbances in biological systems, animals demonstrate different preferences for fluids, minerals, food, sleep, sexuality, locomotion, etc. All this reflects an altered biologic state, which is associated with physiological changes of various types. Animals also have homeostatic and repair mechanisms of various sorts that allow them to deal with negative alterations in function. These animal analogues of the human form illness are outcomes of coded instructions or genetic programs in the animal. It is upon such archetypal "roots" of illness that social and cultural influences come to bear. Such kinds of influences have produced human illness forms; these get played out behaviorally and prompt social activities aimed at understanding and control.

From the standpoint of the way in which social systems have always functioned, then, illness is and always has been a compelling eventuation since and because it is actualized and signaled in behavior. This fundamental feature of illness is graphically visible today. Physicians in medical practice, or those working in public health programs concerned with spreading biomedicine, are everyday witnesses to the fact that individuals will *seek* and *accept* care when they are hurting, that is, when the *behavioral expressions* of disease are salient. Problems in medical care arise when treatment actions are required on a continuous basis in the absence of the behavioral grounds of disease. Stated differently, failure in the compliance with medical regimens can be explained partly as a result of the fact that such regimens need to be implemented when the biologic compellingness of "disease" is not present. Biologic compellingness of "disease" equals those evolutionarily derived and genetically encoded routines and programs that have as their outcome behavioral disruptions. It is precisely because illness has this link with behavior that social systems have been able to deal with it so effectively. Indeed, the difficulty of inducing "preventive" health behavior stems from the same kinds of considerations: the requirement of motivating a person toward *medically relevant actions* in the absence of an illness, that is, in the absence of activation of those organismic signals and motives that make the pursuit and acceptance of medical care compelling and "natural."

This way of viewing illness and disease is clearly only part of the picture. Quite obviously, social and cultural factors can override and replace those inherited dispositions that become activated during illness, as any physician who has tried to "help" a member of another culture or of different religious sects (e.g., Jehovah's Witnesses) knows. But this merely underscores the powerful types of influences that come to bear on human behavior. It reemphasizes, as it were, the biocultural nature of man. In short, in the view developed here the practice of medicine and the pursuit of optimal health care programs must be approached with emphasis given to human social and cognitive factors that influence them.

Among the present problems facing the disciplines of medicine, that of motivating people to orient to disease (or to its possibility) under conditions during which its behavioral components are dormant (in the absence of illness) must be viewed as critically important. Our social system has given us a view of "disease" and a capacity for dealing with it that was obviously not present in earlier evolutionary epochs. Biomedical knowledge and insights were not then selective factors in human evolution, but they are *now*. Man's development and evolution increasingly partakes of selective factors that are operative in a sociocultural environment, and in this one, biomedical insights and knowledge need to be heeded. With regard to medical care and policy, then, a problem for the social system is to train, motivate, and condition individuals to handle their psychobiologic systems, even when these are not overly (behaviorally) diseased, with the compellingness with which natural selection has conditioned them to deal with illness. It requires as it were, the internalization of culturally selective factors: prudent and healthful behaviors need to be ingrained so that deleterious ones can be warded off and minimized.

There is an interesting irony implicit here. Man began by viewing, responding to, and handling what we term *disease* on behavioral grounds— that is, purely as illness phenomena. Undesirable discontinuities in the way a person functioned, it would seem, have until contemporary times always served as key attributes of a medical problem. It was in social and cognitive behavior that such a problem showed itself and where it was arbitrated: this rendered the expression of the problem as illness compelling, it occasioned concern, it prompted social action, and it seemed "naturally" to validate therapeutic actions. Biomedicine has given man a way of dealing effectively with medical problems on the requirement that they be viewed, responded to, and handled nonbehaviorally, i.e., as an abstract and technological "thing." A concomitant of this state of affairs is that in order to avoid this nonbehavioral disease man has to begin to program his own behavior in line with directives he himself uncovers. Inherited dispositions vis-à-vis illness, products of natural selection, are no longer sufficient to accomplish the task; compliant and preventive behaviors are needed.

One final and related point can be made here. One notes that as a result of cultural advances made possible by the scientific and technological revolutions, man is now living under conditions that make it prudent that health and medically related actions be undertaken in the absence of those behavioral changes that have compelled individuals toward treatment in the past. Indeed, health-promoting life-styles now have appeared as the critical variables for optimizing well-being, and such styles encompass social, emotional, and physical factors. The modern unified or systems view of personhood and illness serves to justify scientifically this course of action. It has as its logical consequence the need for balanced and moderated life routines in order that illness and disease be controlled and its eventuation made improbable. But this, interestingly, is and always has been the cornerstone of the theories of illness of "primitives," whether non-Western or Western (i.e., the Greeks). Behavior was for them the domain of medical problems, a domain directly open to observation, the one directly subject to their control and modification, and the one that is grounded in evolutionarily accumulated insights. The limitation of primitive and Greek theories of illness was not just an outcome of its emphasis on the wrong causes (i.e., preternatural assumptions) or its relative lack of emphasis on cause. The limited success of these theories was an outcome of their approaching illness as natural (i.e., behaviorally compelling) phenomena and within the boundaries set by their level of understanding. The preternatural view of illness may be seen as the result, not the cause, of their limited control over the cause of illness. In his pursuit of the control of medical problems, contemporary man is now shifting to this unified holistic view of illness and personhood that was and still is the cornerstone of primitive medical theories. The irony referred to above reappears in a disguised form. A problem in fully embracing and implementing this ancient truth about illness, in addition to the requirement that health and medical matters be attended to in the absence of behaviorally compelling grounds, has been man's own biomedical achievements. The success of bacteriology and of surgery has provided man with a closed unicausal view of disease: one determinate and concrete thing *causes* or *accounts* for disease, and the eradication of this "thing" involves cure. Clearly, the power and the pervasiveness of the influence of bacteriology and surgery (among other accomplishments of civilization) have persuasively ingrained a view of disease in many ways inconsistent with the ancient one that contained inherited wisdom. This is but an example of how man's own creations act as models or molds for his description and orientation toward phenomena. Some of these acquired views are facilitative and adaptive, others are not, or at least, need to be tempered. In a sense, we are now forced to relearn and implement the ancient or original view of illness and to partially unlearn or dampen or moderate the closed unicausal one with which our own biomedical system has persuaded and lured us.

References

Argyle, M. Nonverbal communication in human social interaction. In R. A. Hinde (Ed.), *The Non-verbal communication*. Cambridge: Cambridge University Press, 1972, pp. 243–268.

Chevalier-Skolnikoff, S. Facial expression of emotion in nonhuman primates. In P. Ekman (Ed.), *Darwin and facial expression (A century of research in review)*. New York: Academic, 1973, pp. 11–89.

Deets, A. C., Harlow, H. F., Singh, S. D., & Blanquist, A. J. Effects of bilateral lesions of the frontal granular cortex on the social behavior of rhesus monkeys. *Journal of Comparative Physiological Psychology*, 1970, 59, 195–204.

Dimond, S. J., & Blizard, D. A. (Eds.). *Evolution and lateralization of the brain.* New York: Annals of New York Academy of Sciences (Vol. 299), 1977.

Eibl-Eibesfeldt, I. Similarities and differences between cultures in expressive movements. In R. A. Hinde (Ed.), *The Non-verbal communication*. Cambridge: Cambridge University Press, 1972, pp. 297–314.

Ekman, P. Universal and cultural differences in facial expressions of emotions. In J. K. Cole (Ed.), *Nebraska symposium on motivation, 1971*. Lincoln: University of Nebraska, 1972.

Ekman, P. Cross-cultural studies of facial expression. In P. Ekman (Ed.), *Darwin and facial expression (A century of research in review)*. New York: Academic, 1973, pp. 169–220.

Fabrega, H., Jr. Medical anthropology. In B. Siegel (Ed.), *Biennial review of anthropology*. Stanford: Stanford University Press, 1971, pp. 167–229.

Fabrega, H., Jr. *Disease and social behavior: An interdisciplinary perspective.* Cambridge, Mass.: M.I.T. Press, 1974.

Fabrega, H., Jr. The function of medical-care systems. *Perspectives in Biology and Medicine,* 1976, 20, 108–119. (a)

Fabrega, H., Jr. The biological significance of taxonomies of disease. *Journal of Theoretical Biology,* 1976, 63, 191–216. (b)

Field, M. The concept of the "health system" at the macrosociological level. *Social Science and Medicine,* 1973, 10, 763–785.

Franzen, E. A., & Myers, R. E. Age effects on social behavior deficits following prefrontal lesions in monkeys. *Brain Research,* 1973, 54, 277–286. (a)

Franzen, E. A., & Myers, R. E. Age effects on social behavior: Prefrontal and anterior temporal cortex. *Neuropsychologia,* 1973, 11, 141–157. (b)

Harlow, H. F. *Learning to love.* San Francisco: Albion, 1971.

Kelman, S. The social nature of the definition problem in health. *International Journal of Health Services,* 1976, 5(4), 625–642.

Levy, J. The mammalian brain and the adaptive advantage of cerebral asymmetry. In S. J. Dimond & D. A. Blizard (Eds.), *Evolution and lateralization of the brain.* New York: Annals of New York Academy of Sciences (Vol. 299), 1977.

Mason, W. A. Environmental models and mental modes: Representational processes in the great apes and man. *American Psychologist,* 1976, *31,* 284–294.

Miller, R. E. Social and pharmacological influences on the nonverbal communication of monkeys and man. In L. Krames, P. Pliner, & T. Alloway (Eds.), *Nonverbal communication* (Vol. 1). New York: Plenum, 1974, pp. 77–101.

Miller, R. E., Caul, W. F., & Mirsky, I. A. Communication of affects between feral and socially isolated monkeys. *Journal of Personality and Social Psychology,* 1967, *7*(3), 231–239.

Myers, R. E., Swett, C., & Miller, M. Loss of social group affinity following prefrontal lesions in free-ranging macaques. *Brain Research,* 1973, *64,* 257–269.

Passingham, R. E., & Ettlinger, G. A comparison of cortical functions in man and other primates. *Brain Behavior and Evolution,* 1974, *7,* 337–359.

Suomi, S. J., Harlow, H. F., & Lewis, J. K. Effects of bilateral frontal lobectomy on social preferences of rhesus monkeys. *Journal of Comparative Physiological Psychology,* 1973, *71,* 448–453.

Young, A. Some implications of medical beliefs and practices for social anthropology. *American Anthropologist,* 1976, *78,* 5–24.

3

Sickness as Cultural Semantics: Issues for an Anthropological Medicine and Psychiatry

Arthur Kleinman

> Human data are of a conceptual order, so they are destroyed if this pre-existing order is disrupted. In social science, one can explain only if one can describe, and this one can do only if one has grasped the concepts embodied in human action. (Crick, 1976, p. 93)

Introduction

One of the chief contributions of several decades of anthropological research is the recognition that culture exerts its most powerful effect on health and sickness through the categories it creates to label and explain behavior (cf. Eisenberg, 1977; Fabrega, 1974; Good, 1977; Kleinman, 1977a). Those cultural categories guide the labeling of behavior as normal or deviant, and, if the latter, determine whether it is labeled medical or nonmedical deviance (Waxler, 1974). When a sickness label is affixed to a person's behavior, cultural categories engender the distinctive conceptualizations the patient, his family, and his caregivers employ to name, valuate, and decide upon a treatment response, often in quite different and at times even conflicting ways. Indeed, much recent medical anthropological research demonstrates

Arthur Kleinman • Department of Psychiatry and Behavioral Sciences, School of Medicine, University of Washington, Seattle, Washington 98195.

that the sick individual's "illness behavior" reflects the influence of cultural categories on conceptions of the body and its functions, perception and expression of symptoms, the social sanctioning of a particular type of sick role, and the significance attributed to the sickness (Fabrega, 1974; Kleinman, 1977b).

It is perhaps most accurate to think of cultural categories as conferring specific *meaning* on sickness experiences, meaning that has both symbolic and instrumental significance. That is, the meaning context applied to sickness makes it over from a "natural" occurrence into a social construction and in so doing provides practical behavioral options for available treatments.

From this anthropological perspective, sickness is viewed as an inherently semantic subject that is inseparable from the conceptions of it held by patients and practitioners. Because 70–90% of all sickness episodes are treated *only* in the context of the family or social network (Hulka, Kupper, & Cassel, 1972; White, Williams, & Greenberg, 1961), and because of those sickness episodes treated outside the popular health domain, choices of which practitioner to consult, whether or not to comply, and how to evaluate therapeutic outcomes are most frequently based on personal and family decisions (Chrisman, 1977), the cultural *meanings* applied to sickness are of considerable practical importance for both health care consumers and providers. Oddly enough, the "biomedical model" that dominates contemporary clinical medicine and psychiatry fails to conceptualize this central aspect of health care, and for this reason is inadequate in itself as an explanatory framework for training health professionals and for conducting clinical practice and research (Eisenberg, 1977; Engel, 1977).

This chapter will review concepts of sickness and care that emerge from an "ethnomedical model," a model, I shall argue, that provides a necessary complement to the biomedical framework. To date most ethnomedical research has dealt with non-Western societies or with ethnic minorities in the United States and other Western societies. I shall argue, however, that this alternative analytic and comparative framework also can be applied to the mainstream of our society. That is, in order to derive a more adequate understanding of our popular *and* professional domains of health care, we must analyze their cultural categories. This means, moreover, that we need also to examine biomedicine from an ethnomedical point of view and must compare it with indigenous systems of medical practice.

In this short space it is not feasible to examine these questions thoroughly.[1] All that can be done is to illumine several key issues that emerge from a cultural analysis of patient and practitioner conceptualizations of

[1]The anthropological approach sketched in this chapter is presented in detail in Kleinman (1979). The practical implications of this approach for clinicians is outlined in Kleinman, Eisenberg, and Good (1977) and in Kleinman (1977c).

sickness, and their interactions, and to suggest that these issues call for a new *anthropological* medicine and psychiatry.

The Social Construction of Illness

Ethnomedical findings offer strong support for the contention that all sickness is socially constructed, not just mental disorders as some claim. Chinese culture, where I have conducted field research, offers striking examples of this general effect of cultural categories.

In Chinese communities, mental illness is very highly stigmatized. Because it is commonly believed it has a hereditary basis, marriage with the normal children of a family with a mentally ill child is in "theory" proscribed. In fact, the only labels of mental illness routinely employed among Chinese populations are those for flagrant psychosis and for mental retardation. Minor psychiatric problems, such as depression, anxiety neurosis, hysteria, or psychophysiological disorders, are usually legitimated with a medical, rather than a psychiatric, sick role.

The most commonly applied term is *neurasthenia* (*shen-ching shuai-jo*), which is used in the same sense it was given at the turn of this century in the West, in Osler's textbook of medicine for instance, as a socially acceptable "physical" problem of vague characteristics covering with a somatic mantle the various kinds of minor psychiatric problems listed above (Pickering, 1974, p. 166). Indeed, this term was introduced into China by Western medical missionaries and medical educators, and largely replaced indigenous terms that had served much the same purpose (Kleinman, 1975a). This sickness label, furthermore, is applied not only by patients but by Western and indigenous practitioners. A case vignette should serve to illustrate this cultural use of medical knowledge.

Case 1. Mr. Chu is a 40-year-old middle-class Taiwanese family head who presented in the Psychiatry Outpatient Clinic at National Taiwan University Hospital with a history of insomnia with early morning wakening, loss of appetite, and 15-pound weight loss, loss of interest in work and sex, tiredness, and irritability of 6 months' duration. A college graduate who had no prior history of psychiatric problems, Mr. Chu was referred to the clinic by his wife and neighbors following several months of unsuccessful treatment by Western-style and Chinese-style doctors, who had labeled his disorder neurasthenia.

Several weeks prior to the onset of his symptoms, Mr. Chu changed jobs in order to secure a higher wage. In his new position as manager of a large vegetable market, Mr. Chu soon began to feel "inadequate" to the tasks of managing about 100 workers, responding to daily crises, and dealing with a demanding boss who became increasingly critical of his performance. He felt incompetent and frustrated and worried constantly about his work, which he came first to fear, then to hate. Mr. Chu was unable to return to his former position or find new work. He felt trapped, because he was entirely dependent on the income from his work to support his family and therefore had to continue in the job, yet found the work "intolerable."

Shortly thereafter, Mr. Chu began to experience the various symptoms listed above. He denied feeling depressed at this time, however, and both he and his family regarded his disorder to be a "physical sickness," Mr. Chu first treated himself with patent medicines and tonic, then with special diet and local herbs, and finally consulted both Chinese-style and Western-style doctors. Both kinds of doctors diagnosed his disorder as neurasthenia and treated him with many types of medicines over several months. During that time Mr. Chu's condition steadily worsened. Eventually he became tearful and overtly despondent but neither openly talked about dysphoric affect nor would entertain a diagnosis of mental illness. He accepted referral to the psychiatry clinic solely because his condition had deteriorated to a point at which he could no longer perform his work and was faced with dismissal by his boss if he did not improve.

Mr. Chu responded well to a course of antidepressant medication with disappearance of his symptoms and improvement in his behavior. Near the end of his treatment, he admitted for the first time feeling "depressed" and suffering from a "psychological problem." With the help of the clinic's staff he was able to persuade his boss to give him a less demanding job, but he felt compelled to find work elsewhere because of "losing face."

From the standpoint of psychiatry, Mr. Chu was suffering from a depressive syndrome masked by somatic complaints. Whereas psychiatry views this disorder as a psychological experience, Mr. Chu's illness experience was principally a vegetative one. Only after being successfully treated in the psychiatry clinic did Mr. Chu and his family give up their conceptualization of his sickness as a "medical" disorder. At that point they discarded the culturally approved category of neurasthenia and the medical sick role that went along with it. In Taiwan, patients who have depression label its somatic concomitants as the disorder, a physical one, and suppress or fail to experience the dysphoric effect. In one study, for example, 70% of patients attending a psychiatric clinic there, who were later determined to be suffering from psychiatric problems, complained either primarily or solely of physical symptoms (Tseng, 1975). My own investigations have shown that this marked propensity to somatize is found among all social classes, though it is less common in highly Westernized college graduates. Alternatively, it can be reasoned that the tendency of Westerners with depression to experience it as almost entirely a psychological problem is an instance of the "psychologization" built into contemporary Western sickness categories (cf. Marsella, 1977). We can analyze this process as the sanctioned use of different cultural idioms (somatic, psychological) to express personal and interpersonal problems. Each idiom reflects different conceptualizations and in turn creates distinctive sickness experiences.

The impact of native categories upon sickness experiences has been well demonstrated for Hispanic-American patients (Fabrega & Manning, 1973; Rubel, 1964), Iranians (Good, 1977), Japanese (Caudill, 1976), Puerto Ricans (Harwood, 1977), and Papua New Guineans (Lewis, 1975), among many other groups. Medical anthropologists have elaborated a conceptual distinction in order to generalize from this very large literature on differences in sickness beliefs and behavior in different cultures. Hence, they distinguish *disease* (the underlying biological and/or psychological malfunctioning or maladaptation) from *illness* (the reaction of patient, family, community, or practitioners to the disease, by which they label and attribute particular significance to it). *Illness,* it is held, is always a social construct, a symbolic form amid a culture's range of symbolic meanings. Thus, culture-bound syndromes can be thought of as universal diseases that have undergone extreme cultural patterning of the illness experience. Similarly, any chronic sickness (asthma, arthritis, schizophrenia) can be analyzed in terms of its disease and illness components. These in turn affect each other reciprocally, such that in a given chronic sickness the psychosocial dimensions of the illness experience might be responsible for the recrudescence of the underlying disease process, and vice versa. This conceptual distinction is merely an analytic shorthand for describing the complex and powerful effect of cultural meaning systems on sickness that we have discussed.

A useful model for thinking about this influence is the "semantic network" model advanced by Good (1977), based upon the linguistic paradigm of the same name. In ordinary words, this model states that sickness terms function to provide a loose semantic tie between beliefs about sickness causation and treatment options. Like semantic networks in natural language, sickness networks relate theoretical knowledge to pragmatic action. They provide a logic for choosing among available therapies and therapists, and criteria for evaluating treatment outcomes (cf. Chrisman, 1977; Schwartz, 1969). In addition, sickness networks relate popular conceptions about bodily functions and symptoms associated with particular sicknesses with popular conceptions about typical social problems that are believed either to predispose to or to be worsened by particular sicknesses. The upshot is popular semantic fields concerned with a limited number of illness categories that tend to crosscut or relate only tangentially with established biomedical concepts about disease. These networks set out a field of culturally constituted meaning around each sickness term. In the main, sickness networks have a greater impact on lay health and health care than do biomedical categories. But in technologically advanced societies such as the United States it is probably also the case that sickness networks increasingly draw upon biomedical concepts and practices. Although semantic network analyses are most useful for illumining the popular arena of health care, it is apparent that they can be applied as well to professional systems of health care, where they disclose that biomedical disease categories, no less than popular illness categories, are social constructs (cf. Freidson, 1970; Shryock, 1969). An extremely important question, which at present is far from being solved, turns on how such cultural categories serve particular sociopolitical and socioeconomic ends of profession, class, and corporate state (cf. Navarro, 1976). Comparative studies of non-Western medical systems have contributed some valuable ideas on how such an analysis might be conducted, even if they have not yet yielded many specific data (cf. relevant chapters in Kleinman, Kunstadter, Alexander, & Gale, 1975; Leslie, 1976).

Culturally Constituted Clinical Realities

Investigations of the social context of health care reveal three separate arenas of health care in society: popular or lay, professional, and folk (healing specialists who do not belong to licensed professional organizations) (Kleinman, 1978). Each of these arenas possesses its own explanatory models, social roles, interaction settings, and institutions, all of which may be and frequently are quite distinct.

For the same episode of sickness, the different arenas apply different explanatory models and thereby create different evidence, sickness categories, and treatment goals. Consequently, transactions between patients and practitioners can be thought of as transactions between different conceptualizations that may engender discrepant and even conflicting values and expectations. Inasmuch as each of these conceptualizations is anchored in a particular social structural position in the health care system, we can regard them as necessarily entailing different views of the clinical process, views that represent the "interests" of the different arenas of care. Through these conceptualizations cultural norms and social interests play an essential part in determining what is wrong and what should be done. I shall refer to the products of this process as culturally constituted clinical realities. Clinical realities may vary cross-culturally and across the separate domains of health care in the same society. Obviously, political, economic, social class, educational, and religious factors also influence clinical reality, but in this discussion we are concerned with its cultural determinants.

Several case vignettes should illustrate how conflicts between clinical realities affect patient care.

Case 2. Mrs. Smith is a 45-year-old American housewife with chronic low back pain who has sought out the help of a noted orthopedic surgeon at a university hospital. Her conceptualization of her sickness is that it has a definite relationship to psychological and social stress as well as to physical exertion. She believes it important to understand what is wrong and to participate in planning her treatment course. She places considerable value on the quality and time spent communicating with doctors. She was disappointed with the care she received from this orthopedic surgeon, primarily because he spent little time with her, did not offer her a detailed explanation of what was wrong, and told her that all she need concern herself with was taking the medicines and carrying out the exercises as prescribed. Interviews with this doctor revealed that he did not recognize explanations to patients as essential and played down the role of psychosocial stress, which he believed fell outside the purview of surgical treatment.

Mrs. Smith first failed to comply with her regimen and soon discontinued care completely. She later consulted a chiropractor, whom she characterized in very positive terms as meeting the expectations she had of a caregiver. She reported symptom improvement under his care, whereas she had experienced no such improvement while undergoing treatment from the orthopedist.

In this case, lay and surgical explanatory models created divergent clinical expectations, expectations that led to failure to comply and poor care.

Case 3. Mr. Hsu is a 40-year-old first-generation Chinese-American cook with a history of several years' duration of "spells" consisting of palpitations, dizziness, and sweating, worsening over the previous 3 months. He visited the internal medicine clinic at a large urban hospital, where repeated physical examinations, electrocardiographic studies, treadmill tests, and analyses of blood chemistry disclosed no abnormalities. Mr. Hsu was told by the clinic's doctors that he had no "medical disease" and that his problems were "all in the head." He was referred to that hospital's psychiatry clinic for psychotherapy but did not follow through and dropped out of care. He complained bitterly about undergoing an expensive work-up but not receiving any treatment. In Taiwan, where he had lived before coming to the United States, doctors are paid, he said, solely for treatment. He denied having psychological problems and angrily rejected the notion that it was "all in the head." And, he added, he and his family and friends did not see how talk therapy could be of any help in itself. Mr. Hsu reported an alternative belief about sickness. He thought that he was suffering from a "cold" disorder owing to loss of *yang* (male principle, and therefore "hot") from too frequent intercourse with his wife, whom he had married 5 months earlier and who was 14 years younger than he. He disclosed the fear that either he would not be able to fulfill his wife's sexual needs or his sickness would worsen because of continued diminution of *yang* through loss of *ching* (semen).

Mr. Hsu and his doctors not only held different views of his sickness but also held conflicting treatment expectations. In Taiwan, as Mr. Hsu noted, the patient pays for the treatment, not for the diagnostic work-up. Moreover, psychotherapy is frequently held by Chinese to be worthless, whereas somatic treatments are believed to be effective. Although from a psychiatric perspective, Mr. Hsu was suffering from acute bouts of anxiety neurosis, precipitated by his recent marriage, from his perspective his problem was a culturally specific disorder based on Chinese cultural categories that he knew were not shared by Americans. Here we see two conflicting culturally constituted clinical realities that had a negative influence on treatment because they remained tacit.

An excerpt from a doctor–patient encounter in Taiwan, but one that could just as well have occurred in the United States, should help demonstrate that biomedicine often constructs clinical realities that exert a strongly negative effect on patient care because those realities systematically fail to confront the personal and social "meaning" of sickness:

> Patient (a 20-year-old male college student suffering from a severe case of nephrotic syndrome): How am I doing?
> Western-style doctor: All right. Your blood and urine tests are the same as last time. (He then goes on to ask the patient about specific symptoms.)
> Patient: When will I be able to return to school?
> Western-style doctor: We shall see. I'm sorry I have to go now. I can't answer any more questions. Why don't you speak to the nurse.

This patient was deeply dissatisfied by this interview. Because the doctor was a well-known specialist who had been following his case over several months, he felt unable to change doctors. Furthermore, he knew from experience that most Western-style doctors would behave in a similar way. The patient was terrified by his disorder. He had read several medical texts dealing with this renal disease and knew that one could die from it. He had been trying for several weeks to learn from his doctor how serious his disease was and what the prognosis was. He could not make plans. And his family members were unable to get more information out of the doctor than he had. In six sessions with the doctor, the doctor had merely reviewed his laboratory tests and prescribed medicines or diet. On no occasion had he been willing to tell the patient the prognosis. Nor had he responded to the patient's very evident fear. When I finally asked this doctor why he did not answer the patient's questions, he told me: "The patient's questions don't matter. He is ignorant of medical concepts. All he has to do is listen to me and follow my advice. Nothing is gained from talking with him, except getting him to take the medicine properly and follow the right diet. It is much more important to study the laboratory findings. They show what is *really* [emphasis added] going on inside his kidneys." There is no need to comment on these remarks other than to highlight them as a remarkably frank expression of the "veterinary" tendency of the biomedical approach, a "cultural" approach that this doctor could so callously employ only because of the sociopolitical power structure that supports it as the sanctioned professional method for treating sickness.

I shall now try to show how the concepts I have advanced in this chapter—especially the *disease/illness* dichotomy and conflicts among culturally constituted clinical realities—can be used by health professionals in clinical teaching and practice. First, I list several key issues generated by these concepts, and then I outline strategies that can be applied in primary care. In the concluding section of the chapter, I return to the notion of the cultural semantics of sickness to draw certain policy implications.

Clinically Relevant Issues Generated by Anthropological Studies

1. In those sicknesses where only "disease" is treated, care will be less satisfactory to the patient and less clinically effective than where both "disease" and "illness" are treated together.

2. Medical legal problems, poor compliance, poor clinical care, and special clinical management problems that result from difficulties with doctor–patient relationships most often are due to hidden discrepancies in views of clinical reality.

3. Where modern health professionals are trained routinely to treat both disease and illness, and to uncover discrepant views of clinical reality, there will be improved compliance, patient satisfaction, and other measurable components of health care, including fewer management problems and better treatment outcomes.

4. Biomedical science tends to blind health professionals to questions of illness and differing versions of clinical reality, so that behavioral-social science teaching is necessary for health professionals to acquire competence in dealing with these essential, but nonbiomedical, aspects of clinical practice. Thus, clinical science, to be adequately conceptualized, must be thought of as both a biomedical and a social science.

The Application of Clinical Social Science Strategies in Primary Care

If we think of the clinical encounter as a transaction between patient and practitioner conceptualizations of sickness and "clinical reality," then a core clinical task becomes making these explanatory models explicit and thereafter translating and negotiating between them. Elsewhere I have discussed patient and practitioner explanatory models in terms of five topics, all or some of which they may discuss (Kleinman, 1975b). These are conceptualizations of (1) cause, (2) onset of symptoms, (3) pathophysiology, (4) course of sickness (including beliefs about type of sick role and severity), and (5) treatment goals. The models also frequently contain specific expectations about style of doctor–patient interaction, therapeutic behavior, and what successful treatment ought to look like. Crucial to patient conceptualizations is the significance of the sickness. The meaning the health problem holds for patients can be crudely evaluated using Lipowski's (1969) paradigm that illness experience may represent (a) threat, (b) loss, (c) gain, or (d) no significance. But the meaning is usually more complex and detailed than this and, as we have already seen, may include cultural as well as personal dimensions. Moreover, patient and family assessments of significance of the sickness are frequently unalike or conflicting, as may be their responses to the other issues covered by explanatory models. Psychosocial gain often is apparent only after considerable contact with a patient and cannot be evaluated through direct questioning. Patients may not be aware of psychosocial gain from sickness.

The clinical tasks health professionals perform should include (1) elicitation of the patient's model (and, where feasible, the family's model, too); (2) formulation and communication of the medical model in a nonjargonistic, lay idiom with information provided about the five clinical issues of chief concern listed above; (3) open comparison of patient and practitioner models so as to recognize divergent views of disease/illness and clinical reality; and (4) express negotiations with patients about discrepant conceptualizations, especially regarding contradictory expectations and therapeutic goals.

The following questions are provided merely to illustrate how this strategy can be applied in the clinic. Doubtless, the casting of appropriate questions will vary for different clinicians, patients, and problems. The first five questions should serve to elicit the patient's model. Patients are frequently hesitant, at least at first, to disclose their models to clinicians. Therefore, clinicians need to persist and to demonstrate to patients that they are genuinely concerned with learning patient models because they believe them to be essential for good clinical care.

1. What do you think has caused your problem?
2. Why do you think it started when it did?
3. What do you think your sickness does to you? How does it work?
4. How severe is your sickness? Will it have a short or long course?
5. What kind of treatment do you think you should receive?

Several other questions will elicit the patient's therapeutic goals and the psychosocial and cultural meaning of his illness, if these issues have not already been incorporated into his answers.

6. What are the most important results you hope to receive from the treatment?
7. What are the chief problems your sickness has caused for you?
8. What do you fear most about your sickness?

Based upon elicitation of the patient's conceptualizations, the caregiver can record the *illness problems* as a complementary list to the *disease problems* evaluated from the perspective of the biomedical model. Similarly, *illness interventions* can be outlined along with *disease interventions*, and the outcome of each can be described. Effective care, then, would be assessed in terms of both lists of problems and interventions. In the same way, particular discrepancies in views of clinical reality could be recorded along with the negotiations aimed at resolving them. Negotiation might at times require the clinician to mediate between patient and family models. Rather than detail a single method of conducting such a clinical negotiation, I would like to emphasize my impression that simply entering into a negotiation and helping the patient to recognize the value of such a negotiation often is enough to resolve discrepancies in clinical reality. Such a negotiation demands that the practitioner be willing to recognize that his conceptualizations may be inappropriate or for other reasons require changing.

The chief purpose served by this clinical social science approach is to widen the biomedical framework to routinely take account of the semantic structure of sickness and care, and thereby to provide better care.

Policy Implications

What has been proposed above is more than a new technique to be added to the existing therapeutic repertoire. Instead it is a call for a major structural change in clinical medicine and psychiatry, a change that would, in effect, create an anthropological medicine and psychiatry. This call is based upon the premise that if the intrinsically semantic nature of sickness and health care is neither recognized nor responded to, then there will be predictable inadequacies in the teaching and practice of clinical care, and, equally, in scientific investigations of that subject. Because the biomedical framework fails to deal with "meaning," it profoundly disorts the cultural and personal dimensions of sickness, and, as we have seen, this can (and frequently does) produce a demonstrably negative effect on care.

Conversely, an anthropological medicine and psychiatry would take as its subject matter the way patient, family, community, and practitioner conceptualizations routinely influence the labeling of sickness, patient careers, treatment choices, patient–practitioner transactions, and evaluations of treatment outcome. It would make the everyday context of sickness in the lay arena of health care a key research issue, and would train health professionals to be as systematic in their evaluation of the crucial social and cultural determinants of sickness behavior as they are in their assessment of biomedical factors. As we have seen, effective clinical communication, treatment of "illness," and resolution of conflicts between views of clinical reality would be its practical contributions to patient care. For anthropological medicine and psychiatry, moreover, health beliefs and health maintenance practices would also acquire salience. Indeed, such an approach would almost certainly come to view the lay or popular health arena (i.e., self-care and family-based care) as *the major* form of health care, and consequently would insist that popular care be rationalized and its positive effects strengthened.

I am sure I need not push this logic further in order for the reader to recognize the large-scale transformations that might result from this approach. To exert such an impact, however, anthropological medicine and psychiatry would require a major reallocation of research funds, faculty positions, curriculum time in health sciences training programs, and considerable support of clinical application in primary care. It is doubtful whether such a basic shift in support could be accomplished unless it received considerable political backing. But it is equally doubtful that without some such far-reaching change, any significant improvement will occur in the human quality of medical and psychiatric care.

Stated simply, the chief policy implication emerging from anthropological studies of the cultural semantics of sickness is that the biomedical program in the health sciences requires fundamental reform. As now constituted, it is an inappropriate foundation for clinical science. What is needed is the addition at all levels of clinical teaching and practice of a complementary but radically different anthropological program, one that takes for its core subject the context of cultural meaning within which sickness and care are conceptualized and experienced. A forceful anthropological program in the health sciences would also widen their scientific paradigm, theoretical interests, and research issues. For clinical medicine and psychiatry this would mean that in addition to the usual biomedical questions, researchers would begin a serious investigation of the cultural semantics of sickness that would attempt to determine, among other things, the ways conceptualizations of sickness may affect psychological and physiological processes and how the context of meaning within which sickness is socially constructed may contribute to the placebo effect and the efficacy of psychotherapy.

References

Caudill, W. The cultural and interpersonal context of everyday health and illness in Japan and America. In C. Leslie (Ed.). *Asian medical systems.* Berkeley: University of California Press, 1976, pp. 159–177.

Chrisman, N. The health care seeking process. *Culture, Medicine and Psychiatry,* 1977, 1(4), 351–378.

Crick, M. *Explorations in language and meaning: Towards a semantic anthropology.* New York: Halsted Press, 1976.

Eisenberg, L. Disease and illness: Distinctions between professional and popular ideas of sickness. *Culture, Medicine and Psychiatry,* 1977, 1(1), 9–24.

Engel, G. The need for a new medical model: A challenge for biomedicine. *Science,* 1977, 196, 129–136.

Fabrega, H., Jr. *Disease and social behavior: An interdisciplinary perspective.* Cambridge, Mass.: M.I.T. Press, 1974.

Fabrega, H., Jr., & Manning, P. K. An integrated theory of disease: Ladino-Mestizo views of disease in the Chiapas Highlands. *Psychosomatic Medicine,* 1973, 35, 223–239.

Freidson, E. *Profession of medicine: A study of the sociology of applied knowledge.* New York: Harper and Row, 1970.

Good, B. The heart of what's the matter: The semantics of illness in Iran. *Culture, Medicine and Psychiatry,* 1977, 1(1), 25–58.

Harwood, A. Puerto Rican spiritism: Description and analysis of an alternative psychotherapeutic approach. *Culture, Medicine and Psychiatry,* 1977, 1(1), 22–48.

Hulka, B. S., Kupper, L. L., & Cassel, J. C. Determinants of physician utilization. *Medical Care,* 1972, 10, 300–309.

Kleinman, A. Medical and psychiatric anthropology and the study of traditional medicine in modern Chinese culture. *Journal of the Institute of Ethnology, Academica Sinica,* 1975, 39, 107–123. (a)

Kleinman, A. Explanatory models in health care relationships. In *Health of the family.* Washington, D.C.: National Council for International Health, 1975, pp. 159–172. (b)

Kleinman, A. Depression, somatization and the new cross-cultural psychiatry. *Social Science and Medicine,* 1977, 11(1), 3–10. (a)

Kleinman, A. Rethinking the social and cultural context of psychopathology and psychiatric care. In T. Manschreck & A. Kleinman (Eds.), *Renewal in psychiatry: A critical rational perspective.* Washington, D.C.: Hemisphere, 1977, pp. 97–138. (b)

Kleinman, A. Clinical relevance of anthropological and cross-cultural research, *American Journal of Psychiatry,* 1977, 135, 427–431. (c)

Kleinman, A. Concepts and a model for the comparison of medical systems as cultural systems. *Social Science and Medicine,* 1978, 12, 85–93.

Kleinman, A. *Patients and healers in the context of culture: An exploration of the borderland between anthropology, medicine and psychiatry.* Berkeley: University of California Press, 1979.

Kleinman, A., Kunstadter, P., Alexander, E. R., & Gale, J. L. (Eds.). *Medicine in Chinese cultures: Comparative studies of health care in Chinese and other societies.* Washington, D.C.: U.S. Government Printing Office for the Fogarty International Center, N.I.H., 1975.

Kleinman, A., Eisenberg, L., & Good, B. Culture, illness and care: Clinical lessons from anthropological and cross-cultural research. *Annals of Internal Medicine,* 1978, 88, 251–258.

Leslie, C. (Ed.). *Asian medical systems.* Berkeley: University of California Press, 1976.

Lewis, G. *Knowledge of illness in a Sepik society.* London: Athlone, 1975.

Lipowski, Z. J. Psychosocial aspects of disease. *Annals of Internal Medicine,* 1969, 71, 1197–1206.

Marsella, A. Depressive experience and disorder across cultures. In H. Triandis & J. Draguns (Eds.), *Handbook of cross-cultural psychiatry* (Vol. 5): *Culture and psychopathology.* Boston: Allyn and Bacon, 1977, pp. 30–72.

Navarro, V. Social class, political power and the state, and their implications in medicine. *Social Science and Medicine,* 1976, 10, 437–458.

Pickering, G. *Creative malady.* London: George Allen and Unwin, 1974.

Rubel, A. The epidemiology of a folk illness: Susto in Hispanic America. *Ethnology,* 1964, 3, 268–283.

Schwartz, L. R. The hierarchy of resort in curative practices: The Admiralty Islands, Melanesia. *Journal of Health and Social Behavior,* 1969, 10, 201–209.

Shryock, R. *The development of modern medicine.* New York: Hafner, 1969.

Tseng, W.-S. The nature of somatic complaints among psychiatric patients: The Chinese case. *Comprehensive Psychiatry,* 1975, 16, 237–245.

Waxler, N. Culture and mental illness: A social labelling perspective. *Journal of Nervous and Mental Disease,* 1974, 159, 379–395.

White, K., Williams, T. F., & Greenberg, B. G. The ecology of medical care. *New England Journal of Medicine,* 1961, 265, 885–892.

4

The Dimensions of Medical Rationality: A Problematic for the Psychosocial Study of Medicine

Allan Young

Medical Rationality

Social anthropologists work to understand why people behave as they choose to behave and why types of behavior (e.g., medical behavior) are often remarkably different from society to society. Much of their thinking on this subject has been shaped by a set of premises that originated in the utilitarianism of Hobbes and Locke and is reflected today in the anthropologists' discourse on the nature of rational man and the universality of rationally determined behavior (e.g., Barth 1966; Frankenberg, 1967; Prattis, 1973; Sahlins, 1976; Wilson, 1970). The first of the premises contends that in every society man is capable of calculating his interests. He is inclined to choose rationally among what he believes are his alternatives, and to set priorities on his different wants, placing self-preservation over the pursuit of physical pleasure, for example. Second, although rational choice presupposes coherent beliefs about the world, there are important differences between how populations perceive and appraise objects and events. These differences are determined by the particular cultures and experiences of the populations. Third, material (technoenvironmental) circumstances limit the

Allan Young • Department of Anthropology, Case Western Reserve University, Cleveland, Ohio 44106.

kinds of alternatives from which people are able to choose. Finally, even after we take into account a population's particular perceptions and circumstances, we are sometimes left with a residuum of behaviors that do not appear to be the product of calculation.

The notion of "medical rationality" refers to how people evaluate, compare, and choose practices intended to prevent, identify, ameliorate, cure, or cause sickness. The social anthropologist's interest in medical rationality has developed relatively recently. It reflects the rejection of earlier approaches to medicine, especially the uncritical borrowing of the assumptions of disease-oriented Western medicine and the appeal to spurious psychological mechanisms; the influence of certain seminal studies, including E. E. Evans-Pritchard's (1937) *Witchcraft, oracles and magic among the Azande,* Thomas Kuhn's (1963) *The structure of scientific revolutions,* and Robin Horton's (1967) "African traditional thought and Western science"; and the adoption of a suitable social-epidemiological framework within which people's medical beliefs and practices can be studied and understood. This framework incorporates the social arrangements and forces that determine differential access to particular kinds of medical services; the ecological, nutritional, and socioeconomic factors that determine people's exposure and vulnerability to sickness-inducing circumstances; and the demographic patterns that are associated with the distribution of at-risk populations (Lieban, 1973; Wellin, 1977).

It is by locating medical beliefs and practices within this framework that the student of medical rationality is able to ask his key questions: Why do people believe that a particular medical practice produces its putative effect? Given a choice of practices, why do people choose a particular one rather than another?

Standards of Efficacy

In order to answer these questions, it is necessary to recognize first that efficacy of proof can be judged by at least three different kinds of standards, i.e., empirical, scientific, and symbolic.

A proof is *empirical* when it is confirmed through events in the material world and explained by coherent sets of ideas. Even though empirical proofs are standards of rational behavior, sometimes they are underwritten by contradictory beliefs. For example, some of the beliefs used to explain what happened during sickness episode X may contradict beliefs explaining episode Y. The paradox of rational but contradictory beliefs is accounted for in two ways:

1. The goal of empirically oriented behavior is to control and interpret particular lived-through events, such as sickness episodes. Ideas tend to be

invoked contingently, with reference to more or less immediate needs, rather than abstractly or systematically. So long as there is no episode in which these mutually contradictory ideas are invoked simultaneously, the condition of coherence is not violated. The thinking of the Thulung Rai (Nepal) is typical in this regard: "One can attempt . . . to pick on particular [sickness-causing] agencies and explore their properties, but to start from the totality of possibilities and try to subdivide it would be to impose a system alien to local patterns of thought" (Allen, 1976, p. 529).

2. When contradictions are called to people's attention, they are accounted for by auxiliary hypotheses or appeals to esoteric knowledge. Auxiliary hypotheses invoke special circumstances to explain why a general principle has not worked in a particular case. For example, Amhara (Ethiopia) explain the failure of an amulet to protect its wearer by supposing that its written text (sewn inside and inaccessible to inspection) has been effaced through exposure to perspiration or rain, or the text is incorrect, or the container is made of the wrong material, and so on. Esoteric explanations suppose that only experts possess the knowledge necessary to resolve contradictions. In some societies, there are also sanctions, such as stigmatization as a magician, which inhibit laymen from seeking out esoteric explanations (Young, 1975, 1976).

Scientific proof sets more stringent standards for confirmation (e.g., hypotheses must be falsifiable) and specifies appropriate and inappropriate classes of ideas (e.g., natural causes are acceptable, anthropomorphized ones are not). Science also insists that coherent systems of beliefs explain broad phenomenological domains—e.g., "medical science"—and not simply particular events, that each of these belief systems be consistent with all the others that collectively describe the natural world, that each system of ideas and facts be pooled and publicly exposed within the appropriate professional community, and that no appeals to esoterism (i.e., "reductionism") be allowed between professional communities (Young, 1978).

Instances of symbolic efficacy should be distinguished from scientific and empirical forms. "Symbolic" can be defined broadly as referring to the ordering of what would otherwise be adventitious collections of objects and events. Through contrasting and connecting objects and events, coherence and meaning are produced. Order and meaning are preconditions for planning and rational action, and in this sense all three kinds of efficacy are constituted symbolically. But there are also important differences in how connections are made in each case. In the instance of scientific proofs, for example, the discovery of order and coherence (e.g., that A is responsible for the onset of B, so that B appears only after A) occurs together with a critical concern over the limits and validity of this discovery (e.g., whether A is a necessary but not sufficient condition for the onset of B, whether the link between A and B is better accounted for by another explanation depending on fewer auxiliary hypotheses). Symbolic efficacy stands at the opposite pole, where critical concern over objects and events is absent.

At the symbolic pole, efficacy is largely equivalent to ordering events and objects, and practices persist because they enable people to *manage* sickness episodes and *orient* themselves to threats of sickness. Thus, while the form in which scientifically and empirically efficacious practices persist ultimately depends on how they are believed to affect the sick or those threatened by sickness, the persistence of symbolically efficacious practices depends on how they affect *all* the people who participate in sickness episodes. These people include sick persons' kin, proxies, healers, and their assistants.

Many symbolically efficacious practices work by giving medical, cosmological, and social contexts to disturbing events (Young, 1977). For example, divinatory techniques, by identifying etiological events and pathogenic agents, work to circumscribe unbounded danger, transform anxiety into fear, and make it possible for people to organize the course of sickness episodes. Other symbolically efficacious practices mainly organize interaction among participants. In the West, for example, there are behaviors enabling the "professional dominance" of physicians over other staff and of medical professionals over laymen (Freidson, 1970). There is also evidence that certain symbolically efficacious practices play a more or less direct part in shaping outcomes. In an intensive follow-up study of 12 cases treated by a shaman-healer in Taiwan, Kleinman and Sung (1976) observed that 10 patients judged themselves at least partially cured even though, according to the observors' appraisals, there had been no change in several cases and symptoms had worsened considerably in one case. Kleinman and Sung trace these positive evaluations of therapeutic efficacy to the shaman's symbolically efficacious practices and the behavioral and social gains they made possible for his clients.

Some Empirically Efficacious Practices

In less developed countries it is generally the case that (1) sickness patterns are dominated by infectious and parasitic diseases, malnutrition, and traumatic injuries; (2) a major portion of sickness episodes consists of self-limiting sicknesses (Joseph, 1977; Morley, 1973; Puffer & Serrano, 1973); and (3) medical rationality is not determined by scientific standards of proof (but see Leslie, 1976, for comments on the great traditions of Asian medicine). These circumstances help explain some of the success of indigenous healers and the persistence of traditional medical beliefs and practices.

The natural course of events in self-limiting sicknesses is

onset of symptoms → outcome,

where the outcome is either a spontaneous remission of symptoms or death. But in every society people have compelling reasons for reshaping this course of events through medical intervention, so that

onset of symptoms → intervention → outcome.

Medical intervention can take various forms, such as the use of medicaments, the propitiation of causal agents through sacrifice and prayer, and changes in diet and regimen. People's reasons for intervening include their inclination to play all reasonable options against unwanted physical, social, and economic outcomes; the desire to exculpate themselves of responsibility for deviant or disvalued behavior (e.g., where deviance means failing either to legitimate "symptomatic" behavior through diagnosis and therapy, or to try actively to avoid unwanted outcomes); and their need to mitigate or disarm sickness's challenge to their ontological security (Young, 1976).

In these circumstances, the fact that many sick people recover is evidence of the intervention's efficacy.

Empirically efficacious intervention against self-limiting sicknesses is an example of medical practices that take credit for events that are going to happen anyway (i.e., spontaneous remissions). Included here are the prophylactic practices (e.g., amulets, dietary regimens, propitiatory behaviors) that consume a major portion of health-related expenditures and efforts in many traditional societies.

Another instance of this class occurs when medical belief systems incorporate etiologies that, according to the scientist's judgment, confuse pathogenic agents with innocuous or less pathogenic ones. For example, Amhara peasants do not distinguish effectively between rabid dogs and some nonrabid dogs that behave erratically and are indiscriminately aggressive. Both kinds of dogs are lumped into a single category of animals that are believed to cause rabies, and they are exterminated as soon as they have been identified. In this way, peasants conflate these different courses of events:

(a) rabid bite → symptoms → death
(b) nonrabid bite ——————→ no disease.

Amhara know the train of events characterizing episodes of rabies, (a), and conclude from this knowledge that untreated victims are likely to die unless a cure is completed before the onset of symptoms. From the scientists's point of view, Amhara are reshaping (a) and (b) into

(c) bite → intervention ⟨ pathogen eliminated → "cure"
                          symptoms ——————→ death

Western medical treatment for rabies is accessible to only a very small number of Amhara peasants, but even people who have heard of this treatment have no reason for supposing that it is more effective than traditional techniques. From an empirical point of view they are correct, since bite victims are brought to clinics only after traditional cures have proven ineffective, i.e., the onset of hydrophobia. At this point, clinics must either refuse to treat the doomed patient or offer only sedation.

The point that traditional practices persist because people believe they are efficacious should not be pushed too far, however. Even in traditional communities there are occasions when people are not wholly convinced by empirical evidence, and the persistence of certain medical practices owes more to the absence of alternatives than to people's strong beliefs in their efficacy (e.g., Forge, 1970, p. 264). Second, to say that a practice persists because people believe it is efficacious implies only that when it fails to bring hoped-for results this event does not contradict people's explanations of why the practice has a *potential* for bringing these results. Efficacious practices persist, in spite of unwanted outcomes, for a variety of reasons: Because a sickness episode is composed of a series of practices, unwanted outcomes can only diffusely raise issues about the efficacy of any single practice. We have already noted that failure can be explained away by auxiliary hypotheses (e.g., Allen, 1976, p. 528). Third, the course of sickness episodes is explained in terms of a clash between particularistic forces —i.e., where pathogenic agents or healers can turn out to have a special animus or "luck" for a particular individual (e.g., see Djurfeldt & Lindberg, 1975, pp. 211–212, on *rasi* in south India)—and the effectiveness of a practice cannot be learned before the fact, but only contingently as it engages a particular pathogenic agent. In some systems, it is assumed that the power to affect sickness and health is undifferentiated, in the sense that the same sources sicken people as well as cure, and an agent who heals in one episode may cause sickness in another. If the sick person recovers, the causal agent was the weaker antagonist; if he fails to get better, the healer and his therapy were the weaker; in either event, the outcome can only confirm the premise of efficacy (Young, 1975).

Modes of Medical Belief

So far our study of medical rationality has focused on the way standards of proof affect people's appraisals of medical events and the efficacy of medical practices. Medical rationality also reflects people's schemes for interpreting these events and determining these practices. Westerners rely on an interpretive scheme that carries highly particularistic assumptions about sickness and health. These assumptions, if they are left unexamined, place a serious obstacle in the way of uncovering the rationality of other medical belief systems. And so, before proceeding, it is necessary to reject the positivist faith that the assumptions of Western medicine simply identify the true nature of medical events, and to make the implications of these assumptions clear. We shall do this by comparing polar types of interpretive schemes (see Young, 1977).

It is possible to sort any community's medical beliefs into notions about (1) pathogenic agents: whether purposive or nonpurposive; (2) places where events responsible for the onset and course of sickness episodes are believed to take place; whether inside or outside the sick person's body; and (3) linkage between and among agents and events: whether related through narrative or through image and analogy.

Something more needs to be said about (3), intrasomatic linkages made through images and analogy. Typically, these are physiological explanations used to link etiological events to the sequence of biophysical and behavioral signs that mark the course of sickness episodes. The physiological notions of many historical and contemporary peoples seem to have developed from their observations of a limited number of biological phenomena, such as the markers separating life from death (e.g., heat, pulsing, and breathing) and imperative behavior that is somehow mediated internally (e.g., hunger/thirst and evacuation) (e.g., Goodfield, 1960; Turner, 1966). Cultures are free, within broad limits, to posit intrasomatic functions through which these biological phenomena can be explained. Even so, we can identify images and analogies that are used by many medical systems to organize these phenomena. Perhaps the most widely used image is represented in the conception of sickness as a disturbed equilibrium. Intrasomatic equilibria are conceived by some systems in terms of static proportions (e.g., Currier, 1966, on the hot–cold balance in Hispano-American folk medicine) and by others as dynamic relations between parts (e.g., Huard & Wong, 1968, on Chinese medicine); by some as exclusively internal relations (e.g., Western medicine); and by others as internal equilibria reflecting cosmic relations (e.g., Beck, 1969, on South Asian medicine).

The ethnographic literature suggests that most medical belief systems explain sickness episodes according to events taking place both inside and outside a person's body (although these explanations are not necessarily combined within particular episodes). For the points we have to make, however, it will be useful to concentrate on polar types of medical beliefs, i.e., where the choice of medical action against serious sicknesses is dominated by a single kind of explanation, whether "externalizing" or "internalizing."

Externalizing belief systems concentrate on making etiological explanations for serious sicknesses (e.g., Evans-Pritchard, 1956, pp. 99–100, 104

–105, 177–196, 222; Fabrega, 1970; Middleton, 1960, pp. 70–80). Here, pathogenic agencies are usually purposive and often human or anthropomorphic. Diagnostic interests concentrate on discovering what events could have brought the sick person to the attention of the pathogenic agency (e.g., grudges repaid by witchcraft, ritual lapses punished by ancestral spirits) in order to identify the responsible pathogenic agent. Often only gross symptomatic distinctions are made, since the intrasomatic link between etiological events and sequences of biophysical signs is either ignored or not elaborated. When intrasomatic processes are used to explain sickness, emphasis is frequently given to the role of notions such as "soul" or "spirit" rather than to biophysical functions. When intrasomatic mechanisms are mentioned, they are often represented by simple conceptions of sickness, such as a reduced natural wholeness (e.g., soul loss in Southeast Asia [Chen, 1975; Tambiah, 1968] and the Arctic [Murphy, 1964], and diminished lifeforce in Africa [Jansen, 1973]). The healer's therapeutic powers are typically expressed in his ability to enter into etiology-narratives in order to compete against purposive agencies and his access to anodynes for symptomatic complaints.

In *internalizing systems,* physiological explanations are indispensible for organizing medical strategies. Even though etiological information is sometimes diagnostically important, diagnosis ultimately relies on the healer's ability to interpret symptoms whose form and place in the sequence of symptoms are explained physiologically.

Medicine in contemporary Western society is an instance of the highly developed internalizing belief systems that originated in the literate, state societies of Europe, Asia, and North Africa. It is unique among internalizing systems because its explanations and therapeutic strategies are organized around microlevel processes and complex machine models (Hall, 1969), and it is used in communities where the power to cure, legitimate, and explain sickness is nearly monopolized by healers and teachers who have been socialized into recognizing only an internalizing, "biomedical" conception of sickness (Freidson, 1970). Other internalizing systems, such as Ayurvedic and Unani medicine in South Asia, concentrate on larger scale organic processes (e.g., humors, *doshas*) that are linked to important extrasomatic influences (e.g., astrological), and must coexist with "folk traditions" incorporating shamanistic and externalizing explanations (Obeyesekere, 1976).

Between the internalizing and externalizing extremes are medical belief systems whose therapeutic strategies depend on both etiological and physiological explanations, although the latter are often weakened by accommodating the motives and purposiveness of causal agencies and the broadly defined character of the agent's pathogenic modes (e.g., when Amhara speak of pathogens "cutting" someone's heart or "eating" his viscera [Young, 1977]).

Symptoms and Syndromes in Externalizing Systems

By uncovering the logic of medical belief systems—functional in the case of internalizing systems, etiological in the case of externalizing ones—we can explain how many non-Western peoples can frequently ignore or confuse what Western medical professionals believe are the obvious symptoms and nosologies of particular diseases. An analogy from language may help here. Internalizing systems incorporate a functional (physiological) model that can encode sequences and combinations of symptoms; symptoms "speak" in grammatical and meaningful ways. Because externalizing systems lack functional models, symptoms are often unarticulated and mute; from a medical point of view they are exclamations and not parts of sentences.

The next paragraphs concentrate on two important products of the externalizing logic—namely, perceptualizing symptoms and fusing syndromes.

When externalizing explanations dominate over internalizing ones, it is common for people to perceptualize the symptoms of some diseases. Symptom perceptualization occurs when people believe that a particular behavior or physical sign is a symptom of sickness, but recognize this symptom only as a percept—i.e., discrete, not articulated in the disease syndromes in which biomedical knowledge incorporates it—rather than as a concept (Lewis, 1976, p. 76).

Symptom perceptualization contributes to the empirical efficacy of cures by fragmenting a disease syndrome into individually manageable symptoms, as, for example, when Amhara perceptualize schistosomiasis into three discrete self-limiting "ailments"—bothersome itch, asthmalike attacks, and gastrointestinal discomfort (Nissimov, 1966). These ailments are perceived as following one another adventitiously over a period of several months, and healers know empirically efficacious cures for each of them.

Nosological fusion results when a medical system fails to distinguish what are, from the biomedical point of view, two or more discrete diseases. By classing together ailments that are characterized by different degrees of virulence (in this way similar to etiological mistakes), nosological fusion contributes to the empirical efficacy of medical practices and masks their real impotence against certain dangerous diseases. For example, the Gnau of New Guinea rely on externalizing explanations, and their sickness names concentrate on etiology. They have terms for indicating the site and features of a sickness but do not use these terms ordinarily to define or analyze how someone is sick. Nor do they depend on observing physical signs or symptoms in order to discriminate between illnesses. To take one instance, diseases of the upper respiratory tract are designated by a term glossed as "chest sickness," and particularities of different episodes of chest sickness are distinguished as either "serious" or "mild." Once someone falls ill, he is vulnerable to further attacks by the spirits that caused the original ailment. His best interests are served by displaying symptomatic behavior that will deceive the spirits into believing they have nearly destroyed him, since this is their goal. And so, Gnau "give a general uniformity to the outward show of illness and tend to mask the different and distinguishable signs or symptom complexes" (Lewis 1976, pp. 65–66, 71–72, 76–77, 82–83, 85).

The Impact of Western Medicine

The introduction of Western medicine into a community inevitably affects people's exclusive dependence on indigenous medicine. However, at the same time that Western medicine's rapid and successful action against many acute ailments displaces some traditional cures, these successes may also contribute to people's confidence in (or at least their reliance on) other traditional cures. For example, Djurfeldt and Lindberg (1975, pp. 178–179), writing about their research in south India, describe how practitioners of Western medicine tend to siphon off many of the sickness episodes against which traditional healers are least successful, i.e., episodes that have become severe and have poorest prognosis are generally taken to practitioners of Western medicine. (See also Gould, 1957, for comments on the disinclination of Indian laymen to seek out Western practitioners for ailments in which manageable illness components dominate over unmanageable components.) One consequence has been that the differential rate of remissions is now more favorable to indigenous medicine than to Western medicine. Calculations of the relative efficacy of cures is complicated when people utilize traditional cures first and then turn to Western medicine. Nichter (1978), also writing about south India, describes the tendency of many people to give credit to Western medicine for suppressing sickness symptoms and to traditional medicine for eliminating the cause of sickness.

Elsewhere, the advantage of traditional practices may be a product of their superior symbolic efficacy. Arthur Kleinman reports that out of a sample of 100 cases treated by non-Western healers in Taiwan, 89 fell into the following categories: self-limiting diseases; non-life-threatening chronic diseases (e.g., arthritis, asthma); and somatized complaints where physical ailments are being presented as "a metaphor for psychological or interpersonal problems." The high proportion of somatized complaints reflects the successes of Western medicine on the one hand and the role of certain sociocultural circumstances on the other: "In Chinese cultural settings, where mental illness is highly stigmatized, minor psychiatric problems are most commonly manifested by somatizing . . . and are managed by providing a socially-sanctioned sick role." It is also interesting that many of the remaining cases in the sample involve non-life-threatening chronic diseases "in which the management of psychological and social problems relating to the illness were the chief concerns. . . ." (Kleinman, Eisenberg, & Good, 1978).

When we write above about "traditional" or "indigenous" medicine in Taiwan, India, or other places, we intend these terms only as conventions for distinguishing non-Western from Western medicine. In no sense should they imply rigid and unchanging systems of medical beliefs and practices. Indeed, it is the adaptability of traditional systems that partly explains their persistence in regions where Western medicine is also practiced (Leslie, 1976).

For example, laymen with whom I spoke in the Kathamandu Valley made a very clear set of distinctions between Western and Ayurvedic drugs and practices. Ayurvedic treatment is considered most appropriate for a delimited variety of complaints, particularly problems connected with digestion (which, in terms of ethnosymptomatology, takes in much ground), genital and urinary functions, loss of vigor, and jaundice. Ayurvedic medicines, as my informants perceived them, are characteristically slow-acting and must be taken over long periods; they have few or no side effects; and their efficacy depends on being able to follow a prescribed dietary regimen. Western medicines, on the other hand, are characterized as powerful, working quickly, and convenient. It is for these reasons, laymen contend, that Western medicines are preferred over Ayurvedic ones, even though it is also believed that Ayurvedic medicines are safer, less expensive, and, if used properly, perhaps more likely to produce permanent cures. One consequence has been that Ayurvedic practitioners, impressed by the demonstrated successes and popularity of Western medicine, have adapted their practices to satisfy their clients. Many Ayurvedic practitioners and medicine sellers now package their medicines to resemble Western drugs, employing gelatin capsules and foil-wrapped tablets, for example. Some practitioners also combine Ayurvedic medicines and treatments with Western drugs, particularly antibiotics. Finally, many private and government-trained Ayurvedic health workers have adopted the clinical use of certain conspicuously Western practices, including blood pressure cuffs, stethoscopes, thermometers, X-ray photographs, and the reports of laboratory tests of blood, urine, and stool specimens. Practitioners explained to me that these borrowed instruments are ways to confirm or accelerate diagnoses they would otherwise make through conventional techniques (e.g., pulsing, examining eyes and mouth, collecting medical histories organized around traditional humoral interests) and accommodate their clients' expectations of what constitutes expert medical services.

Standards of Efficacy in Western Medicine

Western medicine consists of instrumental behaviors that are rationalized and organized by specifically biomedical explanations of disease. It
includes both the research-oriented behaviors of Western *medical science*
and the pragmatic behaviors of Western *medical practice.* These are two
distinctive ways of producing knowledge about sickness and health: Medical science is dominated by scientific standards of proof, and knowledge is
produced for and evaluated by the community of medical professionals and
researchers. In the case of medical practice, on the other hand, knowledge
tends to be produced for the occasion; clinical exigencies and other circumstances often make scientific standards of proof impracticable and unnecessary; and much dosing and treatment is against illness (people's experiences of changes of being and in social function)—e.g., as anodynes against
symptomatic complaints—rather than against disease (abnormalities in the
structure and function of particular body organs and systems) (Eisenberg,
1977; Young, 1978).

Although various factors separate Western medical practice from scientific standards, it will be sufficient to single out three of these. First, there
are occasions when a practitioner must choose a course of action even
though the medical information available to him (e.g., regarding the appropriateness of a particular therapy) is incomplete or ambiguous, or he is
insufficiently trained or experienced to properly decode this information.
Recent studies dealing with the clinical use of drugs illustrate this point.
When a sample of Swedish general practitioners was asked to choose
among alternative drugs for pneumonia (according to decision criteria of
curing effect, side effect, and cost), 65% of the decisions were judged
inappropriate when measured against the opinions of experts in pulmonary
disease (Lilja, 1976). The physician's difficulties are enhanced by the tendency of drug companies to proliferate minor chemical variants of existing
successful drugs. The marketing strategy is to capture a part of the market
by claiming greater therapeutic benefits and fewer adverse effects for the
new drugs, even though the advantages may be negligible in fact. Partly
because of this strategy, the total number of drugs on the market is very
great and, as a recent study of Canadian physicians suggests (Biron, 1973,
cited in Waldron, 1977), doctors are frequently unfamiliar with the constituents of the combination drugs they prescribe and often depend on the
readily available advertising literature (Waldron, 1977). At least in the
United States, government regulations determine that manufacturers' literature lists relatively few indications for which each drug can be used, and
gives counterindications and potential reactions in detail. In Latin America,
on the other hand, legal constraints on marketing drugs are much less
effective. A recent study of 28 prescription drugs marketed in the Americas

by multinational companies indicates that the manufacturers' literature informed Latin American physicians of far more indications for each drug, and often minimized or ignored serious hazards. Thus, while physicians in the United States can easily compare the drugs according to their specificity and calculate a drug's payoff versus its risk, these evaluations are difficult for the Latin American physicians to make (Silverman, 1977).

Second, institutional constraints and rewards that determine the conditions of a healer's career advancement or personal advantage often make scientific standards impracticable in clinical settings. This point is illustrated by Scheff's (1963) analysis of how legal and professional cost-benefits encourage private physicians to adopt the risk-taking strategy of "if in doubt, diagnose sick." Daniels (1972) describes the obverse strategy in the patron-dominated practice of military psychiatry. A final example is the strongly client-dominated practice of parts of Asia, where practitioners of Western medicine must actively compete with one another for clients who expect powerful and rapid-acting drugs. Practitioners often comply by providing unnecessary and dangerous doses of antibiotics and steroids (Martin, 1975; Unschuld, 1976).

Laymen and other nonprofessionals make up a third category of people who, while working within the Western medical system, tend to rely on empirical and symbolic standards for evaluating their prophylactic and therapeutic practices. These practices include (1) the ways laymen dose themselves with patent medicines, vitamins, and home remedies, or treat themselves with exercise and dietary regimens, or attempt to control their exposure to putatively pathogenic circumstances; (2) the ways laymen utilize the drugs and therapeutic programs that medical professionals have prescribed for them (i.e., from the professional's point of view, the patient's degree of "noncompliance"); and (3) the services provided by healers working outside the institutions of professionalized medicine (e.g., chiropractors, podiatrists, naturopaths). In India, and probably in many other countries outside the industrialized West, this last category of practitioners constitutes "an underground system of health care providing the bulk of medical treatment . . . [and] a widely pervasive . . . system of medical education. The professors are the drug-detail men from pharmaceutical companies . . . the junior faculty are the pharmacists in the cities. Each pharmacist has a continuing class of practitioners scattered through the neighboring villages (Taylor, 1976, p. 288).

Efficacy and Productivity

At the beginning of this chapter we argued that medical rationality is represented by people's ability to compare and evaluate alternatives according to standards of efficacy and hierarchies of goals. In earlier sections we made the point that judgments of efficacy made by different medical systems can be bracketed together because they are underwritten by certain universal cognitive processes, reflected in people's notions of causality and noncontradiction. Hierarchies of medical goals set by different medical systems, on the other hand, can *not* be bracketed together in this way, since they are socially determined and, therefore, particular to each society (Fabrega, 1978). For example, in traditional communities in South Asia, the well-being of female children is often given lower priority than the health of male children; Western society uniquely gives some priority to preserving biological life after social life has permanently ended; in rigidly stratified societies where the social ethic denies the equality of different groups, the well-being of elites is given precedence over the health of other groups.

In this section we concentrate on hierarchies that give highest value to medical *productivity;* that is, first priority is given to optimizing the health of the greatest number of people in a population, while providing at least adequate medical services for all the people. We focus on productivity, not because it offers any special analytical advantage (since *all* such hierarchies are socially determined), but rather because it is, in one form or another, the priority with which most international health planners and ministries of health in most contemporary nations claim to calculate the distribution of material resources among different segments of the population and against different health threats.

The relationship between productivity and efficacy is complicated in practice because groups or categories of people often disagree about the order of priorities implied by the goal of productivity and, consequently, the standards against which success is to be measured.

Sometimes the disagreement is between the health planner and the people who have the most to gain from accepting his priorities, i.e., the poor and rural populations for whom "promises of increases in . . . curative services apparently appeal more than do increased programs in preventive medicine. . . ." In spite of the fact that "a dollar's worth of resources spent on . . . preventive medicine . . . yields better results than the similar amount spent on curative medicine," a person's preference for curative services is consistent with our assumptions about the rational man. Among other things, his preference may reflect disbelief or unfamiliarity with scientific explanations of how certain diseases are transmitted, exaggerated expectations about the efficacy of Western curative services, and a realistic lack of confidence in preventive programs that depend on the active and sustained cooperation of other families, groups, or classes in his community (Newman, 1973, pp. 17).

Disagreement over priorities also arises from the position taken by national elites in many less developed countries. Many of these people are willing to accept programs for increasing productivity only so long as the programs do not absorb resources needed to achieve or maintain levels of "medical excellence" (i.e., standards set by medical professionals in industrialized states) of which they are the primary beneficiaries (Navarro, 1974). Stated this way, the position of the elites seems less complicated and more cynical than it is in reality, for the proponents of medical excellence are unlikely to accept the view that low productivity necessarily reflects a conflict between the self-interests of elites and the general interest. They explain away low productivity by arguing that as a less developed country progresses economically, the medical advantages now enjoyed by the few will eventually become the standard for the many; as the traditional regions develop socially and culturally, the premodern and presecular attitudes, beliefs, and values that are major impediments to improving health in these regions will gradually disappear (e.g., Benyoussef & Christian, 1977).

Opponents of this appraisal argue that national and global political economies are the necessary frame of reference for understanding the significance of existing medical practices, and that the most important constraint on improving health in many of these countries is people's ability to afford or obtain primary health services, safer water, efficient waste disposal, and adequate nutrition. Because their poverty is the product of the world economic system and the class structure of particular societies, large regions and population sectors will remain impoverished until fundamental changes in national and world political economies alter this situation. Labeling these regions "developing countries" and "traditional sectors" obscures the tenacity and modernity of their circumstances, and ignores the facts that economic improvement is not inevitable for all regions and that the continued affluence and medical excellence of "developed" regions and classes is often predicated on the continued underdevelopment of other regions and classes (Djurfeldt & Lindberg, 1975; Stavenhagen, 1975).

Although each of these three cases is a *rational* argument for its priorities, they are not equally *good* arguments from the point of view of the health planner. He measures productivity as the difference between (1) a medical system's potential for improving or maintaining levels of health, all things being equal (i.e., the efficacy of its practices, judged by scientific standards, against a specific set of etiological challenges), and (2) its achieved impact on mortality and morbidity. Put into other words, productivity measures the extent to which these other things—e.g., sets of clinical behaviors between and among practitioners and clients that facilitate or inhibit the flow of useful information, the sets of social and economic relations that determine the availability and accessibility of adequate medical services, nutriments, drugs, and laboratory equipment—determine that the potential impact on morbidity and mortality is *not* reached. Perhaps this example will help. For the sake of our argument, let us suppose that the technologically sophisticated practice of the profession-centered system of industrialized states has twice the potential efficacy of an intermediate health technology built around nonphysician health workers who are expected to provide mainly primary health services to the population at risk. But let us also suppose that in many less developed countries the technologically sophisticated system achieves only 20% effectiveness for the population as a whole (i.e., it is available and accessible to only one-fifth of the cases for which it would be scientifically efficacious), because its services are concentrated among the urban and affluent minorities and it diverts resources away from improving services for the majority of the population. The intermediate technology, on the other hand, achieves 60% effectiveness. In these circumstances, the intermediate technology will have the greater effect (3:2) on levels of morbidity and mortality, and medical rationality should favor it over the technologically sophisticated version of Western medicine (Frankenberg & Leeson, 1975; Watson, 1976).

Conclusion

Medical rationality refers to how people evaluate and compare what they believe are their alternative courses of action for gaining particular medical goals. It is three-dimensional.

The first dimension judges practices according to their efficacy—that is, their ability to bring about desired results (scientific and empirical efficacy) or to organize and manage the circumstances connected with sickness (symbolic efficacy).

The second dimension judges the desirability of practices according to socially determined hierachies of medical priorities.

The third dimension judges practices according to what the Western medical belief system considers nonmedical standards. These include the material self-interests of medical practitioners and political decision-makers, and what laymen see as the economic and social cost-benefits of particular courses of action.

The conventional wisdom of most Western laymen and medical professionals is that Western medicine is uniquely rational and efficacious among the world's medical systems. But these claims are (1) partly spurious, because people everywhere are capable of behaving rationally; (2) only partly relevant, since efficacy measures only one dimension of medical rationality and is only one determinant of a medical system's effectiveness; and (3) often beside the point, since the claims are predicated on success at preventing or treating disease but overlook the issue of how effectively practices manage illness.

Thus, the mere introduction of Western medical practices into a locality does not guarantee they will achieve their potential impact on levels of mortality and morbidity for the population as a whole. To explain or predict impacts, one must consider the productivity of practices within a community, region, or nation. Once Western and indigenous practices are compared according to their respective costs (e.g., taking into account that expensive programs of Western curative medicine divert scarce resources and attention away from more productive applications and more pressing health needs) and benefits (i.e., their efficacy against both disease *and* illness), the blanket superiority of Western practices becomes problematic.

Conventional thinking about the uniqueness of Western medicine relies on a scientistic premise (Western medicine = scientific medicine), which confuses (1) the organization of medical science with the organization of medical practice, (2) standards of efficacy with measures of productivity, and (3) the uniqueness of scientific explanation with the unique capabilities of internalizing medical belief systems (e.g., the symptom "reading" power of the disease-oriented view of sickness).

The conventional wisdom insulates Western medicine from alternative approaches to sickness and health and, in this way, limits its capacity for adapting to the socially desirable goal of productivity in both developed and less developed countries:

> The term "modern medicine," used in contrast with traditional medicine, encourages the user to confuse inferences from the modernity-traditionalism dichotomy with reality. . . . The dichotomy implies that practitioners of traditional medicine are uniformly conservative and reject opportunities to acquire new knowledge, and yet the limited evidence at hand indicates that the opposite situation prevails. (Leslie, 1976, pp. 6–7)

References

Allen, N. J. Approaches to illness in the Nepalese hills. In J. B. Loudon (Ed.), *Social anthropology and medicine*. London: Academic, 1976.

Barth, F. *Models of social organization*. London: Royal Anthropological Institute, 1966.

Beck, B. E. F. Colour and heat in south Indian ritual. *Man*, 1969, *4*, 533–572.

Benyoussef, A., & Christian, B. Health care in developing countries. *Social Science and Medicine*, 1977, *11*, 399–408.

Biron, P. A. A hopefully biased pilot survey of physicians' knowledge of the content of drug combinations. *Canadian Medical Association Journal*, 1973, *109*, 35–39.

Chen, P. C. Y. Medical systems in Malaysia: Cultural bases and differential use. *Social Science and Medicine*, 1975, *9*, 171–180.

Currier, R. L. The hot-cold syndrome and symbolic balance in Mexican and Spanish American folk medicine. *Ethnology*, 1966, *5*, 251–263.

Daniels, A. Military psychiatry: The emergence of a subspecialty. In E. Freidson & J. Lorber (Eds.), *Medical men and their work*. Chicago: Aldine, 1972.

Djurfeldt, G. Lindberg, S. *Pills against poverty: A study of the introduction of Western medicine into a Tamil village*. Lund, Sweden: Studentlitterature, 1975.

Eisenberg, L. Disease and illness: Distinctions between professional and popular ideas of sickness. *Culture, Medicine and Psychiatry*, 1977, *1*, 9–24.

Evans-Pritchard, E. E. *Witchcraft, oracles and magic among the Azande*. Oxford: Oxford University Press, 1937.

Evans-Pritchard, E. E. *Nuer religion*. Oxford: Oxford University Press, 1956.

Fabrega, H., Jr. Dynamics of medical practice in a folk community. *Milbank Memorial Fund Quarterly*, 1970, *48*, 391–412.

Fabrega, H., Jr. Ethnomedicine and medical science. *Medical Anthropology*, 1978, *2* (2), 11–28.

Forge, A. Prestige, influence, and sorcery: A New Guinea example. In M. Douglas (Ed.), *Witchcraft confessions and accusations*. London: Tavistock, 1970.

Frankenberg, R. Economic anthropology: One anthropologist's view. In R. Firth (Ed.), *Themes in economic anthropology*. London: Tavistock, 1967.

Frankenberg, R., & Leeson, J. The sociology of health dilemmas in the post colonial world: Intermediate technology and medical care in Zambia, Zaire, and China. In E. DeKadt and G. Williams (Eds.), *Sociology and development*. London: Tavistock, 1975.

Freidson, E. *Profession of medicine: A study of the sociology of applied knowledge*. New York: Dodd, Mead, 1970.

Goodfield, G. J. *The growth of scientific physiology*. London: Hutchison, 1960.

Gould, H. The implications of technological change for folk and scientific medicine. *American Anthropologist*, 1957, *59*, 507–516.

Hall, T. S. *Ideas of life and matter*. Chicago: University of Chicago Press, 1969.

Horton, R. African traditional thought and Western science. *Africa*, 1967, *37*, 50–71; 155–187.

Huard, P., & Wong, M. *Chinese medicine*. New York: McGraw-Hill, 1968.

Jansen, G. *The doctor–patient relationship in an African tribal society*. Assen, The Netherlands: Koninkljke Van Gorcum, 1973.

Joseph, S. C. Worldwide patterns of disease. In S. C. Joseph, D. Koch-Weser, & N. Wallace (Eds.), *Worldwide overview of health and disease*. New York: Springer, 1977.

Kleinman, A., Eisenberg, L., & Good, B. Culture, illness and care: Clinical lessons from anthropological and cross-cultural research. *Annals of Internal Medicine*, 1978, 251–258.

Kleinman, A., & Sung, L. Why do indigenous healers successfully heal?: A follow up study of the efficacy of indigenous healing in Taiwan. Boston: Harvard University Medical School, 1976 (mimeograph).

Kuhn, T. *The structure of scientific revolutions*. Chicago: University of Chicago Press, 1963.

Leslie, C. Introduction. In C. Leslie (Ed.), *Asian medical systems: A comparative study*. Berkeley: University of California Press, 1976.

Lewis, G. A view of sickness in New Guinea. In J. B. Loudon (Ed.), *Social anthropology and medicine*. London: Academic, 1976.

Lieban, R. Medical anthropology. In J. J. Honigmann (Ed.), *Handbook of social and cultural anthropology*. Chicago: Rand McNally, 1973.

Lilja, J. How physicians choose their drugs. *Social Science and Medicine*, 1976, *10*, 363–365.

Martin, K. Medical systems in a Taiwan village. In A. M. Kleinman, P. Kunstadter, E. R. Alexander, & J. L. Gale (Eds.), *Medicine in Chinese cultures*. Washington, D.C.: Fogarty International Center, 1975.

Middleton, J. *Lugbara religion*. Oxford: Oxford University Press, 1960.

Morley, D. *Pediatric priorities in the developing world*. London: Butterworths, 1973.

Murphy, J. M. Psychotherapeutic aspects of shamanism on St. Lawrence Island, Alaska. In A. Kiev (Ed.), *Magic, faith, and healing*. New York: Basic, 1964.

Navarro, V. The underdevelopment of health or the health of underdevelopment: An analysis of the distribution of human health resources in Latin America. *International Journal of Health Services*, 1974, *4*, 5–27.

Newman, P. *A conceptual framework for the planning of medicine in developing countries.* World Bank staff working paper 153. Washington, D.C.: World Bank, 1973 (Mimeograph).

Nichter, M. Patterns of resort in the use of therapy systems and their significance for health planning in South Asia. *Medical Anthropology,* 1978, 2 (2), 29–58.

Nissimov, N. Intestinal schistosomiasis. *Ethiopian Medical Journal,* 1966, 4, 67–69.

Obeyesekere, G. The impact of Ayurvedic ideas on the culture and the individual in Sri Lanka. In C. Leslie (Ed.), *Asian medical systems: A comparative study.* Berkeley: University of California Press, 1976.

Prattis, J. I. Strategizing man. *Man,* 1973, 8, 46–58.

Puffer, R., & Serrano, C. *Patterns of mortality in childhood.* Washington, D.C.: Pan American Health Organization, 1973.

Sahlins, M. *Culture and practical reason.* Chicago: University of Chicago Press, 1976.

Scheff, T. Decision rules, types of errors, and their consequences on medical diagnosis. *Behavioral Science,* 1963, 8, 97–107.

Silverman, M. The epidemiology of drug promotion. *International Journal of Health Services,* 1977, 7, 157–166.

Stavenhagen, R. *Social classes in agrarian societies.* New York: Anchor, 1975.

Tambiah, S. J. The ideology of merit and the social correlates of Buddhism in a Thai village. In E. R. Leach (Ed.), *Dialectic in practical religion.* Cambridge: Cambridge University Press, 1968.

Taylor, C. The place of indigenous medical practitioners in the modernization of health services. In C. Leslie (Ed.), *Asian medical systems: A comparative study.* Berkeley: University of California Press, 1976.

Turner, V. Colour classification in Ndembu ritual: A problem in primitive classification. In M. Banton (Ed.), *Anthropological approaches to the study of religion.* London: Tavistock, 1966.

Unschuld, P. The social organization and ecology of medical practice in Taiwan. In C. Leslie (Ed.), *Asian medical systems: A comparative study.* Berkeley: University of California Press, 1976.

Waldron, I. Increased prescribing of Valium, Librium, and other drugs: An example of the influence of economic and social factors on the practice of medicine. *International Journal of Health Services,* 1977, 7, 37–62.

Watson, E. J. Meeting community health needs: The role of the medical assistant. *WHO Chronicle,* 1976, 30, 91–96.

Wellin, E. Theoretical orientations in medical anthropology: Continuity and change over the past half century. In D. Landy (Ed.), *Culture, disease, and healing.* New York: Macmillan, 1977.

Wilson, B. (Ed.). *Rationality.* New York: Harper & Row, 1970.

Young, A. Magic as a "quasi-profession": The organization of magic and magical healing among Amhara. *Ethnology,* 1975, 14, 245–265.

Young, A. Some implications of medical beliefs and practices for social anthropology. *American Anthropologist,* 1976, 78, 5–24.

Young, A. Order, analogy, and efficacy in Ethiopian medical divination. *Culture, Medicine and Psychiatry,* 1977, 1, 183–199.

Young, A. Mode of production of medical knowledge. *Medical Anthropology,* 1978, 2 (2), 97–124.

5

Psychosocial Factors and Health: New Program Directions

World Health Organization

Introduction

At the World Health Assembly in May 1974, member states of WHO adopted a resolution emphasizing the need to explore the role of psychosocial factors affecting health and health care. They requested the organization to develop proposals for strengthening activities in this field.

In order to identify appropriate points of entry for an effective program, a review was made of the existing state of knowledge on the topic, including information derived from such sources as previous WHO activities; responses to a questionnaire sent to member states and nongovernmental organizations in official relations with WHO; the recommendations of the WHO Advisory Committee on Medical Research; the experience and contributions of the WHO Collaborating Centre for Research and Training on Psychosocial Factors and Health, in Stockholm; and the results of consultations at national and regional levels, with members of expert advisory panels and with a provisional Steering Committee composed of public health administrators.

World Health Organization • Paper presented by the Director–General, World Health Organization, to the Twenty-ninth World Health Assembly; prepared by T. W. Harding, A. Jablensky, E. E. Meyer, J. Moser, and N. Sartorius of the Division of Mental Health; published with permission of the World Health Organization.

This chapter presents a summary of the review, together with the program proposals made to the World Health Assembly in May of 1976. The proposals were endorsed by the Assembly and the program is now under way.

A Selective Review of Psychosocial Factors, Health, and Health Services, with Particular Reference to WHO Activities

Psychosocial Influences on the Incidence of Disease

Social class is defined differently in different societies and by different investigators. Nevertheless, however defined, it correlates highly with economic conditions, education, way of life, attitudes and expectations, and exposure to different types and degrees of stress. In a review of the literature it has been suggested that, although the social classes may not differ significantly regarding the total amount of stress experience, the types of stress and, more importantly, the availability of external resources and internalized coping mechanisms protecting the individual from developing a pathological response to stress differ among the social groups. The relationship between health programs and socioeconomic development has been reviewed in earlier WHO publications (Economics of Health and Disease, 1971; Interrelationships, 1972; Myrdal, 1952). Class-related living conditions may explain findings indicating that low socioeconomic status is associated with a shorter expectancy of life at birth, an increased risk of developing some mental disorders, poorer indices of growth and health in childhood, higher infant mortality, and prematurity and/or low birth weight (WHO Technical Report No. 217, 1961). Class-related behavioral patterns (e.g., age at marriage, fertility) have also been suggested as possible reasons for the higher prevalence of cervical cancer among women in lower socioeconomic groups and of breast cancer and cancer of the corpus uteri among women in middle and upper socioeconomic strata.

Cultural change, migration, urbanization, and industrialization can have widely varying consequences—positive and negative—for the health of different population groups and individuals. Adverse effects are usually observed in situations of rapid change, which strip away the habitual supports and protections with which traditional culture surrounds the individual. Overall morbidity and mortality rates for lung cancer (even when smoking habits are excluded) have been found to be increased for first-generation migrants from rural to industrial areas, as compared with second-generation individuals of the same origin.

A study in Africa found that adherence to traditional beliefs and values was associated with lower blood pressure in members of extended rural families, but individuals who maintained such beliefs after having moved to the city had an increased risk of hypertension. Evidence exists suggesting that populations of the same ethnic and, presumably, the same genetic stock can exhibit very different morbidity patterns if exposed to different cultural influences; for example, compared with the general population in Japan, the Japanese living in the United States of America have an excessive death rate from cardiovascular and cerebrovascular diseases but, as noted in a WHO expert committee report (WHO Technical Report No. 365, 1967), lower death rates from gastric cancer.

The earlier interest in identifying specific constellations of external events, physical and mental constitution, intrapsychic conflicts, and hypothetical "mental mechanisms" that trigger off maladaptive physiological responses and produce specific psychosomatic disorders involving tissue change (such as bronchial asthma, peptic ulcer, or ulcerative colitis) has been noted by a WHO expert committee, which recommended more emphasis on approaches focusing on the general, nonspecific effects of psychosocial variables on the risk of developing a variety of illnesses. (WHO Technical Report No. 275, 1964). It has been pointed out that in developed countries the majority of episodes of illness of all kinds that occur over a period of time in a population tend to cluster within a relatively small proportion of individuals, and the theory has been propounded that these individuals may have in common some psychosocial characteristics, such as experience of the environment as threatening. The epidemiological method of standardized recording and counting of units of "life events" affecting the individual has demonstrated that the onset of different conditions (such as tuberculosis, myocardial infarction, schizophrenia, or depressive illness) is preceded by an excess of life events that may facilitate in a nonspecific way the occurrence of the disorder.

Occupational stress and strain are a problem of growing concern. A WHO study group (WHO Technical Report No. 183, 1959) has reviewed the mental health consequences of automation. The incidence of ill health in a variety of occupations has been found to be associated with job dissatisfaction, uncertainty about the future, boredom, low participation, and poor social support from co-workers and supervisors. A current WHO project is concerned with the health consequences of shift work in industry. Research on the pathogenic mechanisms and health effects of exposure to different stressors, especially in relation to working conditions, is being carried out by the WHO International Research and Training Centre on Psychosocial Factors and Health, in Stockholm.

The association between psychosocial stress factors and cardiovascular disorders has been studied particularly extensively. Following observations on "epidemics" of hypertension in situations of continuous stress (e.g., in combat conditions or during the siege of Leningrad), hypertensive responses have been found to occur more frequently in minority groups, among recent migrants from rural to urban areas, and in a variety of occupational situations, especially those characterized by high noise levels. Evidence, however, that such hypertensive responses to stress may be the prelude to chronic hypertensive disease is limited. Some studies have demonstrated that periods of psychological tension are accompanied by increased blood cholesterol levels, and a large number of observations suggest links between sociocultural factors and coronary heart disease. The effects of stress in the urban environment on the occurrence and outcome of cardiovascular disorders are the subject of WHO studies in Europe (Kaunas, USSR, and Rotterdam, Holland) and in the Western Pacific region.

An important perspective has been opened by multidisciplinary research based on the concept of stress that emphasizes the role of general, presumably phylogenetic, adaptive responses to a large variety of external stimuli mediated through neuroendocrine mechanisms. In a series of multidisciplinary symposia organized in collaboration with the University of Uppsala and the WHO Collaborating Centre on Research and Training in Psychosocial Factors and Health, Stockholm, a detailed review was carried out of current knowledge about the role of psychosocial stimuli as stressors. The symposia dealt with the psychosocial environment and psychosomatic diseases, childhood and adolescence, female and male roles and relationships, and working life (Levi, 1971, 1975, 1978, 1979). An important topic discussed in these symposia was that of behavioral "coping strategies" for dealing with stress that could be of particular importance in the prevention of morbidity and disability. A number of these coping strategies have been described which seem to facilitate adjustment to stress. The degree to which coping strategies are universal or even similar in different cultures is not known.

Behavior and attitudes conditioned both by culture and by the physical environment play a direct role in the inception and spread of widely prevalent noncommunicable conditions, like malnutrition, and communicable diseases. This has been recognized, for example, in the WHO project on schistosomiasis in the Lake Volta area, which demonstrated that a sociological approach to the health-related behavior of individuals can suggest specific ways to increase the effectiveness of prevention of a communicable disease.

Psychosocial Influences on the Course and Outcome of Disease

Recovery or failure to recover from illness is also related to psychosocial influences. The different mortality rates for the same disease conditions that have been reported for various social groups and whole societies reflect particularly the importance of differences in social and economic conditions for the outcome of disease. The significant demographic shifts that have followed economic development in industrialized countries have resulted in a different pattern of morbidity characterized by a high proportion of chronic disorders such as old-age diseases (WHO Technical Report No. 507, 1972) and disability. In addition, the introduction of new technology has resulted in psychosocial consequences that were not the focus of attention before, as noted by a WHO study group that considered the mental health aspects of the peaceful uses of atomic energy.

The stigma society attaches to certain diseases—for example, mental disorders (WHO Technical Report No. 177, 1959), epilepsy, (WHO Technical Report No. 130, 1957), and leprosy (Hasselblad, 1974)—has been described in WHO and other publications as a major contributor to disability resulting from such conditions, regardless of their clinical severity. Even in the absence of stigma, social factors such as the complexity of the modern urban environment play an important role in the genesis of disability.

Social conditions and psychosocial factors also play a direct role in the process leading from acute to chronic disease and impairment, and then to disability. This has been clearly recognized in the development of the WHO program on disability prevention, in the proposals for the inclusion of separate codes for impairments and handicaps in the International Classification of Diseases, and in a recent WHO-supported study in Belgrade (Slater *et al*, 1974).

Sociological studies have pointed to the importance of the expectations, prescribed patterns of behavior, and value concepts inherent in each society's stereotype of the "sick role." Complex interactions occur between the symptoms of disease and their perception by the individual and the social environment that result in the adoption, maintenance, or rejection of the "sick role."

The aspects of the problem have been clearly demonstrated particularly in relation to some of the mental disorders. The importance of community attitudes toward the mentally ill was reviewed by a WHO expert committee on mental health over 19 years ago (WHO Technical Report No. 177, 1959). Schizophrenic patients discharged from the hospital are at different levels of risk of relapse, depending on the amount of emotional tension in the family to which the patient returns. The term *social breakdown syndrome* has been suggested to describe the deterioration of personal habits and the loss of activity, aspirations, and ability to communicate that accompany chronic disorders and constitute the nucleus of social disability.

Fairly consistent findings in different cultures suggest that the characteristics of the individual's immediate social environment, e.g., participation in a cohesive family and the availability of group support, can function as buffers against influences that cause disease or disability. Thus, first admission rates for psychiatric disorders in the United States of America have been found to be lower for members of larger households and higher for members of small households (Kramer, 1969). At the same time, families in which one member has a psychoneurotic or other behavior disorder show a disproportionately large share of illness, accidents, and chronic disorders; this further confirms the contention that the family is the focal point of important influences on individual health. On the other hand, family structure affects the health of its members, as shown, for example, in WHO's collaborative study on social and psychological factors affecting breast-feeding behavior and in a recent review of influences of "cycles of disadvantage" on the health of the child.

Evidence from a number of studies suggests that both on physical conditions and in serious mental disorders, factors related to the social and cultural environment play a major role in determining the course and outcome of the conditions, and are more accurate predictors of recovery or lack of recovery from illness than clinical symptoms alone. The follow-up phase of the WHO collaborative project, the International Pilot Study of Schizophrenia (1973), showed strikingly different course and outcome of schizophrenia of initially similar severity among patients from different countries. The proportion of patients who recovered fully and did not suffer social impairments was considerably higher in the developing countries; the proportion of patients in whom the disorder became chronic and disabling was significantly higher in the developed countries taking part in the study (World Health Organization, 1979).

Behaviorally Determined Disorders

Much attention has been given in recent years to psychosocial factors underlying conditions related to dependence on alcohol and other drugs (including nicotine), which show a trend of increase in many countries; it has been suggested that other behavioral disorders such as inveterate gambling, overeating, and certain sexual perversions may be due to similar underlying causes. The pathogenetic mechanisms are far from clearly understood but are ascribed to a complex combination of psychobiological and sociocultural factors and often are explained as learned responses.

Since problems related to the use of alcohol and the use of other drugs may occur at the same or different times in the same person, and since there are many similarities between their psychosocial causes and the necessary preventive and treatment measures concerning dependence on alcohol and dependence on other drugs, a WHO expert committee (WHO Technical Report No. 363, 1967) has recommended that, at least at the national level, such problems should be considered together for planning purposes. The committee stressed the need for the development of comprehensive programs to meet the physical, psychological, social, economic, and other problems arising in relation to the drug-dependent person, his family, and society in general.

These matters were explored further by a European Regional Office working group on health education programs concerning drug abuse in young people (Working Group, Hamburg, 1973) and by a WHO interregional course in 1971 and seminar in 1972 on national programs on problems of alcohol and drug dependence (Moser, 1974). It was found that parliamentary commissions or coordinating agencies had been established in several countries with representatives from various ministries and other bodies to ensure a multidisciplinary approach to the problems concerned. More recently (1975), a European Regional Office symposium on the planning and organization of services for alcoholism and drug dependence noted the psychosocial aspects of rehabilitation and observed that treatment may be predominantly medical in the initial phase but, as the focus shifts toward reintegration of the individual into his family and community, the emphasis becomes increasingly multidisciplinary.

In preparation for a WHO meeting in 1975, extensive reviews were prepared of the social, psychobiological, psychiatric, economic, and legislative aspects of disabilities related to alcohol consumption. It was shown clearly that whereas a proportion of persons who consume considerable amounts of alcohol develop an alcohol-dependence syndrome, many heavy drinkers do not but are affected by other psychological, social, and physical consequences, which in turn have repercussions on the family and wider community.

Many countries have reported trends toward an increase in alcohol-related problems among women. This may be linked to increasing emancipation, the decline in the size of families, and the increase in female responsibilities, including employment outside the home. At the same time, the age of onset of alcohol-related problems is falling in many areas. A recent report brings evidence of an increase of at least 30% in alcohol consumption between 1960 and 1968 and indicates that changes in the overall consumption of alcoholic beverages have a bearing on the health of the people in any society (Bruun, Edwards, Lumio, Mäkelä, Pam, Popham, Room, Schmidt, Skog, Sulkenen, & Osterberg, 1975). Control of the availability of alcohol thus becomes a public health issue. Therefore, in addition to measures such as public education and early identification and treatment of persons with alcohol-related problems, other preventive strategies have to be considered, such as limitations on the number and type of outlets, the content and types of beverage permitted, and the regulation of hours of sale and of marketing and profit as well as pricing and taxation.

Combinations of psychosocial factors may result in one or another of the dependence disorders. Thus, where the host and environmental factors remain the same, change in the availability of the agent may result merely in change in the type of dependence; and change in the environment alone may sometimes result in apparent remission of the disorder. An illustration of this was seen among United States military personnel returning from Viet Nam, many of whom had become dependent on heroin. On follow-up in their home communities a few months later, only a small percentage were still using heroin; however, for a considerable number the change in environment merely altered their drug use pattern and they became heavy consumers of alcohol. The recently published WHO manual on drug dependence (Kramer & Cameron, 1975) outlines possible action to reduce or eliminate environmental factors related to drug dependence, such as attempts to reduce the social and economic stress, the blocked opportunities, and the sociocultural pressures that encourage the nonmedical use of dependence-producing drugs.

Drugs that have long been in use in certain parts of the world are now creating problems in other parts. Thus, the use of cannabis and opiates has spread in Europe and North America, while alcohol is increasingly being used in India, Pakistan, and some North African and Eastern Mediterranean countries (WHO Technical Report No. 516, 1973). Another notable trend is the change in patterns of use of drugs by individuals from the middle and upper social classes. An increasing tendency to multiple drug use has been observed, involving a wide variety of drugs with different effects (WHO Technical Report No. 516, 1973; WHO Technical Report No. 460, 1970).

Many studies have reported that heavy drinkers are strongly represented among persons who attempt or commit suicide, and a high frequency of alcoholic parents has been found among young people attempting suicide (Prevention of Suicide, 1968). It has been suggested that dependence on certain other drugs may be an alternative to suicide. There appears to be a particularly high risk of suicide during withdrawal from drugs. As among alcoholics and drug-dependent persons, those known to be suicidal do not appear to show any consistent pattern of psychological attributes. Groups with a high risk of suicide include in most areas of the world the aged, especially recently retired males; university student populations; and persons suffering from depressive illness. High suicide rates have been found in geographical areas with high indices of social disorganization (overcrowding; a high proportion of persons living alone, mostly in boardinghouses and cheap hotels; a high incidence of alcoholism, drug dependence, and criminality; and a high population mobility). Findings in relation to attempted suicide have been similar. In the European region the problem of suicide in young people was the subject of a WHO working group held in Zagreb in 1973 (Working Group, Zagreb, 1974) and of a WHO conference held in Luxembourg in 1974 (Conference on Suicide,

1974). Case histories of suicide and attempted suicide show a more frequent history of broken homes in childhood than is seen in the general population; in some countries this is true also of persons dependent on alcohol and drugs.

From some countries, very considerable increases in rates of nonfatal self-poisoning among young people have been reported in the last few years (Suicide and Attempted Suicide, 1974). These are often interpreted as a "cry for help," although on interrogation the young people are frequently ambivalent about whether their intention was to die. The desperate situations in which they find themselves are sometimes related to increased independence at an early age, and in some cases to unpreparedness to accept nonfulfillment of their desires.

The incidence, course, outcome, and consequences—both individual and social—of certain communicable diseases are particularly strongly influenced by psychosocial factors. In many parts of the world alarming increases in sexually transmitted diseases, for example, have been noted. There appear to be clear causal relationships with such psychosocial factors as changes in attitudes toward sexual activity and promiscuity, in part related to the increased availability and use of contraceptive techniques and of treatment for the sexually transmitted diseases (WHO Technical Report No. 572, 1975; Teaching of Human Sexuality, 1974). These matters were discussed at a WHO meeting on health education in the control of sexually transmitted diseases held in Geneva in November 1974 and at the Technical Discussions held during the Twenty-eighth World Health Assembly on "Social and health aspects of the sexually transmitted diseases: Need for a better approach." The Health Assembly recognized the need for a "fuller appreciation of the public health aspects of sexually transmitted diseases" in its resolution WHA 28.58.

The psychosocial aspects of the etiology and management of mental retardation have been considered in several WHO activities (WHO Technical Report No. 392, 1968; WHO Technical Report No. 75, 1954). Among the causes of intellectual retardation, cognitive as well as cultural deprivation has been shown to play an important role. It has been shown further that psychosocial and educational assistance, as well as medical care, can do much to alleviate the condition and help a percentage of the mentally retarded to assume a useful role in society. In their management, stress is being laid increasingly on the "normalization principle," emphasizing the support of the family in the care and training of their mentally retarded members, and on the use as far as possible of general education, health, and leisure-time facilities for the mentally retarded rather than the establishment of separate facilities. Considering that, according to presently available knowledge, mental retardation affects up to 3% of a population, the Health Assembly recognized the need for research in this area in its resolution WHA 28.57, stating that "epidemiological, psychosocial and biological research" in this area should be encouraged.

Road accidents (Norman, 1962; Fatal Accidents, 1974; Symposium on Human Factors, 1967; Road Accidents, 1975) are responsible for more than 250,000 deaths each year and over 30% of all deaths in the 15–25 age group. Contrary to the belief that road deaths are a matter of concern only to the highly industrialized countries, the road accident problem has risen in developing countries. For example, the road death toll per 10,000 vehicles in India is 10 to 15 times that of the United States of America or the United Kingdom; in Kuwait there has been a threefold increase in road accidents in 10 years; and in Kenya road deaths per passenger mile are several times higher than in the United Kingdom and the United States of America. Psychosocial factors are at least as important as physical strain in the causation of accident-proneness. They include decrease in alertness due to the monotony of driving, overstimulation from noise and traffic jams, and emotional stresses caused by marital conflicts, job frustration, and economic problems. Abuse of alcohol and drugs is often a concomitant causal factor, a fact the Twenty-seventh World Health Assembly recognized in resolution WHA 27.59 on the prevention of road traffic accidents. The same is true for occupational accidents, neither the frequency nor the severity of which has diminished in the past few decades, thus indicating the limits of technical prevention.

Psychosocial Factors and Health Services

There has been widespread recognition in recent years of the profound problems involved in providing health care. In developing countries, where the majority of people have no access to basic health services (although there may be many traditional forms of health care), the key issues have been identified as coverage, cost, and acceptability in technical, individual, and social terms. In industrialized countries where medical care has become increasingly costly and technically complex, dissatisfaction with existing systems is now expressed, together with concern over their effectiveness in the relief of human suffering. These problems in which psychosocial factors play a major role have been identified as important areas for WHO action and are reflected in a number of ongoing programs such as those on primary health care, disability prevention, and health manpower development.

Health Workers

Emphasis on teamwork and on a shared, clearly defined, and attainable goal has led to persistently high morale and remarkable levels of work under adverse conditions in the smallpox-eradication campaign and in a series of health programs in China, India, Indonesia, and Tanzania, described in a recent publication by WHO (Newell, 1975). These examples demonstrate clearly that the motivation, attitudes, perception, and social position of the health worker in relation to the community are at least as important as technical skills and knowledge.

Health workers who are socially distant from those they serve may find that their beliefs, values, and goals seem incongruous and unacceptable to ordinary people. They may be seen as outsiders, and communication between them and the people may be distorted by mutual prejudices and fears. In seeking to overcome these barriers there is a danger that health workers will "oversell" themselves and stimulate expectations of health care that cannot be met. The end point of such a process of social and psychological alienation is frequently low morale, frustration, and decreased work output among health workers and low acceptability to and inappropriate use of health facilities by the people. An important indicator of this situation may be a high rate of migration of health workers, a problem investigated in a WHO multinational study of the international migration of physicians and nurses.

The importance of relating the selection and training of health workers to their subsequent roles and taking into account their attitudes, motivation, and satisfaction has been reflected in WHO's program in Health Manpower Development. At present, although selection is clearly a crucial point in determining the psychosocial characteristics of health workers and their suitability for health careers, little or no account is taken of this in practice. Willingness to work in rural areas and under difficult conditions and ability to establish good relations with other health workers and the public may be more important than evidence of academic performance. In a busy public environment such as a factory or marketplace, an outgoing, resilient person may provide a more adequate health service; in family planning services, a sensitive individual with the quality of empathy is likely to function better. Yet educational achievement remains the main criterion of selection, in spite of the availability of knowledge of the importance of such factors as the candidate's personality traits and social bias in selection.

The training milieu and experience profoundly influence the subsequent attitudes and functions of health workers (WHO Technical Report No. 521, 1973). Trainees may adopt inappropriate attitudes and beliefs during their training—for example, an undue preference for a specialist rather than a generalist career or an overemphasis on curative action at the expense of preventive action (WHO Technical Report No. 269, 1964). Social class prejudices may also be acquired during training (Mangin, 1965) as a result of the perception by trainees of the social prestige of their teachers. A recent WHO publication (Training and Utilization of Feldshers,

1974) has underlined the importance attached to the "moral education" of feldshers in the USSR, its aim being to develop a socialistic attitude toward work, a feeling of responsibility for the task assigned, and a sense of collective purpose and discipline.

In addition to knowledge drawn from specific disciplines such as sociology, psychology, and anthropology, the need for a continuous element in medical education devoted to improving skills in human relationships has been stressed (Teaching of Psychiatry, 1961). The place of behavioral sciences and mental health in medical education has been discussed at a number of WHO seminars organized by the WHO Regional Office for Americans/Pan American Sanitary Bureau (AMRO), the WHO Regional Office for Europe (EURO), and the WHO Regional Office for South-East Asia (SEARO). There has also been some increase in recent years in behavioral science teaching in schools of public health (WHO Technical Report No. 533, 1973). These activities could be complemented by others laying more emphasis on the application of psychosocial knowledge to the training of other categories of health personnel. In this way it may become possible to organize training activities that would take psychosocial principles into account, such as ensuring that initiative and practical work are encouraged within the training experience and rewarded as much as academic performance; maintaining the contact of trainees with and their awareness of the community at large and fostering attitudes and beliefs leading to an acceptance of a wide and flexible range of tasks in health work; preserving and enhancing, through practical experience, the ability of trainees to communicate meaningfully with individuals, families, and other social groups and to understand their needs.

In addition, the specific psychosocial skills and knowledge required by particular groups of health workers should be defined in relation to the nature and environment of their future work in the light of, for example, local beliefs and taboos concerning foods for nutrition work; the social welfare provisions for rehabilitation work; and aspects of sexuality for family planning and gynecological work (WHO Technical Report No. 572, 1975).

The principles concerning the selection and training of health workers must also be applied during their subsequent working careers. Health administrators and team leaders need to have considerable skills in human relationships and to be aware of factors contributing to job satisfaction, individual initiative, and the prevention of interpersonal conflicts. Their awareness of the fact that even apparently limited administrative changes may have widespread and unanticipated psychological consequences will help them to predict and monitor such effects and lead to direct application of psychosocial knowledge in policies on posting, length of assignments, and rotation of posts, in devising systems of special allowances, and in defining the roles of health team members. The latter has been carefully considered in an expert committee meeting (WHO Technical Report No. 235, 1962) and in a series of meetings (Working Group, Cracow, 1973; Working Group, Nice, 1974) forming part of the EURO long-term program in mental health.

Exchange of experience between categories of health workers and in-service training are important ways of increasing mutual understanding leading to better working relationships. This can be achieved by regular meetings of staff (at local, regional, and national levels), temporary exchanges of posts (for example, chief nurses in mental hospitals and general hospitals taking over each other's work for short periods), multidisciplinary and team training, and a variety of other measures. The series of multidisciplinary workshops on mental health service organization in Nigeria, held with WHO support, has demonstrated the relevance of these approaches in a developing country (Psychiatry and Mental Health Care, 1971).

Health Interventions

Intensive efforts to rehabilitate disabled people (such as the mentally ill, amputees, and those suffering from leprosy) through individually based efforts (drug therapy, vocational training, prosthetics, surgery, and reassurance) have very limited success unless environmental factors such as society's tolerance of the disabled (WHO Technical Report No. 177, 1959), the attitudes of patient's families, problems of physical access, and the need for opportunities for work are also taken into account. Efforts to prevent smoking or excessive alcohol intake through modifying individual attitudes have been undermined when there are simultaneous commercial campaigns to promote the sale of tobacco and alcohol (WHO Technical Report No. 568, 1975). Provision of waste disposal facilities has achieved little where individuals were not motivated to make use of them (Wagner & Lanix, 1958).

The regulation of fertility is another example of the need to take culturally determined beliefs and attitudes and the felt needs of communities into account in the planning of programs. The establishment of an "Acceptability Task Force" shows the organization's recognition of the need for work on these problems.

Although the importance of psychosocial factors in immunization programs was recognized nearly 150 years ago by Gaen in 1835, many critical issues that limit or increase acceptability are not yet properly understood. Acceptance rates vary widely and a number of useful strategies are available and being used (e.g., the use of trusted local staff rather than outsiders. contact with and support by important and influential local leaders, and quick action to counteract rumors and false information concerning the nature and purpose of immunization).

In the case of very young children, health interventions are directed jointly at the mother and the child. A keen awareness of the strong emotional forces involved in the mother–child relationship is important. The harmful consequences of emotional deprivation in early childhood was the subject of an early and influential WHO publication (Bowlby, 1952).

Seeking or not seeking health care depends on the strength of opposing forces. An individual may perceive a danger or threat to his health or feel discomfort or pain. As a result he will be "pushed" toward health care, but the strength of this push will depend on the amount of discomfort, the degree of perceived danger, and the extent of his belief that these will be decreased through health care. Ease of access, convenience, and the "visibility" of health care facilities (all of which are influenced by cultural factors) have a "pull" effect; they tend to increase the likelihood of an individual seeking health care. This is an important principle in planning health facilities for groups that may have ambivalent attitudes or may be reluctant to seek care (as shown, for example, in the WHO international collaborative study of dental manpower systems).

An administrative structure is a necessary part of health services, but certain structural features are undesirable. The separation of certain kinds of services, for example, into mental hospitals, geriatric hospitals, and leprosaria tends to reinforce negative attitudes (fear, stigma, low status) toward the individuals involved in the separated service (both patients and staff). Such services may also take on the features of a "total institution," with a lack of contact with the outside world and an inflexible and closely controlled internal social structure, so that patients become increasingly dependent and lacking in initiative. Inactivity, low self-esteem, lack of personal possessions, and constant arguments over trivial matters characterize patients in such institutions. Remedying such a state of affairs requires psychosocial skills. The mental health program in Jamaica, supported by AMRO, is an example of a carefully planned attempt to change the image of a large custodial mental hospital by improving facilities within the hospital, phasing down the hospital population, and integrating mental health into the general health facilities on the island.

Another problem that can arise in a health service structure is inequitable distribution of resources, so that central institutions in large towns are better equipped and staffed and enjoy a higher status than peripheral units. Such a pattern inevitably gives rise to dissatisfaction and low morale among staff in the peripheral units, while the centralized units may become increasingly involved in prestige activities that lack relevance to existing health problems. Recent efforts of the organization in promoting the provision of primary health care attack some of these problems, in which political and social measures play a determining role.

The implications for health services of rapid social change have been reviewed elsewhere (Meyer & Sainsbury, 1975; Health Hazards, 1972) and this important subject will be dealt with only briefly. Migration from rural areas to urban centers has given rise to densely populated periurban and urban slums in which the health needs of migrants are often poorly understood and unemployment, poor housing, overcrowding, and other social stresses are common features. The health services, already overextended, have not been able to cope with the needs of the rapidly increasing population. Environmental sanitation in densely populated urban areas poses particular problems and has been the subject of WHO assistance, principally in preinvestment planning, to ensure that the technology used is suited to the country's conditions. WHO has also been involved, in the region of the Americas, in low-cost housing construction projects through the Inter-Institutional Committee on Housing and Urbanization.

Since 1956, when the United Nations first began studying land settlement—because of dam construction schemes to increase agricultural productivity, the settlement of nomads, the spread of deserts, and other causes —the number of such projects has increased exponentially. Resettlement raises health care issues, such as the increased probability of ill health and/ or mental breakdown under conditions of change, stress, or loss of support that have not yet been studied sufficiently. The onchocerciasis control program in the Volta River basin, which involves the resettlement of more than 10 million people, has provided WHO with an opportunity for such studies and for the application of available knowledge about psychosocial factors to a major health program.

Health Action in Other Sectors

Psychosocial factors are of particular importance in health interventions in which coordination between the structured health services and other sectors is of decisive importance. A good example of a setting in which such coordinated approaches are necessary is the working environment where employers, work planners, health and social service workers, labor unions, and the workers themselves must be involved in order to protect health (Human Relations and Mental Health, 1958). If health services ensure full collaboration with and health education of teachers, a wide variety of important health attitudes and behavior (e.g., cleanliness, choice of foods, tooth care, sexual behavior) can be inculcated in schools (WHO Technical Report No. 193, 1960). If handicapped children, including the mentally retarded, attend normal schools, schools can be places where children learn to accept and relate to those who might otherwise be stigmatized. Mental health training for the police, welfare workers, lawyers, and judges (all of whom have frequent contact with deviant and disturbed people) will increase community resources for coping with the mentally ill (WHO Technical Report No. 564, 1975). These issues have been the topic of several EURO activities, including a working group on evaluation of mental health education programs in Nancy, 1973 (Working Group, Nancy, 1974); a study in 1973–1974 (Study on Youth Advisory Services, 1973–1974), and a working group in 1975 on youth advisory services; and a working group on forensic psychiatry in Siena in 1975. Coordination with other sectors is also of great importance in providing health care for groups that health services have difficulty in reaching, such as adolescents who have many health problems (e.g., sexually transmitted diseases, drug abuse) that are closely interwoven with social problems (maturation, seeking independence, establishing an adult role, employment) (WHO Technical Report No. 308, 1964; Bovet, 1951). This interaction of health and social factors was discussed in the EURO working group (Working Group, Helsinki, 1973) and symposium (EURO Symposium, 1974) on problems of deviant social behavior and delinquency in adolescents and young people and in a WHO study group in 1971 (WHO Technical Report No. 516, 1973).

Community Members

Community members are sometimes considered simply as consumers of health services, and this has led to a largely artificial separation between health providers and health recipients. The passive role thus given to members of the community diminishes their independent health-seeking behavior and decreases their active involvement in health action. Health services tend to become inward-looking and may, in turn, fail to be active in seeking links with the community. Such links should be sought, not only with the individual, but also with key social groups, particularly the family, which can form a natural focus for health care (Buckle, Hoffmeyer, Isambert, Knobloch, Knoblochova, Krapf, Lebovici, Pertejo de Alcami, Pincus, & Sandler, 1965).

The importance of two-way communication and mutual understanding between health workers and community members (including lay participation in decision making), a careful analysis of the health beliefs of individuals as they relate to personal health behavior, the active use of the community as a therapeutic tool, and the stimulation of the community's own response to health problems are parts of the psychosocial approach to this problem. The relevance of this approach can be illustrated by three examples.

1. Overuse or inappropriate use of health facilities is of increasing concern to health administrators. Patients attend physicians, hospitals, and

clinics for trivial complaints, reject reassurances, and continue to seek help from a variety of medical services. In some countries where great efforts are being made to establish rural health care, the overuse of hospitals and clinics in town still continues, apparently because patients lack confidence in local health clinics (the so-called bypassing phenomenon). In many cases, expensive and potentially hazardous treatments and investigations may be resorted to (e.g., unnecessary radiological investigations). Contributory factors include unrecognized mental illness, the phenomenon of reinforcement of illness behavior by the inappropriate use of drugs and other medical interventions, and the effect of certain sickness benefits and insurance provisions. In addition, patients may seek medical advice when the health problem itself has been resolved and social problems persist. Improved training in psychosocial skills would allow a better assessment of patients' problems and needs and more effective intervention.

2. The primary health care concept, as evolved by WHO, has as one of its central defining characteristics the idea that communities, at present underserved, would assume increased responsibility for and involvement in their own health care. This raises several social and psychological issues. For health professionals it represents a sharp change in their ways of thinking and, unless action is taken to demonstrate its validity, the concept of primary health care will be discounted and programs undermined. Community involvement can be achieved and maintained only with a proper understanding of social groups (including those who might be excluded from the larger community and be denied access to primary health care), entry points, channels of communication, and sources of resistance.

3. Traditional medicine as a source of health care has been written about and discussed extensively in the past few years, and it is a potent source of controversy, particularly within the medical profession. In many communities various forms of traditional care (and there are many) have been and remain the principal source of relief and care for the sick. The healers are often trusted, accepted, and easily accessible, whereas modern scientifically based medicine is frequently not. Those who have had close and sustained experience with the work of healers have stressed that traditional forms of healing are usually deeply imbedded in the social and cultural structure of society and that ill-considered attempts to control, integrate, or otherwise manipulate traditional healing systems may be seen by ordinary people as undesirable interference. Changes are likely to be slow and to require careful understanding of social issues. Where integration between traditional and modern medical care is sought, proper recognition of the contributions and skills of traditional healing and respect for the healers themselves is likely to lead to a sharing of responsibility for health care.

Program Proposals

General Considerations

The WHO psychosocial program could contribute best to other health-related programs if incorporated into them at the country level. This means that a careful examination of existing and planned health programs to determine which of them could benefit most from a psychosocial input must have high priority and should become an integral part of country health programming. To bring this about, coordination is needed among health administrators, decision-makers in the social sphere, and behavioral scientists at the country level. At the international level, coordination and collaboration would have to be intensified with the United Nations and the members of its system (in particular, ILO, UNESCO, the United Nations High Commissioner for Refugees, the United Nations Research Institute for Social Development, and the United Nations Social Defence Research Institute) and with the appropriate nongovernmental organizations.

There has been widespread reluctance or failure to evaluate the outcome of social measures and decisions affecting health with the same stringency as is usually applied to the assessment of biomedical interventions. The evaluation of psychosocially oriented interventions should therefore be a prominent feature of the proposed program. The results of such evaluation would permit better utilization of resources and stimulate decision-makers to use more rational approaches in dealing with social issues. In order to facilitate evaluation, existing information systems need to be adjusted so that decision-makers have data about the psychosocial factors necessary for the planning and evaluation of health services in a usable form and without delay. For this, the development of adequate social indicators and the simplification and standardization of reporting methods and instruments are a prerequisite. Projects to develop the necessary methodologies coordinated by WHO would therefore be a part of the program.

The psychosocial input into health care delivery has to be provided through the personnel available. To achieve this, decision-makers and health workers should be made aware of the importance of psychosocial factors and of the social and psychological consequences of health action. A necessary feature of the program therefore would be appropriate training and education at all levels of the health care provision system.

In planning and carrying out this work, it is of particular importance to ensure the applicability of concepts and methods to conditions in the countries in which they are used. Most behavioral science has been developed in the industrialized countries of Europe and America. The concepts, methods, and findings of the studies done in these areas may not be applicable in other sociocultural settings, and new strategies and research techniques may be necessary to supplement the approaches to psychosocial problems in the developing countries. Moreover, particularly in a psychosocial program, radical steps must be taken to avoid the donor–recipient relationship in which the developing countries are mere consumers of methods and projects prepared elsewhere. The fact that in many instances researchers in developing countries serve at best as data collectors for outside experts is contrary to the very nature of a psychosocial program, in which the methods, concepts, and approaches must be developed in the setting in which work takes place, by people who understand it and are part of it, and with a full understanding of the temporal and sociocultural dimensions of the problems under study. Projects undertaken in accordance with these principles and directed to the solution of specific problems facing the countries would therefore be undertaken as part of the program.

Objectives and Activities

Three medium-term objectives have been formulated:

The Application of Existing Knowledge in the Psychosocial Field to Improve Health Care. Specific needs for a psychosocial input have been identified in a number of WHO programs, and some projects to provide it have already been started. An important and early function of the proposed psychosocial program would be to provide a focal point that would facilitate coordination of psychosocial projects undertaken in conjunction with various programs of the organization and ensure that knowledge and experience gained in the implementation of such projects are shared and further applied and thus lead to a more rational utilization of resources. Such coordination may facilitate the identification of specific needs for and the provision of psychosocial inputs in other priority programs of the organization.

An important common component of the various projects undertaken in conjunction with other health programs is that of education and training. Concrete projects in this area would be useful as input in country health programs and in a variety of WHO projects. Courses and curricula that provide the necessary psychosocial skills and knowledge and can be incorporated into the training of different categories of health and welfare personnel would therefore be designed and evaluated. For administrators and decision-makers, mechanisms would be developed to enhance their awareness of psychosocial factors relevant to health action and enable them to contribute actively to planning in other sectors. In 1976 a course with this objective was organized by WHO with the assistance of the Swedish government and in collaboration with the WHO Psychosocial Centre, Stockholm. Other practical approaches to promoting rapid and wide dissemination of such information would have to be developed.

The Development of Methodologies through Collaboration with Countries So That Relevant Psychosocial Information Can Be Made Available to Health Planners. If a psychosocial component is to be taken into consideration in country health programming and in the evaluation of the success of health actions, specific information about it will be necessary. The methods now available cannot provide such information on a wide scale; in many instances they have been produced in technologically advanced countries and there is little evidence about their suitability for application in other settings. The same is true for methods for the assessment of community attitudes and for the identification of factors that promote community care and self-care for sick or disturbed individuals.

It would therefore be necessary to assess the usefulness of existing methods and strengthen the capacity of countries to develop or adapt methods to meet their needs. The definition of psychosocial indicators and the elaboration and standardization of techniques for their measurement would also lead to the acquisition of a common language in the psychosocial field that would in turn facilitate the exchange and pooling of information and the application of knowledge. WHO can play a crucial role in such collaboration, which would not only produce specific methods and research techniques adapted to needs of countries but would also develop and strengthen the potential of countries to acquire and apply knowledge in the psychosocial field. Cross-culturally applicable methods of measurement, standardized definitions, and other tools for international collaboration in the psychosocial area are necessary and would be developed through collaborative work coordinated by WHO.

Linked to the development and definition of indicators and of measurement techniques is the need to devise new methods for the collection and utilization of information. At the country level this means developing mechanisms for the rapid feedback of information to the decision-makers. WHO would provide assistance through the compilation of information adapted to consumer needs, collaboration with countries in establishing efficient information systems capable of handling psychosocial data, and wider utilization of the facilities of WHO collaborating centers.

At the international level, the creation of a data bank and information center on published and ongoing work on psychosocial factors and health would make information available to a variety of users and enable countries to benefit from each other's experience. At present the relevant data are spread over several data banks, there is little information about work done in the developing countries or about ongoing projects, and the selection of key words and hierarchies is inadequate for the quick provision of information. Such a data bank could be managed by the WHO Centre on Research and Training on Psychosocial Factors and Health, Stockholm, which has already accumulated a large amount of relevant information.

Acquisition of Knowledge on Which Health Action Can Be Based. The new knowledge necessary for more effective programs can be obtained by a systematic effort to evaluate health actions and learn from failures and successes. In some instances, however, applied research would have to be undertaken to obtain information necessary for dealing with specific health problems. Clearly, priorities for such research would have to vary from setting to setting and country to country. The central goal of WHO's activities concerning research in this area would be to strengthen the capacity of countries to undertake psychosocial research. Only in this way would it be possible to ensure the acquisition of relevant and valid information in countries on a continuing basis.

There are two topics of direct and immediate relevance to the area of psychosocial factors and health: uprooting and family functioning. Interest in studies on these two topics has been shown in many countries, and their importance was recognized during the Technical Discussions at the Twenty-seventh World Health Assembly in 1974, which were concerned with the psychosocial environment. The United Nations, the United Nations High Commissioner for Refugees, ILP, and UNESCO have expressed interest in collaborating with WHO in this study.

Uprooting has been recognized as the common factor in a number of psychosocial high-risk situations such as migration, urbanization, resettlement, and rapid social change. It occurs in most countries of the world and is often associated with meaningless violence, the abuse of drugs and alcohol, criminality, and reactive mental disorders. In spite of the considerable interest and concern about this problem, there is relatively little positive knowledge on which to base intervention programs. Projects would therefore be undertaken to identify high-risk groups among the uprooted populations and to test strategies aimed at reducing specific strains and stresses or providing services and forms of care best suited to the needs of such groups.

Although anthropologists and other social scientists have carried out studies of the characteristics of family functioning in different cultures, relatively little is known about the changes in those characteristics that take place as the result of rapid social transition, stress as a result of sickness, or a move to an urban environment. Data obtained from studies concerned with these issues could be of direct use in a number of health programs and help prevent the untoward consequences of social, economic, or legal action.

The study of family functioning would be collaborative, link the family health and mental health programs, and involve WHO collaborating centers and other institutions. It would be cross-cultural and comparative and aim at assessing the characteristics of the family, including its structural attributes (size, generational composition), its biological and medical characteristics (e.g., fertility, occurrence of physical and mental disorders), and its functioning under conditions of rapid social change, specific stress (e.g., when a family member is sick), and health interventions.

Summary of Program Proposals

Because of the complexity of the psychosocial field, the scarcity of trained manpower, the limited resources in the countries in which the program must be implemented, a pragmatic approach has been adopted in the proposals put forward.

In essence, the program aims at the application of available knowledge through better coordination of projects at the national level and at WHO. This coordination between ongoing projects and between agencies and authorities that can provide a psychosocial input in health programs will be combined with work in the field of education and training, which is the common element of all projects dealing with psychosocial factors. Two additional objectives and the activities leading to their implementation have also been proposed: the development of methodologies to permit a psychosocial input in health programs in the countries, and research on uprooting and family functioning, to provide knowledge needed in a number of priority health programs.

Certain activities would be continuing throughout this period, including the coordination and strengthening of ongoing projects; the identification of programs that would particularly benefit from a psychosocial input and the provision of such an input; and the evaluation of the psychosocial results of health actions undertaken in countries and of activities concerning education and training. In addition, the emphasis in the 1st year of this 5-year period would be on establishing close collaboration with the countries; in the 2nd and 3rd years on the development of methods and on the proposed research; in the 4th year on stimulation and evaluation of health interventions based on new knowledge acquired in the program; and in the 5th year on evaluation of all the program activities.

The recognition in many countries that the human factor is at least as important as the technical factor in overall development, and that there are numerous problems that cannot be resolved without the consideration of psychosocial factors, the need that countries have expressed for a program in this area, and the availability of knowledge necessary for intervention all strongly suggest that a program on psychosocial factors and health is timely, likely to yield practical results, and, therefore, deserving of the support of member states.

Acknowledgments

This material has been prepared by the authors on the basis of many contributions, particularly those made by Dr. L. Levi, director of the WHO

Collaborating Centre on Psychosocial Factors and Health, in Stockholm, Sweden; Dr. M. Bailey, at the time behavioral scientist in the Division of Mental Health; and other staff of the Division of Mental Health and of WHO. These and others have also critically reviewed the document, and the authors want to express their most sincere appreciation for their invaluable help.

References

Bovet, L. *Psychiatric aspects of juvenile delinquency*. Geneva: World Health Organization, 1951. (Monograph Series, No. 1)

Bowlby, J. *Maternal care and mental health*. Geneva: World Health Organization, 1952. (Monograph Series, No. 2)

Bruun, K., Edwards, K., Lumio, M., Mäkelä, K., Pan, L., Popham, R. E., Room, R., Schmidt, W., Skog, O-J., Sulkunen, P., & Osterberg, E. *Alcohol control policies in public health perspective, Helsinki*. Collaborative project of the Finnish Foundation for Alcohol Studies, Regional Office for Europe of WHO, and Addiction Research Foundation, Toronto, 1975.

Buckle, D., Hoffmeyer, H., Isambert, A., Knobloch, F., Knoblochova, J., Krapf, E. E., Lebovici, S., Pertejo de Alcami, J., Pincus, L., & Sandler, J. *Aspects of family mental health in Europe*. Public Health Papers, No. 28. Geneva: World Health Organization, 1965.

Conference on suicide and attempted suicide in young people, Luxembourg, 1974. Copenhagen: WHO Regional Office for Europe, 1975. (Document EURO 5446 III)

The economics of health and disease. *WHO Chronicle*, 1971, *25*, 20–24.

EURO symposium on problems of deviant social behavior and delinquency in adolescents and young people, Bratislava, 1973. Copenhagen: WHO Regional Office for Europe, 1974. (Document EURO 5430 III)

Fatal accidents with detailed information on traffic accidents. World Health Statistics Report, Vol. 24, No. 12, 1971.

Hasselblad, O. W. Psychosocial aspects of leprosy. *Pan American Health Organization Bulletin*, 1974, *8*, 282–288.

Health hazards of the human environment. Geneva: World Health Organization, 1972.

Human relations and mental health in industrial units. Report on the work of an advisory group, Geneva, 17–19 December 1956. Copenhagen: WHO Regional Office for Europe, 1958. (Document EURO 96)

The international pilot study of schizophrenia (Vol. 1). Geneva: World Health Organization, 1973.

Interrelationships between health programmes and socioeconomic development (Public Health Papers, No. 49). Geneva: World Health Organization, 1972.

Kramer, J. F., & Cameron, D. C. (Eds.). *A manual on drug dependence*. Geneva: World Health Organization, 1975.

Kramer, M. *Applications of mental health statistics*. Geneva: World Health Organization, 1969.

Levi, L. (Ed.). *Society, stress and disease—The psychosocial environment and psychosomatic diseases*. Report of a symposium sponsored jointly by the University of Uppsala and the World Health Organization. London: Oxford University Press, 1971.

Levi, L. (Ed.). *Society, stress and disease—Childhood and adolescence*. Report of a symposium sponsored jointly by the University of Uppsala and the World Health Organization. London: Oxford University Press, 1975.

Levi, L. (Ed.). *Society, stress and disease—Female and male roles and relationships.* Report of a symposium sponsored jointly by the University of Uppsala and the World Health Organization. London, New York, Toronto: Oxford University Press, 1978.

Levi, L. (Ed.). *Society, stress and disease—Working life.* Report of a symposium sponsored jointly by the University of Uppsala and the World Health Organization. London, New York, Toronto: Oxford University Press, 1979.

Mangin, W. The role of social organizations in improving the environment. In *Environmental determinants of community well-being* (Scientific publication, No. 123). Washington, D.C.: WHO Regional Office for the Americas, 1965, pp. 41–51.

Meyer, E. E., & Sainsbury, P. *Promoting health in the human environment.* Geneva: World Health Organization, 1975.

Moser, J. *Problems and programmes related to alchol and drug dependence in 33 countries.* Geneva: World Health Organization, 1974. (WHO Offset Publication, No. 6)

Myrdal, G. Economic aspects of health. *WHO Chronicle,* 1952, *6,* 203–218.

Newell, K. W. (Ed.). *Health by the people.* Geneva: World Health Organization, 1975.

Norman, L. G. *Road traffic accidents: Epidemiology, control and prevention* (Public Health Papers, No. 12). Geneva: World Health Organization, 1962.

Prevention of suicide (Public Health Papers, No. 35). Geneva: World Health Organization, 1968.

Psychiatry and mental health care in general practice. Report on a Seminar/Workshop, Ibadan, 20–27 January 1971. University of Ibadan, Department of Psychiatry and Neurology.

Road accidents. *World Health,* October 1975.

Slater, S. B. *et al.* The definition and measurement of disability. *Social Science and Medicine,* 1974, *8,* 305–308.

Study on Youth Advisory Services, 1973–74. Copenhagen: WHO Regional Office for Europe, 1977. (Document EURO 5447 III ICP/MNH 016 III)

Suicide and attempted suicide (Public Health Papers, No. 58). Geneva: World Health Organization, 1974.

Symposium on human factors in road accidents, Rome, 16–20 October 1967. Cophenhagen: WHO Regional Office for Europe, 1967. (Document EURO 0147)

The teaching of human sexuality in schools for health professionals (Public Health Papers, No. 57). Geneva: World Health Organization, 1974.

Teaching of psychiatry and mental health (Public Health Papers, No. 9). Geneva: World Health Organization, 1961.

The training and utilization of feldshers in the USSR (Public Health Papers, No. 56). Geneva: World Health Organization, 1974.

Wagner, E. G., & Lanoix, J. N. Social and psychological implications of rural sanitation programmes. In *Excreta disposal for rural areas and small communities.* Geneva: World Health Organization, 1958. (Monograph Series, No. 39)

WHO Technical Report Series, No. 75. *The mentally subnormal child.* Report of a Joint Expert Committe convened by WHO with the participation of United Nations, ILO and UNESCO, 1954.

WHO Technical Report Series, No. 130. *Juvenile epilepsy.* Report of a Study Group, 1957.

WHO Technical Report Series, No. 177. *Social psychiatry and community attitudes.* Seventh report of the WHO Expert Committee on Mental Health, 1959.

WHO Technical Report Series, No. 183. *Mental health problems of automation.* Report of a Study Group, 1959.

WHO Technical Report Series, No. 193. *Teacher preparation for health education.* Report of a Joint WHO/UNESCO Committee, 1960.

WHO Technical Report Series, No. 217, *Public health aspects of low birth weight.* Third report of the Expert Committee on Maternal and Child Health, 1961.

WHO Technical Report Series, No. 235. *The role of public health officers and general practitioners in mental health care.* Eleventh report of the WHO Expert Committee on Mental Health, 1962.

WHO Technical Report Series, No. 269. *Promotion of medical practitioners' interest in preventive medicine.* Twelfth report of the WHO Expert Committee on Professional and Technical Education of Medical and Auxiliary Personnel, 1964.

WHO Technical Report Series, No. 275. *Psychosomatic disorders.* Thirteenth report of the WHO Expert Committee on Mental Health, 1964.

WHO Technical Report Series, No. 308. *Health problems of adolescence.* Report of a WHO Expert Committee, 1964.

WHO Technical Report Series, No. 363. *Services for the prevention and treatment of dependence on alcohol and other drugs.* Fourteenth report of the WHO Expert Committee on Mental Health, 1967.

WHO Technical Report Series, No. 365. *Epidemiological methods in the study of chronic diseases.* Eleventh report of the WHO Expert Committee on Health Statistics, 1967.

WHO Technical Report Series, No. 392. *Organization of services for the mentally retarded.* Fifteenth report of the WHO Expert Committee on Mental Health, 1968.

WHO Technical Report Series, No. 460. *WHO Expert Committee on Drug Dependence.* Eighteenth report, 1970.

WHO Technical Report Series, No. 507. *Psychogeriatrics.* Report of a WHO Scientific Group, 1972.

WHO Technical Report Series, No. 516. *Youth and drugs.* Report of a WHO Study Group, 1973.

WHO Technical Report Series, No. 521. *Training and preparation of teachers for schools of medicine and of allied health sciences.* Report of a WHO Study Group, 1973.

WHO Technical Report Series, No. 533. *Postgraduate education and training in public health.* Report of a WHO Expert Committee, 1973.

WHO Technical Report Series, No. 564. *Organization of mental health services in developing countries.* Sixteenth report of the WHO Expert Committee on Mental Health, 1975.

WHO Technical Report Series, No. 568. *Smoking and its effects on health.* Report of a WHO Expert Committee, 1975.

WHO Technical Report Series, No. 572. *Education and treatment in human sexuality: The training of health professionals.* Report of a WHO meeting, 1975.

World Health Organization. *Schizophrenia: An international follow-up study.* New York: Wiley, 1979.

Working Group on the health education programmes concerning drug abuse in young poeple, Hamburg, 1972. Copenhagen: WHO Regional Office for Europe, 1973. (Document EURO 5418 IV)

Working Group on problems of deviant social behaviour and delinquency in adolescents and young adults, Helsinki, 27–30 June 1972. Copenhagen: WHO Regional Office for Europe, 1973. (Document EURO 5425 III)

Working Group on the role of the psychologist in mental health services, Cracow, 1973. Copenhagen: WHO Regional Office for Europe, 1973. (Document EURO 5428 I)

Working Group on suicide and attempted suicide in young people, Zagreb, 1973. Copenhagen: WHO Regional Office for Europe, 1974. (Document EURO 5431 III)

Working Group on evaluation of mental health education programmes, Nancy, 1973. Copenhagen: WHO Regional Office for Europe, 1974. (Dcoument EURO 5432 III)

Working Group on the role of the social worker in the psychiatric services, Nice, 1972. Copenhagen: WHO Regional Office for Europe, 1974. (Document 5438 I)

6

The Role of Indigenous Medicine in WHO's Definition of Health

Paul I. Ahmed and Aliza Kolker

The WHO Definition

The goal of adequate health care for all the earth's people, pursued by the leaders of the world's nations in the last three decades, was formulated in the preamble to the constitution of the World Health Organization in 1946. That document defined health as "a state of complete physical, mental and social well-being and not merely the absence of disease and infirmity." This state was regarded as the fundamental right of all human beings "without distinctions of race, religion, political belief, economic or social condition," and the health of all people was declared "fundamental to the attainment of peace and security" (Chasse, 1978). This definition, vague and idealistic as it was, has been used as a focus for health planning guidelines and policies by donor agencies and developing countries alike. In this chapter we will discuss the implications of the WHO definition for health manpower planning and the obstacles that impede its full realization. These obstacles

Paul I. Ahmed • Office of International Health, U.S. Department of Health, Education and Welfare, Rockville, Maryland 20857. Aliza Kolker • Department of Sociology, George Mason University, Fairfax, Virginia 22030. This paper reflects the professional opinions of the writers and does not represent the policy of the U.S. Department of Health, Education, and Welfare. An earlier version of this paper was presented at a conference on public management conducted by the National Institute of Public Management, Mexico, in Mexico City, January 20–22, 1978 and to the Eastern Sociological Conference in New York, March, 1979. A later version was presented to a meeting of the senior staff, Department of Social Services, Birmingham, England, December 4, 1978.

include the general problems of instituting planned change, the shortcomings of the Western medical model itself, and the severe shortages of trained manpower that seem more or less permanent in developing nations. We will contend that the only realistic means for the realization of this ambitious goal is the mobilization of all the resources of recipient nations, including traditional medical personnel, who at present serve many unrecognized functions not being met by the Western medical systems.

The WHO definition of health as a state of "complete well-being" has been attacked as "frankly unattainable":

> Did the framers of the 1946 Preamble seriously intend for all family disputes, political contradictions, and the risk of being run over by a truck to fall within the province of the medical system? I think not. More likely, "health" was redefined in this context as the ultimate social intent. (Guidotti, personal communication, 1978)

Consequently, the usefulness of this definition as a basis for health planning has been called into question (see, for example, Mechanic, 1968).

A careful consideration of the background of the 1946 constitution, however, would lead to a different interpretation (see Chasse, 1978). The goal of pursuing "the complete physical, mental and social well-being" of all the people of the earth, and not only of the privileged few, may be construed as the expression of a precarious ethical consensus of the world's leaders arising out of the chaos and destruction of World War II and the Cold War.

In addition to providing a unifying goal for a conflict-torn world, the WHO definition also gave expression to the uneasy recognition, long growing in the forefront of the medical profession, that modern medicine, for all its spectacular successes, was not ushering in a brave new world; many old problems remained unsolved while new problems were being created. If modern medicine was unable to fulfill the unlimited promise that it had held out, then it was necessary to replace the purely physical definition of good health—the absence of disease—with one that called for the total well-being of persons, so that other disciplines and resources could be mobilized to pursue that goal.

The Western Medical Model

The limitations of the Western medical model have been amply documented (see Engel, 1977; Fabrega, 1975). Briefly stated, the biomedical model, which dominates the concept of disease in the Western world, "assumes disease to be fully accounted for by deviations from the norm of measurable biological . . . variables. It leaves no room within its framework for the social, psychological and behavioral dimension of illness" (Engel, 1977, p. 130). The model is positivist in that it assumes that only objectively measurable phenomena are "real," and reductionist insomuch as it claims that the language of biochemistry will ultimately suffice to explain such sociopsychological and cultural phenomena as "illness."

The biomedical model has dominated the academic study of disease at least since the Renaissance ushered in the scientific approach to the study of man, but it has gained complete acceptance only since the middle of the 19th century, when the causal link between germs and disease was definitively established. This discovery has been considered "the most powerful single idea in the history of medicine . . . the single greatest weapon in the so-called conquest of disease" (Twaddle & Hessler, 1977, pp. 11–12). It has made possible a massive and effective assault on acute disease through immunization and treatment, and ushered in a period of optimism in which it seemed possible to eradicate all illnesses of mankind.

The biomedical model, based largely upon the germ theory of disease, became the basis of medical practice as well as academic medicine at the turn of the 20th century, when medical training was reorganized and put on a scientific basis in the wake of the Flexner report (1910). Both the academic and the clinical branches of the medical profession readily embraced "the notion of the body as a machine, of disease as the consequence of the breakdown of the machine, and of the doctor's task as repair of the machine" (Engel, 1977, p. 131). Indeed, the biomedical model has been so spectacularly successful that in addition to being the only legitimate *scientific* model of disease, it has also become the dominant *folk* model of disease in the Western world. (A folk model, according to Engel (1977), is an effort at social adaptation; it is a culturally specific belief system used to explain disturbing natural phenomena so that some corrective action may be undertaken.)

While the successes of the new model were beyond all expectations, there was a cost involved. Lost was the pregerm theory conception of the individual as organically related to his environment, and of illness as consisting of behavioral and psychosocial components as well as biological ones. In a dramatic shift, the discovery of germs transformed medicine "from a people-oriented to a disease-oriented profession. Physicians became absorbed in the study of disease, and their mission and training shifted from the care of sick people to the diagnosis and cure of disease" (Twaddle & Hessler, 1977, p. 12).

Notwithstanding the spectacular successes of the biomedical model (with the underlying basis in germ theory) in eradicating acute disease and reducing mortality, for at least the last generation many doubts have been voiced about its ultimate adequacy (see Twaddle & Hessler, 1977). The decline in morbidity due to acute disease has been accompanied by an increase in the prevalence of chronic disease such as cancer and diabetes, prompting such noted authorities as microbiologist Rene Dubos (1959) to claim that complete health is a mirage, and that the ultimate conquest of all disease is an unattainable ideal. More recently, a variety of nonbiological factors contributing to disease or correlated with its incidence have been isolated, from environmental carcinogens to accumulated life stresses and the pressures of rapid social change. Consequently, some authors have called for the inclusion of environmental, social, and psychological factors in the study and treatment of disease (King, 1972; Coelho & Stein, 1977; Graham & Stevenson, 1963). Indeed, according to some critics, the biomedical model constitutes an impediment to further advances in health care. This is so because the model has systematically excluded nonbiological phenomena from the category of disease or insisted that these phenomena are ultimately explainable in physiochemical terms, and so it has become a dogma, any questioning of whose basic premises constitutes heresy (Engel, 1977; Fabrega, 1974, 1975).

Some authors have suggested alternative models of disease that do not sacrifice the enormous advantages of the biomedical model while at the same time incorporating sociopsychological and cultural aspects left out by that model. Thus, Fabrega (1975) calls for a theory of human disease that incorporates culturally specific interpretations of disease, immediate and long-term behavioral effects of the disease (i.e., impairments in routine activities and interactions), and the modes of organization used by the social group to deal with disease. Engel (1977) similarly calls for the systematic incorporation of behavioral and psychosocial data (e.g., information about stress-producing life changes) both in diagnosing and in treating disease:

> To provide a basis for understanding the determinants of disease and arriving at rational . . . health care, a medical model must also take in the patient, the social context in which he lives, and the complementary system devised by society to deal with the disruptive effects of illness, that is, the physician role and the health care system. This requires a biopsychosocial model. (p. 196)

If the need for incorporating nonbiological factors in diagnosing and treating disease is perceived as imperative in Western culture, where the biological model is universally accepted, it is even more compelling in non-Western cultures. This is so because a very large gap between the culturally specific folk model of medicine and the scientific model significantly hampers the effectiveness of treatment. Villagers in Gopalpur, India, for example, avoid going to the hospital because they trust the local medicine man more fully (Khare, 1973). Similarly, Indians living on the Modoc reservation in California deeply distrust the modern physician:

> Western medicine fails to provide the close support and attention that native treatment provides and seems determined to alienate the patient from his family,

his land, his culture, and all the other sources from which he draws strength. . . .
Not only are the [Indian] attitudes towards health different, but the collision
of centuries of tribal experience and a discordant aggressive alien society have
produced perceptions and . . . constructs which are interpretable only from
within the patient's own culture. Indians who have retained their traditional
beliefs often see Western medicine as a very superficial, palliative magic which
fails to percerive or deal with the profound disharmony in the universal order of
things which is illness. (Guidotti, 1973, pp. 101–102)

It should be noted parenthetically that a recent effort to establish a Navajo
medical school in New Mexico in order to bridge the gap has been en-
meshed in bureaucratic delays for the past 7 years (Goldberg, 1978).

The Western medical model, then, in addition to encountering the
general problems of technology transfer discussed below, is inhibited by the
prevalence of alternative folk models that prevent a consensus between
doctor and patient, a consensus often considered necessary for effective
medical intervention (see Fabrega, 1975). We feel that if alternative folk
models are incorporated into the Western health care system, instead of
being viewed as competing with it, the chances for effective intervention
will be higher. This is in addition to the current role of folk or traditional
medicine in filling the gaps left by the severe shortage of Western-trained
manpower and facilities.

The Problems of Technology Transfer

The importation of the Western medical system into non-Western
countries, in addition to being hampered by the built-in limitations discussed above, also suffers from the general problems confronting the transfer of technology in any sphere.

Spectacularly successful as the Western medical system has been, its
effectiveness alone is not enough to assure that once available to the people
of a developing country it will be gratefully accepted and widely utilized.
Indeed, as we have learned from four decades of research on planned
change and the utilization of innovations in such diverse spheres as agriculture and education as well as medicine, the mere availability of an innovation whose technical superiority has been demonstrated is rarely enough to
secure adoption (see Havelock, 1971; Rogers & Shoemaker, 1971). Researchers have pointed out repeatedly that the following factors are no less
important:

1. Relative cost. Effective though the innovation may be, its sheer cost
may limit its usefulness. Medical services at the village level, even when
nominally free or available for token fees, are often prohibitively expensive
when bus fare and absence from work are calculated. Press (1978) notes,
for example, that in Third World cities modern physicians, clinics, and

hospitals tend to serve the middle and upper classes, whereas the poorest turn to the much cheaper neighborhood healers. Even more unfortunate is the fact that operating modern, Western-donated facilities in the capital city may drain the nation's health budget and thus result in even poorer service to the rural population (see Ahmed, 1977). Indeed, Foster (1977) and other researchers believe that prohibitive costs rather than cultural resistance to change is the major obstacle to greater utilization of modern health care.

2. Manpower shortage. It is undeniable that even where modern facilities exist, trained manpower is in desperately short supply, and there is no reason to believe the shortage will be alleviated in the near future. In Mali, for example, there were only 108 physicians in 1972 for a population of over 4 million, a ratio of about 40,000 persons per physician. Of these physicians, 82, or over three-fourths, lived in the major cities. The majority of the rural population, therefore, was not served by physicians at all. As Imperato (1975) points out, in the rural areas in Mali modern health facilities are extremely limited, consisting often of a small dispensary with a few diagnostic facilities and a handful of medications rather than a fully staffed dispensary with a well-stocked pharmacy. The situation is no better in other African and Asian countries. Compared to 1 physician per 622 persons in the United States, in Chad there is 1 physician per 44,382 persons, in India 1 physician per 4,162 persons, and in Nepal 1 physician per 36,540 persons (United Nations Statistical Yearbook, 1976). As Foster (1977) points out, "Paradoxically, the growing acceptance of Western medicine is creating a crisis in most developing countries. There are not now, nor will there be in the foreseeable future, sufficient fully-trained health personnel to meet all health needs." It is not surprising, then, that most of the population of the world, especially in rural areas, is served by traditional medicine men, not by modern medical practitioners.

3. Unanticipated consequences of planned change. The benefits of Western medicine in developing countries have been considerable. In Egypt, for example, the crude death rate has dropped from 20 per 1,000 in 1948 to 12 per 1,000 in 1974, with life expectancy at birth increasing from 36 (males) and 41 (females) in the 1930s to 52 (males) and 54 (females) in 1974. In Brazil the crude death rate dropped to 9 and life expectancy increased from 37 (males and females) to 58 (males) and 61 (females). By comparison, the crude death rate in the United States is 9 and the life expectancy 68 (males) and 76 (females) (United Nations Statistical Yearbook, 1951, 1976). Notwithstanding these gains, the importation of the Western medical system has resulted in some disturbing unanticipated consequences. Chief among these have been overpopulation as a result of reduced mortality, various problems resulting from the prolongation of life beyond its economically productive span, an increase in the prevalence of some chronic diseases, and occasionally excessive dependency on drugs.

These have contributed to some disenchantment with modern medicine, in the developing countries no less than in the West.

4. Compatibility. One of the most important factors in the adoption of innovations is the perceived compatibility of the innovation with the user's beliefs, values, and behavioral patterns. A now classic example from the field of agricultural extension is the introduction of hybrid seed corn in New Mexico in 1946 (see Rogers & Shoemaker, 1971). The results were spectacular: The yield from the hybrid seed was double the yield from the old seed and within a year over half the farmers adopted the new seed. During the next 2 years, however, all but three of the farmers who had adopted the new seed discontinued it, although its technical superiority was unquestioned. The reason was that the corn was used to make tortillas for local consumption, not only for animal feed (as the extension agent had assumed), and the farmers' wives did not like the flavor and texture of the new hybrid corn. The innovation had failed despite its undeniable technical superiority because it did not agree with local taste preferences. In another case, as Guidotti (1973) points out in the excerpts quoted above, the incompatibility between Western medicine and the native perceptions of the Modoc Indians in California seriously hampers the utilization of such modern medical care as is available. The Western-trained physician may fail to diagnose or to perceive illnesses that are real to the Indian, or may emphasize diseases that are neither discomforting nor disabling to him. It will be remembered that to the Modoc Indian, as to many millions of the Earth's inhabitants, neither pain nor a slowly killing disease presents a frightening prospect: he has lived with both for countless centuries. A different sort of value clash centers on the importance of privacy, which may prevent the Modoc Indian from revealing his personal affairs to the health worker for fear it might come to the attention of opposing factions in the village and thus be used against him.

The Rockefeller antihookworm campaign in Ceylon (Foster, 1977) revealed another example of the need to overcome perceptual and attitudinal incompatibility before health care can be effectively administered. The campaign to eradicate hookworm failed partly because it was conceived as strictly preventive, and the Ceylonese could not accept the logic of *preventing* disease through environmental sanitation while their more pressing problems—wounds, abscesses, and acute diseases—were going untreated. Fortunately, most medical teams today combine preventive with curative care (Foster, 1977).

A different type of value incompatibility is manifested in the resistance of Western-trained health bureaucracies and professionals to changes that may threaten their position or their cherished role expectations. In this respect of course, they are no different from bureaucracies and professionals elsewhere, or indeed, from human beings and organizations in general.

A common example is the frequent reluctance of physicians and nurses to relinquish some of their tasks to subprofessionals, even when the physicians and nurses themselves are hopelessly overburdened and the change will clearly benefit the client population. This was the case in Tanzania, where a reorganization of mother-and-child health clinics to offer more comprehensive and accessible care was initially opposed by the clinics' staffs (Hart, 1978). As Foster (1977) notes, "Physicians are anxious to use every level of health worker in furthering a health program . . . but the words 'diagnose' and 'prescribe' evoke the strongest feelings of professional possessiveness." Another bureaucratic hurdle to improving health care delivery is the resistance of clinic staffs to combining preventive and curative care, a practice that, as we saw above, is necessary if the people are to trust the government clinics and use them extensively (see Hart, 1978; Foster, 1977). These are but a few examples of entrenched bureaucratic patterns and professional attitudes that, like the traditional values and attitudes of clients, impede change.

These, then, are some of the obstacles to a wider utilization of Western medicine in developing countries, obstacles that prevent Western medicine in these countries from achieving the same spectacular gains as in the West. There is a growing awareness in the international health community that the only way to assure adequate health care in the future is to integrate traditional health resources into the Western medical system and thus to utilize all the country's resources in the service of effective medical care. Such integration must be done on a limited and careful basis, of course, to prevent the abuses of traditional medical practices from being perpetuated.

What are the systems of medicine now serving the majority of the population in developing countries and what are their implications for the Western medical system?

Traditional Medical Systems

The persistence of traditional conceptions of disease and traditional medical practices side by side with a Western medical system has been documented amply. Thus, the Government of India's Report of the Committee on Indigenous Systems of Medicine (1948, p. 78) says, "It is admitted by all that at the present time Indian medicine ministers to more than 80 percent of the population, and that it is perhaps the only kind of care available in the rural areas." That the situation in India is not greatly different today is attested by Dunn (1976, pp. 154–155):

> In modern India, the indigenous systems remain enormously important as providers of medical care, not only in the villages but also in the cities, and there can be no doubt that Ayurveda and Unani [the scholarly medical traditions of India's

past] contribute substantially to the cumulative impact of these systems on Indian health and ill health. . . . There can be little doubt that popular traditional medicine will indefinitely survive, whatever the level of development of cosmopolitan [i.e., Western] health care.

Indeed, as Leslie (1976, p. 1) points out, "the health concepts and practices of most people in the world today continue traditions that evolved during antiquity," although only a few, such as the Chinese, Ayurvedic, and Unani traditions, continue as scholarly as well as popular traditions.

These three Asian systems share in common an overall conception of disease and an overall organization of practice that actually underlie many other traditional systems of medicine (see Imperato, 1975; Kiteme, 1976; Leslie, 1976; Opler, 1963). They are based on a finite number of "humors," which are actually alignments of opposing qualities: hot–cold, wet–dry, male–female, strong–weak, etc. The equilibrium of these qualities maintains health, and their disequilibrum causes illness. Human anatomy and physiology are viewed as intimately bound with the social and physical environment, indeed with the cosmos. Hence, treatment consists of restoring a state of harmony between the body and the environment as well as within the body. This is done by the manipulation of diet, herbal medications, behavioral modifications, and rituals.

It must be emphasized that while many folk curers are charlatans and quacks, of course, much traditional medicine is firmly grounded in ancient traditions of rational learning and requires lengthy periods of formal education before one is allowed to practice. Leslie (1976), for example, rejects the assumption that all non-Western medicine is unscientific:

> By commonly recognized criteria, Chinese, Ayurvedic, and Arabic medicines are scientific in substantial degrees. They involve the rational use of naturalistic theories to organize and interpret systematic empirical observations. They have explicit, orderly ways of recording and teaching this knowledge and they have some efficacious methods for promoting health and for curing illness. (p. 7)

The training of African healers is a lifelong enterprise, often learned from one's father through an arduous apprenticeship. The apprenticeship requires periods of meditation in the forest, communing with the forces of nature, the mastery of over 200 pharmacological herbs, extensive self-mortification, elaborate rites de passage, and a rigid code of ethics. Guidotti (1973) similarly reports that the Achumawi shaman, before being admitted to practice, must undergo a long and rigorous training during which he must master and control a variety of "pains" that are considered the etiological factors of disease. To incorporate these "pains" into his body the shaman must cooperate with an interceding spirit, be instructed by an older shaman, and undergo special initiation ceremonies. Thus, "shamanism was not an arbitrary and disorganized body of belief, although it may have degenerated to this in the hands of some quack practitioners after the white invasion"; indeed, fused with insights obtained from mysticism and altered states of consciousness, shamanism has made major contributions to Western pharmacopoeia (Guidotti, 1973). It is not surprising, then, that in many countries native medical traditions are highly organized in associations of practitioners, teaching institutions, and research institutions. This is particularly true in India and in China, where the governments recognize and support the native traditions (see Leslie, 1976). It is harder to accept or to justify the disdain commonly manifested by some Western-trained medical practitioners toward native practices, particularly in light of the inadequacy of Western medicine at its current level to meet the needs of the people in many developing nations.

That traditional medical systems serve many needs not being adequately served by Western medicine, in addition to filling the vacuum created by the shortage of Western-trained manpower and the high cost of training, is undeniable. These functions are both psychological and sociological, and they differ somewhat between stable traditional societies and those undergoing the dislocations of rapid urbanization and modernization. They include the following:

1. Relief of stress and anxiety caused by the uncertainties of illness. By treating the "whole personality" and by viewing health "as a complex, ecologically contained phenomenon, with natural, super-natural, ritual and social causation" (Ademuwagum, 1969, p. 1087), they operate on the basis of the same cultural premises as their patients and are able to invoke cultural, religious, and psychological support to relieve anxiety. In addition, the medicine men use therapeutic devices that are familiar to the patient, including everyday foods and drinks, familiar taboos and superstitions, and a common language or dialect. This further reduces the anxiety inherent in contact with the unfamiliar world of modern medicine. Khare (1973), for example, reports that in India, villagers are often reluctant to seek medical aid outside the village because they cannot expect the same amount of sympathy and care that they get from the native healer. They also trust the native healer more because he does not use unfamiliar treatment. The hospital in the nearby town remains unvisited, because the care it provides is perceived as cold, dehumanizing, and stress-provoking.

2. Cost and convenience. As we have seen above, modern medical care, even when offered free of charge or for a nominal fee by a government clinic, is expensive and inconvenient when we calculate the cost of transportation for a mother with several children or of a day's unpaid absence from work. Press (1978) estimates that of the low-income clientele of a Bogota clinic, 30%–40% could not be cured either because they could not afford the cost of proper treatment or because their impoverished environment counteracted the effects of antibiotics or other drugs. Women in Moslem societies may be further inhibited from traveling outside their village to seek medical

help because of strong cultural restrictions on women's mobility. By contrast, the traditional healer lives nearby, charges affordable fees, and is available day and night.

3. Primary group involvement. Not only do traditional healers manifest a more particularistic, affective, and diffuse attitude than do Western medical practitioners (i.e., the former are more personally involved with the patient and tend to treat "the whole person"), but they often involve the entire family as well as the community in the process of diagnosis and treatment. This is not only emotionally gratifying to the patient, but it reinforces his motivation to comply with the prescribed treatment (Ademuwagum, 1969).

4. Control of deviance. For the closely knit traditional community, traditional medicine may constitute an important mechanism of social control by diagnosing the cause of disease or ill-fortune and by prescribing corrective measures. An example offered by Opler (1963) is the Indian villager who suddenly became irrational and violent and alarmed his family by loudly criticizing India's national leaders and praising those of Pakistan. A shamanistic rite revealed that the cause of his dangerous behavior was the evil influence of the ghost of a Muslim, and that he was being punished for having stolen an offering to the gods. He was ordered to return the offering, and the deranged behavior, once isolated and condemned, ceased. In this instance the cause of the deviant behavior was diagnosed as supernatural yet ultimately caused by the villager; his dangerous behavior was safely contained. The traditional healer also acts as an agent to control overly lusty appetites, restoring social equilibrium by dramatizing and reinforcing the idea that it is dangerous to covet unattainable wealth and power (see Landy, 1974). Unlike Western medicine, which asks, "How did I get sick?" traditional medicine asks, "Why did I and not my neighbor get sick?" It ultimately provides a satisfying answer couched in terms of some superhuman system of retribution and justice. This imparts a sense of resignation and an acceptance of the inevitable (see Hughes, 1968).

Press (1978) and Landy (1974) note the special, additional functions of traditional healers in transitional societies—healers serving recent urban migrants in the teeming cities of developing countries. These functions include the following:

5. Minimizing the trauma of cultural change: the traditional healer as "cultural broker." Traditional healers help to maintain the personality integration of the rural migrant in a baffling urban milieu by interpreting illness in familiar terms and by exhibiting familiar behavioral, linguistic, and attitudinal patterns. At the same time, the urban folk healer often incorporates scientific terminology into older magical thought patterns, prescribes antibiotics, and refers difficult cases to a government hospital or clinic. He thus helps to ease the migrant's adaptation to modern health usage and to mod-

ern cultural patterns in general. The healer's role, then, in many cases, has been resynthesized to incorporate modern elements; he has become not a change resistor but a change agent, mediating between the old and the new worlds.

6. Alleviating personal stress resulting from social disorganization, uprooting, and anomie. In cities, wider economic opportunities combine with the attentuation of ascribed status and with increased social mobility to raise the aspiration level of recent rural migrants. Inadequately prepared and disadvantageously located, however, migrants commonly fail to attain their aspirations. As Coelho and Stein (1977, p. 392) put it, "Their hopes are dashed by shanty towns, social ghettos, underemployment, isolation, lack of assistance, and nostalgia mixed with frustrations. Little by little the hoped-for well-being turns into daily frustration; family life disintegrates, health is threatened." Traditional medicine, by encouraging displacement of responsibility for failure from self to other sources, rationalizes failure and alleviates the stress resulting from it. This is different from the function of rural healers in *lowering* aspirational levels or minimizing *attempts* to achieve.

7. Fostering ethnic identity. In ethnically heterogeneous cities, traditional medicine provides a focus for group identity by distinguishing between group members and nonmembers. It thus supplements other aspects of the group's culture such as religious and ethnic rituals.

When we consider the diverse functions of traditional medicine in rural as well as in urban societies, it is not surprising that it has survived in spite of the increasingly successful onslaughts of modern medicine. Indeed, it has either survived intact or made a significant comeback even in the present-day United States. As the *New York Times* has recently reported (Vecsey, 1978), spiritual healing, long associated with Pentecostal groups, is rapidly gaining acceptance in Catholic and Episcopal churches. It seems that by appealing to deep-seated psychological cravings, spiritual healing fulfills a need not being met by modern Western medicine even in a society where the dominant folk model is the scientific one. This is much more true in societies with strong nonscientific folk traditions and where Western medicine does not have sufficient manpower to meet the needs of the population.

Conclusions: Toward Integrated Medical Care

In the final account, the WHO definition of health as "a state of total well-being" cannot be met without an integrated effort at rural development, since freedom from disease must be complemented by freedom from hunger, from repression, and from ignorance. It is clear that efforts to improve health care must be accompanied by economic development educational upgrading, and political liberation. The details of such an integrated approach, however, lie outside the scope of the chapter. For the purpose at hand, it is important to emphasize that in order to meet the goal set by the WHO definition, the issues of health manpower needs must be reconsidered in the context of the total national health system. The question to ask is "What kind of health system do we need?" instead of "What kind of health manpower do we need?"

While the question of what kind of health system a country needs depends on its unique sociocultural and economic characteristics, it is possible to establish some general guidelines. It is clear that health care must be oriented toward serving the needs of all people in the country and not only the urban or the more well-to-do. The focus of health planning should be on primary health care in the villages rather than on technologically sophisticated health care in the cities, as has been traditionally the case in hard-pressed developing countries attempting to modernize rapidly. Flahault (1976) suggests an integrated hierarchical approach to structuring national health systems. At the lowest level he envisions village dispensaries providing rudimentary primary health care to local communities. (Primary care, according to Flauhault, 1976, p. 442, "provides simple and effective services that are readily accessible to patients and help to improve the living conditions of individuals and communities." This includes preventing the spread of communicable diseases through vaccination, treatment, and referral; mother and child care; health education for better hygienic and sanitary habits; etc.) Village dispensaries are to be supplemented, supported, and coordinated by rural health centers, by rural hospitals, by district and regional health services, and finally, by specialized national institutes and university hospital centers. At each level of centralization the services provided are more specialized and the level of staff training is more advanced. Thus, while rural hospitals and regional centers are to be at least partially staffed by fully trained medical personnel, village dispensaries are to be staffed entirely by auxiliary health workers. These workers will originate from the community, receive only a few months' training, and continue to work at their usual occupations. They will need to be supervised and assisted regularly by the central organizations. It is at this point that the Western and the traditional medical cultures intersect: the auxiliary health workers may be recruited from the practitioners of traditional medicine who are willing to undergo training and to submit to supervision. This will assure the compatibility of the health workers' approach with the attitudes and perceptions of the clients, and at the same time will incorporate into the Western medical systems alternative folk medical systems that constitute potential sources of resistance to it.

One example of an integrated approach to primary health care is the WHO project in Somalia (see Ahmed & Steinglass, 1978). Following independence in 1960, all practicing physicians left the country. By 1973, there were 193 physicians in the country, of whom 135 were Somali. This meant a ratio of 1 physician for every 15,500 persons. More than 90% of these physicians worked in urban centers. There were only 4 dentists, 770 nurses and midwives, and 74 medical laboratory technicians. Since 1960, health-planning efforts have followed the traditional pattern in developing countries. In the last decade Somalia has devoted a very large portion of its health budget to establishing a medical school, where the teaching, done primarily by Italian doctors, is largely theoretical and academic, and to expanding the three schools for nurses and midwives, thus still leaving the rural population almost without access to modern medical care. By contrast with this familiar pattern of centralizing health resources in urban, hospital-based, high-quality medical care, WHO has undertaken an innovative experiment to improve primary care to the rural population. Community-based village health workers, recruited partly from the ranks of traditional practitioners, are being trained in rudimentary preventive medicine, nutrition, sanitation, and the treatment of common illnesses. After the training (which lasts about 3 months) the auxiliary health workers return to the village, where they continue to work at their usual occupations but are also responsible for community health care. They are supported and supervised by the district staff. To be sure, the project has encountered numerous bureaucratic obstacles, particularly objections to its "alien" origins (it is supported by WHO and thus is not a part of the national health system). It has also created a need for more personnel at the district level to supervise and train the auxiliary health workers, as well as a need for training in community health care at all levels. In any case, the interface between the health bureaucracy and the people it serves has been transformed and the balance has shifted back to the community. For the first time the rural population is being served by Western-trained medical personnel, however rudimentary their training and equipment.

Whether or not traditional medical practitioners can be integrated formally into the national health services, the important point is that health care should be available to all. In order to make "a state of physical, mental and social well-being" available to all people, it is necessary to refocus the efforts of the health care system toward the needs and values of the people in rural communities; it is necessary to bring them into the process of health care that affects their lives.

References

Ademuwagum, F. A. The relevance of Yoruba medicine men in public health practice in Nigeria. *Public Health Reports*, 1969, *84*, 1085–1091.

Ahmed, P. I. *Psycho-social and cultural aspects of international health care assistance to developing countries.* Paper presented to the World Congress of Mental Health, Vancouver, B. C., August 21–28, 1977. (Mimeograph)

Ahmed, P. I., & Steinglass, R. *Syncrisis—The dynamics of health: Somalia.* Washington, D. C.: Office of International Health, U. S. Department of Health, Education and Welfare, 1978.

Chasse, J. D. The role of the WHO definition of health in the planning and analysis of health programs, 1978. (Mimeograph)

Coelho, G. V., & Stein, J. S. Coping with stresses of an urban planet: Impacts of uprooting and overcrowding. *Habitat,* 1977, *2,* 379–390.

Dubos, R. *Mirage of health.* Garden City, N. Y.: Doubleday, 1959.

Dunn, F. L. Traditional Asian medicine and cosmopolitan medicine as adaptive systems. In C. Leslie (Ed.), *Asian medical systems.* Berkeley and Los Angeles: University of California Press, 1976.

Engel, G. L. The need for a new medical model: A challenge for biomedicine. *Science,* 1977, *196,* 129–136.

Fabrega, H., Jr. *Disease and social behavior: An interdisciplinary perspective.* Cambridge, Mass.: M.I.T. Press, 1974.

Fabrega, H., Jr. The need for an ethnomedical science. *Science,* 1975, *189,* 969–975.

Flahault, D. An integrated and functional team for primary health care. *WHO Chronicles,* 1976, *30,* 442–446.

Flexner, A. *Medical education in the United States and Canada, Bulletin No. 4.* Carnegie Foundation for the Advancement of Teaching, 1910.

Foster, G. M. Medical anthropology and international health planning. *Social Science and Medicine,* 1977, *11,* 527–534.

Goldberg, D. Indian medical school snarled in red tape. *Washington Post,* March 19, 1978.

Graham, D. & Stevenson, I. Disease as a response to life stress. In H. I. Lief (Ed.), *The psychological basis of medical practice.* New York: Harper & Row, 1963.

Guidotti, T. L. Health care for a rural minority: Lessons from the Modoc Indian country in California. *Community Medicine,* 1973, *118,* 98–104.

Hart, R. H. Rural health reorganization in Tanzania: The implications of change implementation, 1978. (Mimeograph)

Havelock, R. G. *Planning for innovation through dissemination and utilization of knowledge.* Ann Arbor: Institute for Social Research, University of Michigan, 1971.

Hughes, C. C. Medical care: Ethnomedicine. In D. Sills (Ed.), *International encyclopedia of the social sciences* (Vol. 10). New York: Collier and Macmillan, 1968.

Imperato, P. J. Traditional medical practitioners among the Bambara of Mali and their role in the modern health care delivery system. *Tropical and Geographic Medicine,* 1975, *27,* 211–221.

Khare, R. S. Folk medicine in a North Indian village. *Human Organization,* 1973, *22,* 36–40.

King, S. Social psychological factors in illness. In H. Freeman, S. Levine, & L. Reeder (Eds.), *Handbook of medical sociology.* Englewood Cliffs, N. J.: Prentice-Hall, 1972.

Landy, D. Role adaptation: Traditional curers under the impact of modern medicine. *American Ethnologist,* 1974, *1,* 103–127.

Leslie, C. (Ed.). *Asian medical systems: A comparative study.* Berkeley and Los Angeles: University of California Press, 1976.

Logan, M. H., & Hunt, E. E. (Eds). *Health and the human condition: Perspectives on medical anthropology.* North Scituate, Mass.: Duxbury Press, 1978.

Mechanic, D. *Medical sociology.* New York: Free Press, 1968.

Opler, M. E. The cultural definition of illness in village India. *Human Organization,* 1963, *22,* 32–35.

Press, I. Urban folk medicine: A functional overview. *American Anthropologist,* 1978, *80,* 71–84.

Report of the committee on indigenous systems of medicine. Ministry of Health, Government of India, 1948.

Rogers, E. M., & Shoemaker, F. F. *Communication of innovations.* New York: Free Press, 1971.

Twaddle, A. C., & Hessler, R. M. *A sociology of health.* St. Louis: C. V. Mosby, 1977.

United Nations Demographic Yearbook. New York: United Nations, 1951, 1976. (Published annually)

United Nations Statistical Yearbook. New York: United Nations, 1951, 1976. (Published annually)

Vecsey, G. Spiritual healing gaining ground with Catholics and Episcopalians. *New York Times,* June 18, 1978.

II

Psychosocial Factors in Disease: Some Specific Examples

Introduction

Social-environmental factors affect disease in each of its phases: its etiology, its symptoms, and its outcomes. Actual living conditions, such as poverty, overcrowding, or stress, influence the incidence of disease; cultural norms affect the type of symptoms that will be noticed or reported; and the social structure affects the course and outcome of treatment. In this section we examine some specific nonbiological factors that affect particular diseases. The list could be extended considerably, of course; the articles in this section provide a few examples.

A major link between social-environmental conditions and illness is stress, a condition rooted in the psychophysiological state of the organism. Stress results from the body's straining to cope with disagreeable physical or emotional stimuli, or from the failure to cope with such stimuli. A number of studies have concluded that inability to manage the social, psychological, or emotional demands of life, whether routine or unusual, may increase the body's susceptibility to hypertension, to cardiovascular complications, to asthma, or to other health problems (see, for example, House, 1974; McNeil, 1970; Moss, 1973). Some researchers suggest that the *normal* conditions of 20th-century living, particularly overcrowding and frequent mobility, place new and stressful demands on the adaptive capacities of organisms (Coelho & Stein, 1977). Others suggest that the *accumulation* of frequent life changes, whether "good" or "bad," increases susceptibility to serious illness by multiplying the stress responses that the individual must manage simultaneously (Holmes & Rahe, 1967). Thus, both the magnitude and the rate of change have been associated with disease-enhancing stress responses.

The first article in this section, by House and Jackman, concentrates on the health hazards of one common type of stress—occupational stress. It reviews the literature on occupational stress and provides some provocative insights from the authors' own research. The authors note the reported relationship between occupational stress and such outcomes as alcoholism, coronary heart disease, hypertension, and ulcers; they add, however, that past studies have focused on the direct causation of specific diseases, but have not explored the additive or interactive relationships between stress and chemical or physical disease-producing stimuli. Methodologically, these studies are limited by retrospective data. Longitudinal data are needed to explore how health and illness result from the interaction of multiple causes, biological, chemical, and psychosocial, and how stress may have a *nonspecific* effect on lowering the resistance of the individual to a vardety of infectious and chronic diseases from tuberculosis to cancer.

The authors report other research on the effects of perceived occupational stress on the health of factory workers. They define occupational stress as consisting of excessive work load, role conflict, heavy responsibility, concern about performance, low job satisfaction, low occupational prestige and self-esteem, and inadequate extrinsic and intrinsic rewards. They report a consistent relationship between job pressures and neurotic, ulcer, and coronary symptoms (the traditional "stress diseases") and inconsistent but strikingly suggestive relationships between job pressures, exposure to chemical irritants, and such symptoms as cough and rash.

The authors recommend longitudinal research into the nonspecific causes and effects of stress, and structural improvements in the quality of work life through such measures as supportive supervision, job enrichment, decentralization of authority, and improving the fit between workers' personalities and occupational demands.

The second chapter, by O'Connor and Ahmed, deals with drug abuse from the perspective of ecosystems. Drug abuse may be viewed as one dimension of the continuous process of interaction between the person and his environment. According to the authors, an effective approach to drug abuse must focus on the meaning of the specific behavior (substance abuse) in the total context of the human ecosystem. They point out that the conventional fragmented treatment of drug abusers is doomed to failure because it removes the patient from his usual life space, treats the isolated "deviant" or "ill" behavior in an institutional context, and then returns the individual to the same system. Moreover, the fragmented approach fails because it often ignores the range of personalities and situations found among drug abusers. It is necessary to differentiate, the authors argue, between those who otherwise exhibit normal memberships and behaviors in all groups that constitute their life space and those whose environmental supports are so inadequate or lacking that addiction becomes a habitual behavioral response in efforts to cope. Under these circumstances, attempts to "change" the drug user often meet with the user's resistance and, in any case, leave unchanged the original imbalance between the individual and his environment, making a permanent behavioral change unlikely.

The authors claim that an effective societal approach to drug abuse requires a clarification of the definition of drug abuse in its diverse meanings: as illness, as deviant behavior, and as abnormal behavior. Such a clarification must precede a comprehensive and well-articulated set of interventions on the part of the agencies charged by society with dealing with the problem.

Psychosocial dimensions affect not only the onset of the disease, as the first two chapters illustrate, but also its course and its treatment. In the third article in this section, Hersh discusses the symbolic and psychological implications of cancer. From the vantage point of the treating physician, Hersh offers insights into the dramatic physical and psychological changes that take place in patients as the results of the disease, of the treatment, and of the reactions of the patient and his family. These changes include, in addition to physical morbidity, a painful blow to self-image, social and physical isolation, guilt, stigma, and depression. Hersh traces these painful changes to what he believes to be the most traumatic aspect of cancer—loss of control over one's life and one's body. In citing several poignant case histories, Hersh highlights the theme that the loss of control, and the fear of such loss, constitute the most dreaded aspect of cancer, rather than the fear of death itself.

Hersh suggests some guidelines for dealing with the terminally ill patients and their families, cautioning, however, that these guidelines must be viewed in the context of the limitations of research on various aspects of the problem (including, for example, the issue of the sexuality of the handicapped and of inpatients).

Hersh argues that cancer, "the dreaded disease," will be finally demythologized as we gain more control over its occurrence through preventive measures. Until such time, however, we must learn to accept it as what it is—"a group of related diseases, chronic in their course, usually of unknown etiology, which currently affect someone in every family." We must turn our attention from technologically intensive treatment aimed at prolonging life at any cost to enchancing the quality of the patient's remaining life. This entails preserving the dignity and autonomy of the patient, promoting his continued participation in various social roles such as family and school, and helping the family cope with the stress. In this process, according to Hersh, we will be able "to demythologize the dreaded disease," and to attain a new definition of health for cancer patients.

Of all categories of disease, the one most heavily intertwined with psychosocial dimensions is probably mental illness—itself a category that pertains to behavioral and emotional, rather than simply physiological disturbances. Although the medical profession has pursued the analyses of the physiological or at least the objective psychological correlates of mental illness, no fit between mental illness and the positivist biomedical model has been clearly established (see Engel, 1977). In the last chapter in this section, Robitscher points out that no satisfactory distinction has ever been made between objective manifestations of mental pathology and socially disapproved behavior. Yet, according to Robitscher, notwithstanding the flimsiness of the distinction, the labeling of certain behavioral and personality patterns as mental illness entails potentially disastrous consequences for the patient. Such consequences include the progressive deterioration of personal and work relationships, discrimination in employment, and finally, loss of ability to pay for further treatment.

Robitscher argues that in diagnosing a patient as mentally ill, the psychiatrist faces difficult dilemmas. On the one hand, the psychiatrist is reluctant to subject the patient to the irreversible stigma of such a diagnosis; on the other, he is eager to use the diagnosis broadly in order to help the patient to obtain further treatment, to secure health insurance coverage, or to escape legal responsibilities.

The psychiatrist may also tend, by virtue of the "professional deformity" to overdefine mental illness, a tendency that increases not only his fees but his professional authority. Robitscher reviews the history of the psychiatrist's authority. At various times it has encompassed eugenic sterilization, lobotomy, physical straitjacketing, chemical (tranquilizer) straitjacketing, and institutionalization—in short, far-reaching intrusion into every aspect of the patient's mind, body, and life. Furthermore, the psychiatrist can manipulate the labels at will because no lay person can challenge his authority effectively; the patient himself is trapped into having to accept the label if he is eventually to be discharged as "cured," and because the dividing line between mental illness and "normality" is vague and shifting.

Robitscher highlights the issues of the cultural bias and relativity of psychiatric diagnosis, but rejects the extreme position of such labeling theorists as Goffman and Szasz, who would maintain that there is no objective difference between mental illness and normality. "Hard core" mental illness, manifested in uncontrollable behavior that may harm the individual or his surrounding society, is real enough. But extreme caution is recommended in applying diagnostic labels; such categories are useful as working hypotheses but can be overinclusive labels for making such crucial life-altering decisions as granting or denying parole, employment, or admission to professional school. Robitscher calls for a *narrowing* of the definition of mental illness to those cases where extreme or acute disorders undeniably exist. Such a narrowing would serve both to minimize the harmful consequences to the patient and to avoid the dilution of psychiatry to a parascience that deals with the multitudinous variety of life adjustment problems that are increasingly common in fast-changing modern societies.

References

Coelho, G. V., & Stein, J. S. Coping with stresses of an urban planet: Impacts of uprooting and overcrowding. *Habitat*, 1977, *2*, 379–390.

Engel, G. L. The need for a new medical model: A challenge for biomedicine. *Science*, 1977, *196*, 129–136.

Holmes, T. H., & Rahe, R. H. The social readjustment rating scale. *Journal of Psychosomatic Research*, 1967, *11*, 213–225.

House, J. M. Occupational stress and coronary heart disease. *Journal of Health and Social Behavior*, 1974, *15*, 12–27.

McNeil, E. B. *Neuroses and personality disorders*. Englewood Cliffs, N.J.: Prentice-Hall, 1970.

Moss, G. E. *Illness, immunity, and social interaction*. New York: Wiley, 1973.

7

Occupational Stress and Health

James S. House and Mark F. Jackman

There has been a growing concern with health problems in the United States, not the least of which is the burgeoning national expenditure on medical care. The failure of accelerating expenditures in medical care to produce proportionate gains in life expectancy or other indicators of the quality of health and life has called into question our society's tendency to equate quality of health with quality of medical care. Although improvements in the quality, cost-effectiveness, and distribution of medical care are important and necessary, this equation of health with medical care results in vast amounts of money and energy being directed toward increasingly complex institutions to care for the sick, often at the expense of preventive programs aimed at maintaining the health of the nonsick (Task Force Report, 1973).

Growing awareness of this problem has increased concern with identifying and eliminating health hazards before they cause illness. With chronic rather than acute infectious diseases now constituting the major sources of ill health, preventive efforts must look beyond biological causes of illness to environmental and psychosocial factors that directly or indirectly affect health. Since most American adults spend from one- to two-thirds of their waking life at work, the workplace has recently become a focus of efforts to

James S. House • Institute for Social Research, University of Michigan, Ann Arbor, Michigan 48106. Mark F. Jackman • Department of Sociology, Duke University, Durham, North Carolina 27706. Preparation of this chapter has been supported by Public Health Services Research Grant RO1–MH28902 from the National Institute of Mental Health, as has our current research, which is described briefly here.

identify and eliminate health hazards and to enhance physical and mental health (cf. Ashford, 1976; Task Force Report, 1973). The passage of the 1970 National Occupational Safety and Health Act made healthful working conditions a national goal, although the primary concern of this act and the programs stemming from it have been physical and chemical hazards at work.

In contrast, this chapter, like the volume of which it is a part, seeks to document the impact of varied psychosocial aspects of work, here subsumed under the rubric of occupational stress, on a wide range of health outcomes. Adequate understanding of the source and nature of health and illness requires consideration of psychosocial as well as physical, chemical, and biological aspects of the work situation. Utilizing a paradigm for stress research as its organizing framework, this chapter seeks to review and critique current theoretical and empirical knowledge of occupational stress and health. Earlier reviews of occupational stress and health by House (1974a, b, 1975) serve as points of departure allowing us to focus here on more recent theoretical and empirical knowledge and trends. In particular, the present chapter emphasizes that occupational stress appears to play a role in the etiology of a wide range of health problems, not just those traditionally termed *stress-related* or *psychosomatic*, and that understanding this broad impact of stress requires increased attention to how stress interacts with physical, chemical, and biological factors in the etiology of specific diseases. Adequate understanding of the impact of occupational stress on a broad range of health outcomes has important practical implications. The effects of occupational stress, we suggest, can be reduced and/or alleviated more easily than many other hazards to health since work organizations provide an accessible and potentially powerful mechanism for intervention programs. And the results of such interventions promise broad and substantial improvement in the quality of health and life.

"Stress" and Health: The Promise and the Problems

Over the past few decades the concept of "stress" has played a central role in the development of a broader, more psychosocial, conception of health. The concept is probably most closely associated with Selye's (1936, 1956) pioneering work on the "nonspecific" effects of noxious stimuli, including psychosocial ones, on the internal psychological and especially physiological functioning of organisms. The work of Selye, Cannon, and others showed that full understanding of health and disease requires research and theory that transcends the boundaries of bodily systems and scholarly disciplines (cf. Mason, 1975). One of the major functions of the stress concept, then, has been to stimulate a multi- and interdisciplinary body of work and to serve as an integrative rubric for this vast body of work. However, the multidisciplinary nature of stress research has also led to such a proliferation of understandings and misunderstandings of the term *stress* that Hinkle (1973) and Mason (1975) have suggested abandoning the term altogether, while Cassel (1976, p. 108) has declared that "simple-minded invocation of the word stress has done as much to retard research in this area [i.e., "the potential role of the social environment in disease etiology"] as did the concepts of the miasmas at the time of the discovery of microorganisms."

A Paradigm for "Stress Research"

"Stress" has been used to refer to environmental stimuli or situations, individual cognitions or emotions, and physiological responses. Although there neither is nor can be agreement on a single conceptual or operational definition of "stress," we and others (cf. Levine and Scotch, 1970; Mc-Grath, 1970) still feel that "stress research" constitutes a meaningful body of literature grounded in a distinctive metatheoretical paradigm that helps "the investigator to ask more meaningful questions and to consider variables he might not have looked at had he used a more limited and conventional perspective" (Mechanic, 1970, p. 106). Various authors (French, Rogers, & Cobb, 1974; Levine & Scotch, 1970, pp. 200–231; McGrath, 1970, pp. 15–17) see five classes of variables as necessary in any comprehensive paradigm of stress research: (1) objective social conditions conducive to stress, (2) individual perceptions of stress, (3) individual responses (physiological, affective, and behavioral) to perceived stress, (4) more enduring outcomes of perceived stress and responses thereto, and (5) individual and situational conditioning variables that specify the relationships among the first four sets of factors. Figure 1 presents a model relating these five classes of variables. The arrows between boxes indicate hypothesized causal relationships, while the arrows coming down from the from the box labeled "conditioning variables" indicate that social and individual variables condition or specify the nature of these relationships (as explained below).

The paradigm has important implications for the study of stress (or psychosocial factors, more generally) and health. The paradigm emphasizes that particular objective, social, or environmental conditions do not invariably give rise to particular health outcomes, but rather their impact depends on how these conditions are perceived and responded to by human actors. Stress research deals broadly with how individuals react to situations where their usual modes of behavior are insufficient, and consequences of not adapting are serious—generally situations where the demands made severely test persons' existing abilities or where there are

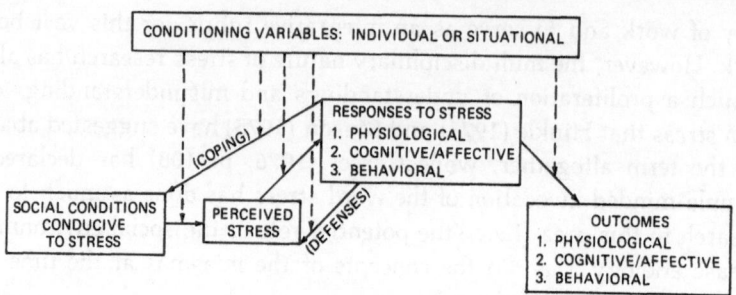

Figure 1. A paradigm of stress research. Solid arrows between boxes indicate presumed causal relationships among variables. Dotted arrows from the box labeled "conditioning variables" intersect solid arrows, indicating an interaction between the conditioning variables and the variables in the box at the beginning of the solid arrow in predicting variables in the box at the head of the solid arrow. (From House, J. S. Occupational stress and coronary heart disease: A review and theoretical integration. *Journal of Health and Social Behavior*, 1974, *15*, p. 130. Reprinted by permission of the publisher.)

substantial obstacles to the fulfillment of strong needs and values (cf. French *et al.*, 1974). But any particular social or environmental condition will be perceived as stressful (i.e., threatening, frightening, overly demanding, etc.) by some persons but not by others, depending on the characteristics of the persons and other aspects of their social situations (the conditioning variables in Figure 1). The perception of stress may lead to somewhat transient behavioral, psychological, or physiological *responses* (e.g., taking an alcoholic drink, feeling anxious or sad, a rise in blood pressure) and ultimately to more enduring health outcomes (e.g., alcoholism, neurosis, essential hypertension). However, perceived stress produces a particular response only for certain individuals or in certain situations, whereas the more enduring outcome of a given response depends on how the response affects the precipitating objective conditions and/or perceptions of stress and whether the person is particularly vulnerable (due to prior medical history problems, genetic weaknesses, lack of social support, etc.) to a given outcome.

Consider a concrete example from the area of occupational stress. High levels of work load and responsibility constitute potential stressors, but people with differing abilities, training, and needs will react differently to these potential stressors—some finding them pleasant challenges and others perceiving them as more than they can handle (i.e., stressful). However, even individuals experiencing the same degree of perceived stress will manifest a variety of responses and, hence, also a variety of health outcomes. Faced with excessive work load or responsibility, one person may do nothing; another will strive to meet the challenge by working harder; another may reorganize his work activities or gain new skills, or call on others for assistance, thus reducing the level of work load and responsibility and the degree to which these are perceived as stressful; another may deny or repress the perception of stress. The pattern of responses will be determined by the interaction of the perceived stress and various conditioning variables (e.g., social supports, personality).

If the objective conditions or the capacity of the person for dealing with them can be changed (arrow labeled "coping" in Figure 1), no enduring deleterious health outcomes are likely. If the objective conditions remain the same, efforts to deny or repress perceptions (defenses in Figure 1) may temporarily relieve anxiety, physiological arousal, and some behavioral responses; but since such responses involve perceptual distortions they are likely to lead ultimately to neurotic problems or to bring on further stresses (as the person becomes less in touch with reality). Unsuccessful coping and/or failure to act at all are likely to produce chronically elevated levels of associated behavioral, psychological, and physiological reactions (e.g., drinking, anxiety, blood pressure) and perhaps even death (e.g., overdose, suicide, heart attack). But whether an initially transient response, even if prolonged, produces a chronic or enduring outcome depends on genetic predispositions, other personal characteristics (e.g., sex, poor nutrition, physical conditions), environmental exposures (to microorganisms and toxins), or other conditioning factors that may increase or decrease the likelihood of a given permanent outcome.

Key Directions in the Study of Occupational Stress and Health

Although this paradigm reflects the thinking of major stress researchers from Selye on, much research on stress and health has not be informed adequately by it. Much of this research has been done, not by students of stress, but rather by students of particular diseases or classes of diseases. Rather than utilizing the stress paradigm above, such researchers have utilized a more traditional medical model:

> Stated in its most general terms, the formulation subscribed to (often implicitly) by most epidemiologists and social scientists working in this field is that the relationship between a stressor and disease outcome will be similar to the relationship between a microorganism and the disease outcome. . . . The corollaries of such a formulation are that there will be etiologic specificity (each stressor leading to a specific stress disease), and there will be a dose-response relationship (the greater the stressor, the more likelihood of disease). (Cassel 1976, p. 109)

The influential psychoanalytic perspective in psychosomatic medicine has similarly emphasized that specific intrapsychic conflicts and personality patterns are associated with specific diseases (Alexander, 1950). Thus, research and theory on the role of stress, and of psychosocial factors more generally, in the etiology of health and illness have been organized around specific diseases. The search has been for the types of stress, personality, or "behavior patterns" that make persons coronary-prone or ulcer-prone or arthritis-prone, etc. Consequently, all reviews of research on stress and psychosocial factors and health have been organized around specific diseases. A variety of factors continue to shape research and theory in these directions (e.g., scientific specialization, research and funding institutes, and publication outlets are often structured along disease-specific lines).

However, Selye (1976), Cassel (1976), Hinkle (1973), and others (Syme, 1967) have emphasized that, properly understood, the stress paradigm embodies a quite different conception of the role of environmental and psychosocial stimuli in the etiology of health and illness. From his seminal article to the present, Selye (e.g., 1976, pp. 53–54) has argued that what he termed *stress* (a pattern of bodily reactions to external demands or noxious stimuli) is *nonspecific* and *conditional* in both its *causes* and its *effects*. These ideas rest in turn on the idea that states of health and illness are always the product of *multiple causes* (cf. Hinkle, 1973). Selye's "stress" reaction or "general adaptation syndrome" represents a broad pattern of reactions of the body's neuroendocrine, immunological, or other homeostatic systems, which, he argues, can be induced by a broad range of physical, chemical, biological, and psychosocial stimuli. Hence, this syndrome is nonspecific and multicausal in that it can both be induced by a wide range of potential stressors and cause or contribute to the development of a wide range of diseases.

Selye (1956) describes the syndrome as involving an initial lowering of bodily resistance or immunity during which a variety of infectious diseases (e.g., tuberculosis) may develop that under normal circumstances would be successfully resisted. There follows an activation of bodily defense mechanisms characterized by arousal of the autonomic nervous systems (with adrenaline discharge; increased heart rate, blood pressure, and muscle tone; and increased digestive secretion coupled with heightened tendencies toward inflammation in the stomach and other bodily tissues). If prolonged, this bodily state can produce a wide range of what Selye termed *diseases of adaptation* (e.g., cardiovascular-renal diseases, rheumatism and arthritis, ulcers, inflammatory and allergic diseases)—that is, diseases caused by the body's own attempts to adapt to stress rather than by any external agent directly. Whether this syndrome is activated, and whether it produces a given enduring disease outcome is *conditional* upon other characteristics of the individuals (e.g., personality, age, genetic predispositions, and medical history) involved and/or their environments (e.g., treatment with drugs or hormones, exposure to infectious agents or environmental toxins, social support from others).

It should be noted that there are some critics (e.g., Mason, 1975; Williams, 1975) of the concept of *absolute* nonspecificity of causes and effects of stress as put forth by Selye. Mason (1975) notes that when psychological factors (e.g., anxiety aroused by a novel or strange situation) associated with laboratory experiments on some *physical* stressors (e.g., heat, fasting) are controlled and minimized, these stressors no longer evoke the hormonal responses charasteristic of Selye's stress syndromes. Hence, he argues, Selye's stress syndrome is, in fact, elicited only by stimuli that produce *emotional arousal:* ". . . the apparently non-specific physiological responses in Selye's triad were largely a reflection of the ubiquity of emotional arousal superimposed upon the general tendency for most endocrine systems to respond to multiple stimuli." This qualification, if true (cf. Selye, 1975, 1976), constitutes a substantial criticism of Selye's theory but is of little concern for those like ourselves whose concern is largely with the effects of psychosocial factors that produce emotional arousal and consequent physiological responses. However, Williams (1975) finds that social or environmental situations that demand sensory intake (e.g., vigilance) and sensory rejection (e.g., intense concentration), both of which may be perceived as stressful, produce somewhat different physiological responses. Still, for our purposes, the important thing is that effects of stress upon health appear to be at least *relatively* nonspecific, even if not absolutely so. One hopes that future research will help clarify this argument.

In sum, the stress paradigm has been increasingly seen to require study of how multiple psychosocial, physiological, and physical-chemical factors combine (both additively and interactively) to produce a wide range of diseases. Any given objective occupational or potential stressor can be perceived in multiple ways, and any given perception of occupational stress can produce multiple short-term responses and long-term health outcomes. Thus, there are not stress-related diseases and non-stress-related diseases. Rather, occupational stress can be involved in the etiology of almost any disease, provided that stress might affect any of the psychological or physiological processes necessary to produce the disease. This is not to say that occupational stress and other psychosocial factors may not be more important in the etiology of some diseases than others or that stress phenomena may not on occasion be sufficient to produce disease. However, in general, we would expect occupational stress to interact with other factors to produce disease, although considerable theoretical and empirical development is still needed to specify and empirically document the nature of these interactions.

Thus, future work on occupational stress and health must increasingly attempt to evaluate how occupational stress relates to a wide range of diseases, and especially to examine the potential interaction between psychosocially induced occupational stress and physical, chemical, and biological hazards to which the worker is exposed. Theoretical and empirical analyses of health and disease etiologies must incorporate both psychosocial or stress factors and more traditional physical, chemical, or biological factors. Such studies are few and far between at this point, but conditions seem ripe for them in the future, and this chapter seeks to stimulate their development.

Empirical Evidence

Earlier papers by the first author (House, 1974a, b, 1975) reviewed the evidence available up through the early 1970s on the effects of occupational stress, especially on coronary heart disease but also on ulcers, arthritis, and general mortality or longevity. As already noted, these reviews largely reflected the position that specific psychosocial stress factors cause specific diseases. Since most studies consider only a single type of health outcome, most existing evidence is disease-specific, and we have no way of knowing whether the stress factors associated with that disease might be associated with other diseases as well. We will summarize briefly the conclusions of these earlier papers here and note the results of more recent research on the role of occupational stress in these diseases. We will turn then to a consideration of theory and evidence from nonoccupational as well as occupational sources suggesting that occupational stress factors may play a role in the etiology of other diseases. Finally, we will review the background and preliminary results of our current research, which looks at the effect of occupational stress on a range of health outcomes.

Most of the evidence discussed here comes from cross-sectional and retrospective studies, rather than prospective or longitudinal studies. We emphasize below that it is essential to move toward more prospective and even applied experimental studies if we are to document more firmly a causal impact of occupational stress on health. Nevertheless, although the results of many individual studies are open to alternative interpretations, the total available evidence from a combination of retrospective, cross-sectional, and a few prospective studies can be interpreted most plausibly as indicating a causal impact of occupational stress on a wide range of health outcomes.

Occupational Stress and "Stress Diseases"

Almost all research on occupational stress and health has focused on specific psychosomatic or stress-related diseases, predominantly on coronary heart disease. Studies reviewed earlier by House (1974a,b, 1975) indicated that two broad classes of objective work conditions and perceived occupational stress—lack of job rewards and excessive job pressures or demands—were associated with higher rates of coronary heart disease (CHD) and/or CHD risk factors (e.g., high levels of blood pressure, cholesterol, and smoking). Lack of rewards at work produces feelings of job dissatisfaction and low occupational self-esteem. Major forms of job pressure include work overload, role conflict, and excessive responsibility. Although only a few studies published since that review have focused directly on occupational stress and dissatisfaction, a variety of studies reviewed by Jenkins (1976) have included work pressures and dissatisfactions in larger indices of general life dissatisfaction and pressure and have found the latter indices to be significantly associated with the prevalence and/or incidence of CHD (although positive findings occur more often when angina pectoris rather than myocardial infarction is the dependent variable). A number of these studies have also shown specific occupational factors such as problems and conflicts with co-workers (Medalie, Snyder, Groen, Neufeld, Goldburt, & Riss, 1973), work dissatisfaction (Theorell & Rahe, 1972), and excessive overtime (Theorell & Rahe, 1972; Thiel, Parker, & Bruce, 1973) to predict a higher incidence of CHD. Our own research, presented in more detail below, has found both lack of job rewards and experience of job pressures to be associated with heightened levels of angina pectoris (assessed by questionnaire) and hypertension and coronary disease risk (i.e., high levels of blood pressure, cholesterol, and smoking) in the blue-collar work force of a large factory. However, Caplan, Cobb, French, Harrison, and Pinnau (1975) failed to find a clear relation between such occupational stresses and heart disease risk factors. Overall, though, the published data continue to suggest a significant role of occupational stress in the etiology of coronary disease.

The best-established psychosocial correlate and predictor of coronary disease is the Type A "behavior pattern" identified by Friedman and Rosenman (1971), the key attributes of which appear to be competitive drive and time urgency or impatience (Jenkins, 1976, p. 1035). Jenkins (1976, p. 1034) emphasizes that the Type A variable "represents neither a stressful situation nor a distressed response, but rather a style with which some persons habitually respond to circumstances that arouse them." This suggests that Type A is an enduring trait that conditions (in the sense of Figure 1) workers' perceptions of, or responses to, occupational stress. However, the nature and history of the Type A concept suggests that it is also closely associated with the experience of potentially stressful objective conditions of work and/or perceived occupational stress. Thus, the impressive body of data on the impact of Type A on coronary disease can be viewed as further indication of the impact of occupational stress (cf. Friedman & Rosenman, 1971; Rosenman, & Friedman 1958).

After heart disease, peptic ulcer is the major physical health problem that has been directly linked with occupational stress. A previous review by House (1974b, p. 160) concluded that interpersonal conflict, responsibility for others, and low occupational self-esteem are associated with higher rates of peptic ulcer. Our current research, described below, provides some further evidence in support of this conclusion, though we measured only self-reported ulcer symptoms.

Measures of perceived occupational stress and of objective conditions conducive to stress (including low status, boring and repetitive work, and to a lesser degree, high levels of pressure) have also been quite consistently associated with poorer mental health, i.e., heightened anxiety, depression, or other neurotic symptoms (Kasl, 1974, pp. 185–186). Again, our current research provides further support for this association, as does the comprehensive study of Caplan et al. (1975). Thus, occupational stress has deleterious effects on mental as well as physical health.

The effects of potentially stressful objective conditions of work and of perceived occupational stress are known to be conditioned by a variety of factors. Social support from others has been increasingly identified in both occupational and nonoccupational settings as a factor mitigating the effects of perceived stress on health (Cassel, 1976; Cobb, 1976). It has also been shown that the effects of objective or perceived job demands and rewards on health vary depending upon the worker's desire or motivation to approach or avoid such demands and rewards—that is, perceived stress and health outcomes are a function of the "fit" between the persons and their objective work environments (Caplan et al., 1975, Harrison, 1978). Finally, House (1972) found that perceived occupational stress increased CHD risk among male workers over 45 years of age but had no effect on those under 45. This may reflect a decline in bodily resilience and resistance with age, which increase workers' vulnerability to environmental stresses, psychosocial or otherwise.

In sum, there is a good deal of evidence that perceived occupational stress and objective conditions conducive to such perceived stress are associated with coronary heart disease, peptic ulcer, and poor mental health—disorders that have traditionally been thought of as "stress diseases," that is, caused at least in part by stress. Obviously, however, such research leaves many questions unanswered. Perhaps most critically we need more prospective studies and/or studies that evaluate the health consequences of planned and unplanned changes in the level of occupational stress. Such research will establish more firmly the causal status of the largely cross-sectional associations just noted. Studies of this nature will also prove useful in analyzing the complex contingencies inherent in the stress paradigm.

Most research has focused on the relation of perceived stresses to health, with little attention to objective conditions of work and to the role of conditioning variables. More attention should be paid in future research to these latter variables, and especially to the nature and effects of *responses* to perceived stress (i.e., coping and adaptation) that have been generally ignored up to this point because they require longitudinal study of the process of stress and reactions to stress. These and other research needs have been more extensively discussed in the earlier reviews by House (1974a, b, 1975). In this chapter, however, we would like to concentrate on how and why the study of occupational stress and health should be extended beyond the traditional confines of psychosomatic or "stress diseases" to all forms of health and illness.

Stress and "Nonstress" Diseases

The passage of the National Occupational Safety and Health Act in 1970 reflected a heightened interest in the effect of work on health in America. Psychosocial forms of occupational stress, however, have never been a primary focus of attention in the developing field of occupational health before or after 1970. Rather, the major concern has been with the effect of physical-chemical work evironments on worker safety and health. Research and public interest have been directed especially toward accidents and physical and chemical hazards productive of fatal or disabling forms of cancer and respiratory disease (e.g., coal dust, cotton, and asbestos fibers). The National Institute of Occupational Safety and Health (NIOSH) and the Occupational Safety and Health Administration (OSHA) have both primarily concentrated their efforts on the physical-chemical work environment, though NIOSH has mounted a small program of psychosocial research. However, Ashford (1976, p. 125) has noted that NIOSH and other researchers in occupational health have not only paid little attention to psychosocial stress, they have also failed to consider the interrelation between psychosocial stress and physical-chemical hazards. Thus, the field of occupational health consists of two quite separate parts: a rather large domain dealing with "nonstress" hazards and nonstress diseases and a rather small part with occupational stress and "stress diseases."

The broadened conception of the stress paradigm presented in the first part of this chapter points, however, to an integration of these two separate parts—one that is beginning to be reflected in empirical research as well as theory. Current medical theory and considerable evidence from animal experiments suggests that psychosocial stress may impair the functioning of the body's immune system, thus making animals and possibly people, through similar mechanisms, more susceptible to infectious diseases, cancer, and autoimmune diseases such as rheumatoid arthritis (Solomon, Amkraut, & Kasper, 1974). Selye (1956) has noted that stress affects the level of substances tending both to enhance and to reduce inflammatory and immune responses and, most importantly, it can disturb the balance between these substances. To the extent that stress reduces immune and inflammatory responses for some period of time, it reduces the bodies' resistance to infectious agents, environmental irritants, and/or the multiplication of mutant cells. To the extent that stress abnormally heightens immune and inflammatory responses for some period, it also can produce autoimmune diseases and/or exacerbate dermatological or respiratory responses to environmental irritants. Thus, stress could contribute to the etiology and/or development of many diseases that have not traditionally been considered "stress-related."

A variety of animal and human studies are beginning to lend empirical support to this idea. Studies reviewed by Solomon *et al.* (1974) show that animals under stress (e.g., experimental crowding, periodic shock, limited feeding) manifested lower levels of antibodies, greater susceptibility to viruses, and increased rates of tumor growth than animals under less stress. For example, Riley (1975) found that mice carrying mammary tumors virus showed a marked delay in the time of onset of tumors if kept in a protected, nonstressful environment compared to mice housed in conventional laboratory facilities. These kinds of experimental findings regarding the immunosuppressive effects of stress have led to increased interest of the National Cancer Institute in studies of psychosocial precursors of cancer (Fox, 1976). Hurst, Jenkins, & Rose (1976) review evidence from human studies indicating that people under stress are more susceptible to illness of all types. The largest body of evidence in support of this proposition has come from studies showing that intense levels and rates of life changes increase persons' susceptibility to a wide range of diseases, from influenza to tuberculosis to coronary disease (e.g., Holmes & Masuda, 1973).

Studies of occupational stress are just beginning to pay attention to nonstress diseases. Our current research is the only occupational stress study we know to have considered nonstress diseases (other than general rates of dispensary visits or sickness absence) in any detail, although similar studies are currently proposed or in planning. We hope a brief description of this research will suggest the potential utility of an approach to occupational health that considers both psychosocial factors and physicial, chemical, and biological ones (Ashford, 1976), as well as indicating the need for and direction of improved future research and application, to which we will turn in the final section of this chapter.

A Study of Occupational Stress and Health

We are currently engaged in a study of occupational stress and health in a large tire, rubber, plastics, and chemicals factory. This study is an offshoot of a larger program of research on the effects of working conditions on health in the rubber industry being conducted by the Occupational Health Studies Group of the University of North Carolina School of Public Health. Our study seeks to determine the impact of occupational stress on a range of health outcomes, and to consider the interplay between psychosocial and physical-chemical factors in determining workers' health. Although the analysis is only partially complete, our data confirm previous findings relating occupational stress to coronary heart disease, ulcers, and neurotic symptoms, and also suggest that in conjunction with exposure to hazardous physical and chemical agents, stress may play a role in the etiology of respiratory and dermatological disorders.

Data and Methods

The data derive primarily from self-administered questionnaires mailed to all hourly workers ($N = 2,856$) in the plant, with response rates of 67.5% ($N = 1,930$) overall and 70% among white males, the group used in the present analyses. Because of their small numbers and relatively poor response rates, black and female workers were excluded from the major analyses reported here. A nonrandom subgroup ($N = 447$) of the total population received medical examinations as part of a study of the effects of vinyl chloride exposure in the plant. This subgroup was composed of workers in the chemicals and plastics division and a small control sample of workers from the rubber division of the plant. Questionnaire data were available on 360 of these workers, allowing the analyses reported below of the association between occupational stress and physiological test or medical examination assessments of health and illness.

From workers' questionnaire responses we have constructed a number of indices of perceived job stress resulting both from excessive demands (i.e., job pressure) and from lack of rewards. The questionnaire data also yield self-reported symptom indices of (1) angina pectoris (the questionnaire of Rose, 1965), (2) peptic ulcer (questions from Dunn & Cobb, 1962), (3) neurotic symptoms (the Health Opinion survey of MacMillan, 1957), (4) persistent cough and phlegm (from Great Britain, Medical Research Council, 1965), and (5) dermatological symptoms (two items written for this study asking whether workers frequently experience itching or rash on their skin during or after work). Each of these measures was dichotomized for our analysis (cf. House, McMichael, Wells, Kaplan, & Landerman, 1979 for details on all measures in the study). For our medical examination subgroup, we have actual physiological tests or medical diagnoses relevant to major coronary heart disease risk factors (blood pressure, cholesterol, smoking), respiratory disease (lung function tests and symptoms from stethoscopic examination), and dermatological problems (physician observation of the presence of dermatitis). The questionnaire measures are the best available but only imperfectly reflect the presence of medically diagnosable illness. Previous validation studies and analyses of our own data reveal that the questionnaire measures are significantly predictive of medical diagnoses and tests, but that the agreement is far from perfect (the questionnaire measures generally exhibit 90% or better specificity, but their sensitivity ranges from as low as 25% to as high as 90%). Ideally, we would hope to observe stress affecting comparable questionnaire and medical measures in similar ways. In fact, this occurs in some cases but not in others. Where the two types of measures do not yield very similar results, especially if we observe relationships, between stress and our questionnaire health measures but not between stress and the medical examination data, the results must be regarded as only suggestive.

Using multiple regression and correlation, we have analyzed the relationship of each health outcome to each of the following perceived stress variables: (1) work load, (2) role conflict, (3) responsibility, (4) conflict between job demands and nonjob concerns (e.g., family), (5) quality concern or worry over not being able to do one's work as well as one would like, (6) job satisfaction, (7) occupational self-esteem, (8) intrinsic rewards, (9) extrinsic rewards (e.g., pay, fringe benefits, good hours), and (10) prestige and importance rewards (low levels of the last five variables are considered stressful). We have also tested the relation to health of a five-item index of Type A traits derived from Sales (1969). In each of these analyses we have controlled for any potential confounding variables that might spuriously produce an association between stress and the health outcomes. Age, education, cigarette smoking, and self-reported exposure to physical and chemical agents were held constant in all analyses involving questionnaire health measures. In the case of the physiological and medical variables, we controlled for any of the following factors that had a significant relationship with the dependent variable: age, obesity, cigarette smoking, physical effort involved in one's job (i.e., exercise), and self-reported exposure to physical and chemical agents. Because results of multiple regressions with dichotomous dependent variables are problematic in certain ways, we have utilized cross-tabular and multiple logistic function analyses to confirm our regression results. We reach essentially the same conclusions by all methods, and the regression results are easiest to present and interpret. House, McMichael, Wells, Kaplan, & Landerman (1979) provide a fuller analysis and presentation of data from our study and related methodological issues. The basic conclusions, however, are consistent with those presented here.

Results

Our data are consistent with earlier findings that stress is associated with higher rates of coronary heart disease, ulcers, and neurosis. The rele-

Table I. Partial Metric Regression Coefficients from Regressions of Health Variables on Each Perceived Stress Variable Controlling Confounding Variables[a]

Stress variable (and range)	Neurotic symptoms ($N = 1,706$)	Ulcer symptoms ($N = 1,648$)	Angina symptoms ($N = 1,578$)	CHD risk ($N = 333$)
Responsibility (0–12)	.012[d]	.005[b]	.005[d]	.029[b]
Quality concern (0–12)	.018[d]	.007[d]	.006[d]	.009[b]
Role conflict (0–12)	.022[d]	.010[d]	.004[d]	.031[b]
Job versus nonjob conflict (0–12)	.024[d]	.009[d]	.003[b]	−.004
Work load (0–12)	.012[d]	.002	.001	.052[c]
Type A (0–30)	.004[d]	.002[b]	.003[d]	−.006
Job satisfaction (0–10)	−.028[d]	−.007[d]	−.001	−.081[d]
Occupational self-esteem (0–18)	−.011	−.007[d]	.000	.004
Intrinsic rewards (0–24)	−.006[d]	−.002[d]	.001	−.005[b]
Extrinsic rewards (0–12)	−.014[d]	−.003	.001	−.015[c]
Importance rewards (0–15)	−.004[c]	−.001	.001	−.001

[a] Age (in years), education (in years), cigarette smoking (number per day), and self-reported exposure (0–3 scale) to physical-chemical hazards were controlled in analyses predicting neurotic, ulcer, and angina symptoms. Age (in years) and rated requirement of physical effort demanded by job (1–5) were controlled in analyses involving CHD risks, while obesity (quetelet ratio) was found to have no effect on the CHD risk index and hence did not need to be entered in the regression analyses.
[b] $p \leq .10$ (one-tailed).
[c] $p \leq .05$ (one-tailed).
[d] $p \leq .01$ (one-tailed).

vant data are presented in Table I. In the case of ulcers and neurosis, we have only questionnaire measures of self-reported symptoms. In the case of coronary disease, our self-reported questionnaire measure of angina is supplemented by an index of coronary heart disease risk derived from the medical data (assessing whether or not a person manifested elevated levels of *two* or more of the following risk factors of coronary disease: systolic blood pressure $\geq$ 150 mg, serum cholesterol $\geq$ 280 mg/ml, and smoking a pack or more of cigarettes per day).

The data show that with one exception job pressures (i.e., responsibility through work load) always related positively to the rate of symptoms of ill health; while job rewards (job satisfaction through importance rewards) are with one exception always negatively related to rates of neurotic and ulcer symptoms and heightened CHD risk but are essentially unrelated to angina symptoms. Most of the relationships are also statistically significant. Our measure of Type A behavior patterns is positively associated with angina symptoms, as would be expected, but not with CHD risk. Although Type A has been associated with elevated risk factors in Friedman and Rosenman's work, it has also been associated with CHD (including angina) even with risk factors controlled (cf. Jenkins, 1971, 1976). Thus, the present data generally accord with prior research, while also showing Type A associated with neurotic and ulcer symptoms.

The coefficients in Table I are metric regression coefficients that indicate the change in the proportion with each form of ill health for each 1-unit change on the stress measure. For example, the coefficient in the upper left corner indicates that the predicted proportion with marked symptoms of neurosis rises .012 for each rise of 1 unit on the scale of responsibility pressure. Given the range of the responsibility index (0–12), this means that the predicted proportion with "marked" neurotic symptoms is about .144 (.012 × 12) greater at the highest level of responsibility versus the lowest. In comparing the effects of different perceived stress indices on a given health outcome, one should compare the products of regression coefficient multiplied by the range of the stress variables, since the metric coefficients are necessarily smaller as the range increases (all other things being equal).

Overall, these coefficients indicate moderate to very sizable effects of perceived stress on both questionnaire and medical examination indicators of health. The data are largely consistent with results of previous research on individual psychosomatic or "stress" diseases and also indicate that most perceived stresses increase the probability of manifesting symptoms of a range of such diseases. Previous research suggests that angina and other forms of coronary disease may have different psychosocial predictors (Jenkins, 1971, 1976). Thus, it is not surprising that angina and CHD risk show a somewhat different pattern of association with the stress variables, yet it is compelling that both self-report and biomedical indicators of cardiovascular disease vary directly with levels of perceived occupational stress.

A quite different, less consistent, but highly suggestive pattern of findings emerges from our analyses of the effects of stress on symptoms of respiratory and dermatological disorders. Exposure to physical and chemical agents is a major occupational cause of such ailments. Further, the stress paradigm advocated in the first part of this chapter implies that perceived stress should exacerbate effects of physical-chemical hazards on these disorders, or alternatively, that the relation of perceived stress to these disorders should be minimal among workers not exposed to physical-chemical hazards but should increase in strength as level of exposure to physical-chemical hazards increases.

To test this hypothesis, we have utilized a measure of workers' self-reported exposure to "dust," "fumes," and "chemicals" they believed to be hazardous to their health. This index merely counts the number of agents to which a worker reports being exposed, but it correlates quite well with objective assessments of levels of exposure across various areas of the plant. Using regression analysis, we have tested whether the impact of stress on health outcomes measures varies across levels of exposure to hazardous physical-chemical agents. In analyses of the entire set of respondents, the results are striking. There is no significant variation across levels

Table II. Partial Metric Regression Coefficients for Regression of Cough and Phlegm and Itch and Rash Symptoms on Perceived Stress (Controlling for Confounding Variables)[a] at Different Levels of Exposure to Physical-Chemical Agents[b]

| | Number of agents exposed to | | | | | | | |
| | Cough and phlegm symptoms | | | | Itch and rash symptoms | | | |
Perceived stress	0	1	2	3	0	1	2	3
Responsibility	.003	.003	.007	.012	−.001	.011[d]	.017[d]	.019[d]
Quality concern	*.000*	*.005*	*.010*	*.020[e]*	.002	*.013[d]*	*.019[e]*	*.024[e]*
Role conflict	−.003	*.005*	*.017[e]*	*.032[e]*	.001	*.013[d]*	*.013[c]*	*.017[c]*
Job vs. nonjob conflict	−.003	*.000*	*.009[c]*	*.017[e]*	−.002	*.015[e]*	*.021[e]*	*.030[e]*
Work load	.003	.006	.010	.016	*.000*	*.012[e]*	*.020[e]*	*.028[e]*
Type A	.000	.001	.003	.006[c]	.002	.000	.001	.000
Job satisfaction	−.003	−.010[d]	−.013[c]	−.016[c]	*.001*	*−.007[d]*	*−.021*	*−.035[e]*
Occupational self-esteem	.004	.000	−.001	−.003	−.005	−.005	−.007	−.010
Intrinsic rewards	.001	−.002	−.002	−.005[c]	−.002	−.002	−.005	−.008
Extrinsic rewards	*.003*	*−.006[d]*	*−.007[c]*	*−.017[e]*	−.008	−.008	−.012	−.018
Importance rewards	.003	−.001	.000	.001	−.002	.000	−.004	−.007

[a]Age (in years), education (in years), cigarette smoking (number per day), and level of self-reported exposure to physical-chemical agents are controlled in each analysis.
[b]Coefficients that are italicized constitute a significant ($p < .10$, two-tailed) interaction effect between the stress variable and exposure to agents in predicting health. The significance levels of the individual coefficients are for tests of whether the coefficient is significantly different from the same coefficient under exposure to no hazardous physical-chemical agents.
[c]$p \leq .10$ (two-tailed).
[d]$p \leq .05$ (two-tailed).
[e]$p \leq .01$ (two-tailed).

of exposure to agents in the effect of stress on our questionnaire measures of angina, ulcers, or neurotic symptoms. However, we find a strong and consistent pattern of variation in the cases of persistent cough and phlegm, and itch and rash.

Table II presents the metric regression coefficients for the regressions of each of the two health outcomes on each of the eleven stress variables within levels of exposure to hazardous physical-chemical agents. In no case does stress manifest a significant relationship with cough and phlegm or itch and rash symptoms among workers who feel they are not exposed to any hazardous physical-chemical agents (cf. left-hand column of each panel of Table II). The impact of almost every stress variable on these health outcomes increases (in the predicted direction) as the number of agents to which a worker reports being exposed increases. The overall interaction between stress and exposure to agents is statistically significant ($p < .10$, two-tailed) in the case of 4 stress variables with respect to each health outcome. In a number of other cases there is a significant difference between the highest and lowest levels of exposure, even though the overall interaction is not significant.

The results are strikingly consistent with the idea that stress can affect a wide range of diseases not traditionally considered "psychosomatic" or "stress-related" by making the body more susceptible to the effects of noxious physical, chemical, or biological agents. However, we must note that we have been unable to replicate clearly this pattern of results in our medical subgroup using more objective medical diagnoses of respiratory or dermatological problems. These results may indicate that our findings with respect to self-reported respiratory and dermatological symptom measures are somehow an artifact of the self-report nature of these data. But it is also true that the medical indicators of respiratory (i.e., symptoms from stethoscopy and lung function tests) and dermatological problems (physician diagnosis of dermatitis) tap somewhat different patterns of physiological symptoms and functioning than the questionnaire measures and may have their own errors and biases. Thus, the discrepancy between the results in Table II and those we obtain with our biomedical indicators do not necessarily indicate that either set of results is invalid. Still, the findings in Table II should be treated as only suggestive of the potential interplay between psychosocial and physical-chemical job hazards on the determination of occupational health problems. We hope future research by us and others will provide more definitive results.

Summary and Conclusions

Most previous research and much theory on stress and health have posited that particular potential stressors or perceived stresses cause particular "stress diseases," even in a dose–response relationship. And our review finds good evidence that perceived occupational stress and objective conditions conducive to this perceived stress are associated with coronary heart disease, gastrointestinal disorders (in particular peptic ulcer), and poor mental health—all of which have been traditionally viewed as stress-related diseases. Yet much of the theoretical literature on stress suggests that all types of stress increase susceptibility to all types of disease outcomes, with the particular disease outcome (or lack thereof) depending on various conditioning variables. A growing body of laboratory experiments, primarily on animals, supports the notion but little research has been done that examines the full range of potential disease outcomes in human populations.

Research Needs

Thus, the most obvious need in future research is for a focus on the relationship of stress to a wide range of diseases, and occupational settings are particularly promising for such research. Studies of occupational stress, and of psychosocial stress more generally, must begin to consider a wide range of health and disease outcomes, including both ones that have and ones that have not been traditionally considered stress-related or psychosomatic in origin. This, however, is only a first step. More important, researchers need to specify more clearly the social, psychological, and physiological processes that produce various diseases and the impact that stress might have on such processes. If stress does interact with physical, chemical, and biological agents or processes in producing a given disease, then we will obtain maximal predictive power with respect to that disease only if we measure both stress and the physical, chemical, or biological causative factors and analyze their separate and joint effects. Thus, for example, we know that stress and a variety of other factors (family history of CHD, lack of exercise, high cholesterol diet, smoking, etc.) may increase a person's risk of CHD and/or its risk factors, yet there have been no analyses of the degree to which stress may interact with these other factors in producing CHD or CHD risk. Similarly, if we think that stress exacerbates the effects of certain physical-chemical irritants to the skin or respiratory tract, we should directly measure persons' exposure to both stress and the specific irritants in order to test our hypotheses. Finally, if we think stress increases susceptibility to infectious disease, we need to assess both stress and exposure (and levels of immunity) to the viral or bacteriological causes of specific diseases.

In sum, it is necessary but not sufficient to show that stress has effects on a wide range of diseases. If understanding of psychosocial stress is to enhance our ability to predict and hence reduce disease, we must gain firmer theoretical and empirical knowledge of how specific forms of psychosocial stress and of noxious physical, chemical, or biological agents interact with each other in the production of disease. This kind of specification has been lacking in our own and other research to this point. We hope this chapter will stimulate efforts to remedy this deficiency in the future. Such work will not be easy, since it requires increased multidisciplinary collaboration, interchange, and training among the social, psychological, and biomedical sciences. Further, in occupational settings we often lack adequate knowledge of the effects of environmental hazards and can measure workers' levels of exposure to them only imprecisely. Yet, despite the many limitations in the current state of research on both psychosocial and physical-chemical aspects of occupational health, we can and should begin to bring these two bodies of knowledge into closer conjunction.

Our knowledge of the nature and effects of occupational stress *per se* can also be strengthened in other ways, which have been noted above and in prior articles by House (1974a, b, 1975). For two reasons, there is a critical need for more longitudinal and/or field) experimental designs in work on occupational stress and health. First, such designs are needed to more firmly establish the degree to which occupational stress is a cause or precursor of health and disease. Second, the crucial, but currently neglected, role of more transient responses to stress (i.e., coping, defense, adaptation) as a link between potential stressors or perceived stress and enduring health outcomes can be adequately studied only in longitudinal or experimental designs that capture the *process* of adaptation over time. Such designs are very costly in time, manpower, and money and are methodologically complex. Thus, they should be undertaken judiciously, but they must be undertaken.

The Need for Experimental Application

Although the existing body of research on occupational stress and health is modest and much remains to be learned, it is appropriate to begin thinking about applications of this knowledge. Existing theory and evidence suggest that alleviating occupational stress and/or buffering people against its effects could decrease people's risk of developing a wide range of physical and mental health problems. Elimination of *excessive* occupational stress can also be considered a step toward more positive mental health, regardless of its impact on disease. Finally, efforts to reduce occupational stress and/or to buffer people against its effects are likely to produce other desirable social outcomes, such as reduced turnover and absenteeism and perhaps higher productivity, while involving few substantial risks (House, 1974b, O'Toole, 1974). Thus, there are good reasons for government and private employers to consider implementing programs to reduce occupational stress and/or to buffer people against it effects.

In other analyses from our study of rubber workers, social support from supervisors and spouses (i.e., the perception that these persons are interested in, and able to help with, work-related stresses) virtually eliminated the impact of stress on health (House & Wells, 1978; Wells, House, McMichael, & Kaplan, 1977). These data suggest the value of including efforts to enhance the social supportiveness of supervisors in programs of supervisory selection and training. Given our conception of perceived stress as resulting from the fit between workers and their work environments, stress reduction efforts can attempt to change individuals, change environments, or improve the fit between individuals and environments. Job selection and placement procedures should endeavor to prevent very bad fits between workers and their jobs and/or to facilitate workers moving out of jobs they find distressing. Most organizations ordinarily specify some probationary period during which a worker in a new job may be found unsatisfactory for that job. Could and should not workers have a similar right, without negative sanction, to decide during this period that the job is not satisfactory to them? Organizations could also help to facilitate the acquisition of skills helpful in coping with occupational stresses among persons who initially lack such skills, rather than allowing persons largely to sink or swim on their own. Finally, efforts can be made to alleviate major situational sources of pressure. The *Work in America* report (Task Force Report, 1973) describes a number of experiments in job redesign and enlargement intended to reduce job dissatisfaction—one form of occupational stress reflecting lack of rewards in work. Similar efforts might be made to reduce situational sources of job pressures such as role conflict and excessive work load and responsibility. Decentralization of task performance and decision making from persons who may be overutilized to those who are underutilized represents one possible strategy in this direction. In some cases, however, there may need to be more extensive organizational changes, such as adding new positions to take on some of the activities that create excessive conflict, work load, or responsibility for incumbents of existing positions. These are just some examples of progressive action that could be undertaken by organizations to internalize and account for the costs individuals and society now incur, either directly or indirectly, by their operations.

We would not presume to contend that from our current knowledge we could suggest a number of simple steps for reducing occupational stress or mitigating its impact. However, we do have sufficient knowledge to suggest that efforts in this direction are both feasible and potentially beneficial to individual health, organizational performance, and societal quality of life. What we would encourage is a spirit of *social experimentation* in which efforts are made to reduce and/or mitigate occupational stress. It is important to utilize a balanced approach to the solution of these problems by taking into account both organizational and individual factors (e.g., Katz & Kahn, 1966, Chap. 13). The effects of such efforts on individual health and other individual and organizational outcomes should be monitored carefully and information gained should be applied as feedback into the experimental process. The kinds of measures we have suggested for reducing stress and improving health may be undertaken primarily for organizational purposes (e.g., improving productivity, reducing turnover), but their effects on health and stress could and should still be evaluated. Such experimentation and evaluation also promises to provide the kind of knowledge of the causal impact of stress that we noted has been lacking in the research literature. In sum, a spirit of social experimentation will improve both scientific and practical understanding of the complex interplay between occupational stress and health. Other societies, especially Sweden and Norway, have already demonstrated that research and practice can be integrated in a program of social experimentation to reduce occupational stress and improve the quality of working life (cf. Davis & Trist, 1974). We would hope that the United States might move more in this direction.

ACKNOWLEDGMENTS

We are indebted to the editors and especially to Redford Williams, M. D., for comments on a previous draft.

REFERENCES

Alexander, F. Psychosomatic medicine. New York: Norton, 1950.

Ashford, N. A. Crisis in the workplace: Occupational disease and injury (A report to the Ford Foundation). Cambridge, Mass.: M.I.T. Press, 1976.

Caplan, R. D., Cobb, S., French, J. R. P., Harrison, R. V., & Pinnau, S. R. Job demands and worker health. U. S. Department of Health, Education and Welfare Publication No. (NIOSH) 75-160, 1975.

Cassel, J. C. The contribution of the social environment to host resistance. American Journal of Epidemiology, 1976, 104, 107-123.

Cobb, S. Social support as a moderator of life stresses. Psychosomatic Medicine, 1976, 38, 300-314.

Davis, L. E. & Trist, E. L. Improving the quality of work life: Sociotechnical case studies. In J. O'Toole (Ed.), Work and the quality of life. Cambridge, Mass.: M.I.T. Press, 1974.

Dunn, J. P., & Cobb, S. Frequency of peptic ulcer among executives, craftsmen, and foremen. Journal of Occupational Medicine, 1962, 4, 343-348.

Fox, B. H. Premorbid psychological factors as related to incidence of cancer: Background for prospective grant applicants. Unpublished paper, Field Studies and Statistic Program, National Cancer Institute, 1976.

French, J. R. P., Rogers, W. & Cobb, S. Adjustment as person–environment fit. In G. V. Coelho, D. A. Hamburg, & J. E. Adams (Eds.), Coping and adaptation. New York: Basic, 1974.

Friedman, M., & Rosenman, R. H. Type A behavior pattern: Its association with coronary heart disease. Annals of Clinical Research, 1971, 3, 300-312.

Great Britain, Medical Research Council, Committee on Etiology of Chronic Bronchitis. Definition and classification of chronic bronchitis for clinical and epidemiological purposes. Lancet, 1965, 1, 775-779.

Harrison, R. V. Person–environment fit and job stress. In C. L. Cooper & R. Payne (Eds.), Stress at work. New York: Wiley, 1978.

Hinkle, L. E. The concept of "stress" in the biological and social sciences. Science, Medicine and Man, 1973, 1, 31-48.

Holmes, T. H., & Masuda, M. Life change and illness susceptibility. Reprinted from Separation and depression, AAAS, 1973, 161-186.

House, J. S. The relationship of intrinsic and extrinsic motivations to occupational stress and coronary heart disease risk. Unpublished doctoral dissertation, University of Michigan, 1972.

House, J. S. Occupational stress and coronary heart disease: A review and theoretical integration. Journal of Health and Social Behavior, 1974, 15, 12-27. (a)

House, J. S. The effects of occupational stress on physical health. In J. O'Toole (Ed.), *Work and the quality of life.* Cambridge, Mass.: M.I.T. Press, 1974. (b)

House, J. S. Occupational stress as a precursor to coronary heart disease. In W. D. Gentry & R. B. Williams, Jr. (Eds.), *Psychologic aspects of myocardial infarction and coronary care.* St. Louis: C. V. Mosby, 1975.

House, J. S., & Wells, J. A. Occupational stress, social support and health. *Reducing occupational stress: Proceedings of a conference.* DHEW (NIOSH) Publications No. 78-140, 1978.

House, J. S., McMichael, A. J., Wells, J. A., Kaplan, B. H., & Landerman, L. R. Occupational stress and health among factory workers. *Journal of Health and Social Behavior,* 1979, *20,* 139–160.

Hurst, M. W., Jenkins, C. D., & Rose, R. M. The relation of psychosocial stress to onset of medical illness. *Annual Review of Medicine,* 1976, *27,* 301–312.

Jenkins, C. D. Psychologic and social precursors of coronary disease. *New England Journal of Medicine,* 1971, *284,* 307–317.

Jenkins, C. D. Recent evidence supporting psychologic and social risk factors for coronary disease (parts I and II). *New England Journal of Medicine,* 1976, *294,* 987–994; 1033–1038.

Kasl, S. V. Work and mental health. In J. O'Toole (Ed.), *Work and the quality of life.* Cambridge, Mass.: M.I.T. Press, 1974.

Katz, D., & Kahn, R. L. *The social psychology of organizations.* New York: Wiley, 1966.

Levine, S., & Scotch, N. A. *Social stress.* Chicago: Aldine, 1970.

MacMillan, A. The health opinion survey: A technique for estimating the prevalence of psychoneurotic and related types of disorder in communities. *Psychological Reports Monograph Supplement,* 1957, *7,* 325–339.

Mason, J. W. An historical view of the stress field (Parts 1 and 2). *Journal of Human Stress,* 1975, *1,* 6–12; 22–36.

McGrath, J. (Ed.). *Social and psychological factors in stress.* New York: Holt, Rinehart & Winston, 1970.

Mechanic, D. Some problems in developing a social psychology of adaptation to stress. In J. McGrath (Ed.), *Social and psychological factors in stress.* New York: Holt, Rinehart & Winston, 1970.

Medalie, J. H., Snyder, M., Groen, J. J., Neufeld, H., Goldburt, U., & Riss, E. Angina pectoris among 10,000 men. *American Journal of Medicine,* 1973, *55,* 583–589.

O'Toole, J. (Ed.). *Work and the quality of life.* Cambridge, Mass.: M.I.T. Press, 1974.

Riley, V. Mouse mammary tumors: Alteration of incidence as apparent function of stress. *Science,* 1975, *189,* 465–467.

Rose, G. A. Chest pain questionnaire. *Milbank Memorial Fund Quarterly,* 1965, *43* (part 2), 32–39.

Rosenman, R. H., & Friedman, M. The possible relationship of occupational stress to clinical coronary heart disease. *California Medicine,* 1958, *89*(3), 169–174.

Sales, S. M. *Differences among individuals in affective, behavioral, biochemical, and physiological responses to variations in work load.* Unpublished doctoral dissertation, University of Michigan, 1969.

Selye, H. A syndrome produced by diverse noxious agents. *Nature (London),* 1936, *138.*

Selye, H. *The stress of life.* New York: McGraw-Hill, 1956.

Selye, H. Confusion and controversy in the stress field. *Journal of Human Stress,* 1975; *1,* 37–44.

Selye, H. Forty years of stress research. Principal remaining problems and misconceptions. *Canadian Medical Association Journal,* 1976, *15,* 53–56.

Solomon, G. F., Amkraut, A. A., & Kasper, P. Immunity, emotions and stress: With special reference to the mechanisms of stress effects on the immune system. *Annals of Clinical Research,* 1974, *6,* 313–322.

Syme, S. L. Implications and future prospects. In S. L. Syme & L. G. Reeder (Eds.), *Social stress and cardiovascular disease, Milbank Memorial Fund Quarterly,* 1967, *45,* 175–181.

Task Force Report to the Secretary of Health, Education and Welfare. *Work in America.* Cambridge, Mass.: M.I.T. Press, 1973.

Theorell, R., & Rahe, R. H. Behavior and life satisfaction characteristics of Swedish subjects with myocardial infarction. *Journal of Chronic Diseases,* 1972, *25,* 139–147.

Thiel, H. G., Parker, D., & Bruce, T. A. Stress factors and the risk of myocardial infarction. *Journal of Psychosomatic Research,* 1973, *17,* 43–57.

Wells, J. A., House, J. S., McMichael, A. J., & Kaplan, B. H. *The effects of social support on the relationship between occupational stress and health.* Paper presented at the meeting of the Southern Sociological Society, Atlanta, April 1977.

Williams, R. B., Jr. Physiological mechanisms underlying the association between psychosocial factors and coronary disease. In W. D. Gentry & R. B. Williams, Jr. (Eds.), *Psychological aspects of myocardial infarction and coronary care.* St. Louis: C. V. Mosby, 1975.

8

Psychosocial Dimensions of Drug Abuse

William A. O'Connor and
Paul I. Ahmed

It is easy to assume that health and illness are objective states that can be defined clearly in any society. But our confusion with respect to drug abuse challenges that assumption. Our current response to drug abuse in the United States is to simultaneously treat it as an illness, punish it as a crime, and attempt to control it as a social event.

The purpose of this chapter is to suggest a more consistent view based on a psychosocial perspective. The core of such an approach is to view behavior, including drug abuse, as a continuous process of interaction between person and environment. This psychosocial system, like any ecosystem from the entire earth to the complex microscopic communities in a single raindrop, must be understood as a living unit before it can be broken into its parts. Such an ecosystem model provides a context in which to define illness and healing in a particular society. To begin to acquire this perspective, let us for the moment examine the focus of healing systems in several cultures.

William A. O'Connor • Department of Psychology, School of Medicine, University of Missouri, Kansas City, Missouri 64110. Paul I. Ahmed • Office of International Health, U.S. Department of Health, Education and Welfare, Rockville, Maryland 20857.

The Healing Process: Four Cultures

Wallace (1959), in his classic study of Iroquois religious psychother-apy, described the process as "mazeway resynthesis." The illness of the individual is assumed to arise from a lack of integration between the pa-tient's behavior and the laws of the spiritual and social worlds. What the individual wants and needs does not fit what the society expects and de-mands in exchange for its resources. The healer must understand both the unique personal world of the patient and the complex, subtle norms of the social context. This maze is resynthesized by a focus on the patient's aware-ness; the healer slowly draws the conscious attention of the patient to previously unrecognized personal feelings and conflicting contextual norms until these are again integrated.

In other cultures, this gap between person and context may be diag-nosed and treated differently. For example, the intervention may be focused more on the community than on the patient. Holland and Tharp (1964) have described the healing processes in Mayan communities as focused on the community itself. The culture is organized largely on a kinship basis, with illness viewed as resulting from a lack of harmony in family, interpersonal, or spiritual relationships; healing therefore occurs in the context of the total kinship community. The elaborate ceremonies of the healer include sugges-tions for modified behavior on the part of the patient, but they also achieve a consensus among the community with regard to the acceptable behavior of the patient and the support with which the community will respond to behavior changes.

At times, the therapeutic intervention may be an almost forcible attack on the community at large. Kennedy (1967) has described zar therapy in Ethiopia in a social-system context. Patients are usually women of low status, a role so stressful in that society that it provides extreme difficulties at a daily survival level. While the zar ceremony contains a considerable degree of catharsis and emotional support, it also invests the patient with membership in the zar cult, creating a degree of status, group membership, continuing support, and power within the Ethiopian community. The re-sponse of the community to the patient may be based less on personal regard than on fear of the possible destructive consequences of failure to placate the person's djinn or personal spirit ally.

Newman (1964) describes a response to "wild man" behavior in the New Guinea highlands in a manner suggesting that intervention may even take place without formal illness or healer. Wild man behavior is character-ized by an acute onset of "psychotic" behavior among young married men, who in the New Guinea highland society are recognized as fulfilling highly responsible and stressful roles. The response of the community is not rejec-tion but an attitude bordering on celebration. The wild man is encouraged in his demanding and bizarre behavior by the whole community, with gentle and tactful interventions only when he might injure himself or another. Within a few days, the behavior appears to exhaust itself and the wild man disappears into the forest for a short time. Upon his return, the wild man assumes a fully normal role, and the community behaves as if the episode had never occurred. But what is central to the process is the recognition of the stress under which the individual operates and the increased level of community support.

The Healing Process: Drug Abuse in the United States

Our contemporary American efforts in the area of drug abuse contain elements noted in each of these four cultures: intervention is sometimes focused on the abuser, sometimes on the community, and sometimes even lacks formal definition of problem and response. But each of the examples is based on a clear recognition of the psychosocial nature of the process: person and setting form a human ecosystem in which behavior has meaning in its context. Such an approach is more difficult in the extraordinarily large and complex organizational framework of contemporary American culture. We have a tendency to ignore context, to remove the "patient" from his usual life space, provide treatment in an institutional context, then return the individual to the same system in which the difficulty emerged. We perceive behavior in a fragmented fashion—responsibility is divided so that blame is placed on the client while authority is vested in the healer. This, in turn, reveals a peculiar orientation in our culture; we often confuse health and power. The norms by which we judge others are organized around amounts of property and numbers of people controlled. Drug abuse covers an extremely wide range of chemical use patterns, types of individuals, and social situations; but research tends to focus on a grouping of drug users who are identified primarily by legal status and whose deficits alone are measured. To begin to clarify the drug abuse process, we must begin with some basic definitions reflecting behavior and context.

Person and Context: Psychosocial Definitions

The interaction between person and context may be of two types: the person's behavior may first be *ecounit-specific*. In each specific social setting, the person occupies an ecological niche. The niche consists of a person who is expected to perform specific activities and resources that the environment provides in return (Wilkinson & O'Connor, 1977). Nonconforming behavior is termed deviant. *Deviance*, therefore, is always ecounit-specific;

that is, an individual becomes labeled as deviant by violating specific norms in a particular kind of setting—e.g., a criminal can be formally labeled only by the legal system. Deviant behavior involves a specific role that the individual does not necessarily experience as dysfunctional; rather, it is the community that defines deviance.

Illness is also ecounit-specific, but it involves one area of dysfunction that is mutually defined by patient and healer. An illness is a specific impairment of the person's ability to function. When an individual feels sick and is diagnosed, the individual gives up a degree of responsibility and may be exempted from some duties. The community provides resources to treat and cure the individual's illness.

A person's behavior, however, also occurs in the *total social context.* The individual's ability to organize a total life-style pattern is termed ecosystem competence. *Normalcy* reflects this total life-style pattern: the individual's contribution to the cohesion of the system as a whole. The "normal" individual's behavior and membership in all groups is typical of patterns in the total community. A particular group of individuals may differ from the general norm without being deviant, sick, or in a state of poor health; for example, their ethnic or religious or occupational identification may be such that they function in an unusual and very distinctive fashion. At the same time, an individual could be perfectly "normal" in virtually every respect while suffering from a cold, being convicted of income tax evasion, or experiencing a general decline in health.

Health also reflects a total system pattern. Health is measured in terms of the individual's ability to expend energy and be actively involved in all the groups and interactions that are desired. Health is considered impaired or poor where the individual cannot meet the demands of the environment in a general sense: to be self-actualized, to give, or to produce. Even in medical terms, we distinguish between a person's general state of health and specific illnesses. An individual can be generally healthy and specifically ill— e.g., an active and energetic individual with an allergy to peanuts, a dental cavity, or a sprained left ankle. On the other hand, an individual may not be actively healthy but also may not have a specific illness (see Figure 1).

Drug Abuse: Definition and Response

It is unlikely that drug efforts will become substantially more effective as long as the definition of the problems and the assignment of remedies remain chaotic. The reality of drug abuse—that it does not exist as a single "illness" but as many types of problems in a heterogeneous population in varied contexts—suggests some obvious directions.

The first step in such a process is to organize treatment systems by

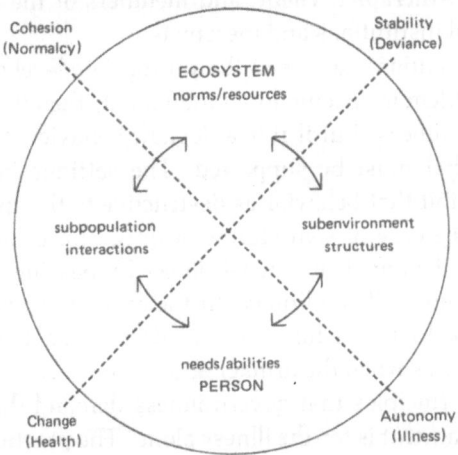

Figure 1. Ecosystem and person.

specific problems and solutions. This means treating only what is legitimately defined as an illness. This process is clear with heroin antagonists for definitely established addiction and medical detoxification techniques. For the remainder of what is now seen as illness, "treatment" is actually focused on social functioning: vocational training programs, community resource centers, remedial educational programs, and the like. The best of scanty evidence to date suggests that drug use patterns are so embedded in life-style and community system interactions that the labeling of the problem as drug abuse probably obscures the most critical problems of the person and limits the most effective community response to those who must first present a drug "illness" to obtain help.

Drug abuse may more often be a response to an environment in which it is unhealthy to be normal. The second step in a more effective response requires distinguishing between treatment and social control. The evidence again suggests that we prefer to call drug abuse an illness, but our treatment is not congruent with an illness model. A patient voluntarily accepts help and is not sanctioned or restricted by legal means as a form of treatment. If, in reality, we wish to penalize drug abuse, then it is a crime; it is not a cure that is at issue. Much of the treatment-outcome research is disappointing only if the myth of illness is maintained.

Third, if resynthesis of person and community are a goal, then responsibility cannot be fragmented as a means. Either drug abuse is the responsibility of the abuser or it is a legal/political problem. Therapists have failed consistently to effectively heal their clients when they are limited to a role as agents of the social regulatory system. The healing contract is by its nature between persons—therapist, client, and members of the community. It is not between social institutions and therapists.

Fourth, intervention must be at the appropriate level of system organization. If the problem is specific to an individual, then it can be diagnosed and treated as an illness. But if it is a deviant behavior, then it is effective social cohesion that must be supported. The settings in which deviance occurs must prohibit that behavior as destructive to the specific function of that system. In the case of some forms of drug abuse, we have defined a deviant behavior, then made it a quasi-illness by passing laws against it in *all* settings and under all conditions. In the case of alcohol, the definition varies; it is a crime to drive while intoxicated, a normal behavior at cocktail parties, and an illness when the drinker and healer so contract.

Finally, the principles that govern illness demand that any treatment does no harm; treatment is for the illness alone. The practice has escaped us in the drug abuse treatment system. We must treat, regardless of outcome, since the problem is defined by the community. It then becomes acceptable to control the problem even at risk to the quasi-patient.

What, then, would provide an effective model in which to define the problem and organize responses? Viewing drug abuse from an ecosystem perspective requires stating clearly basic assumptions about the nature of the process itself.

Ecosystem and Drug Abuse

A psychosocial ecosystems approach would view drug abuse in a manner similar to the mazeway resynthesis approach presented by Wallace. Such an approach views person and community as a biological unit or energy system. The approach is based on three key assumptions (O'Connor, 1977).

Assumption 1: *Drug abuse and treatment occur in a context.* The interaction process occurs in a very specific way. The total ecosystem is divided into groups of interacting individuals in specific social structures or environments - "ecounits." The norms and resources of the total ecosystem or community are thus distributed through regular patterns of behavior and specific social organizations. The individual is both a member of groups and an inhabitant of a variety of environments, the total pattern representing an individual life-style.

Where the individual is identified and treated as having a drug abuse illness, therapist and client and setting form a single and complementary unit: without client, without therapist, and without a community that believes that drug abuse is an illness and its treatment is a necessity, the unit cannot occur. Just as therapist and client play complementary roles, pathology and treatment are complementary functions in the total ecosystem in which they are embedded. Just as therapist and client have mutual role expectations with the treatment system, each is engaged in a series of expectations and confrontations with the community at large. Cultures that do not accept a particular behavior as involving illness do not support the healing process. In the final analysis, it is the interactive system as a whole that demands the presence of both. This in turn suggests a second basic ecosystem assumption.

Assumption 2: *Drug abuse is a function of energy input and distribution in the total ecosystem.* The distribution of community resources and expectations through specific ecounits allows the total community to function in a manner that is both stable and cohesive: the society is predictable and organized so that its members can work in a coordinated fashion. But at the same time, each individual's interaction with the environment allows choices to be made and changes to be initiated in the system as a whole. It is the unique perception and the decision-making capability of the interacting individual that continually modifies and impacts the system as a whole. At a total community level, therefore, there is a balance in the interaction process between stability and change and between cohesion and autonomy. While the total system attempts to maintain its balance, the individual operates a catalytic force.

Assumption 3: *The drug abuse process and its treatment is a function of person, environment, and specific interactions of person and total community.* Such an assumption suggests that pathology exists when group structures do not distribute resources to meet the needs of all inhabitants or where individuals do not interact to meet their needs within the limits of expected behaviors. In this sense, deviance is a function of normalcy; when normal roles do not allow effective and conventional behavior, other roles and behaviors emerge. Treatment systems then become a mechanism for the ecosystem as a whole by which it can correct the imbalance between system and occupant needs. The system can treat itself by the same process with which it treats its clients.

In order to account for the discrepancy between adequate resources and total populations, niches may be generated in which resources are rigidly controlled, such as the welfare and the social security systems. Further, econiches may be created that are occupied by complementary role pairs requiring fewer total resources. Thus, crime occupies both criminals and those who control criminals, and illness occupies both doctor and patient.

It is fascinating to observe, in the economics of public mental health treatment systems, that the difference between the annual income of the patient population and the average income of the community served by the system often produces a dollar figure roughly equal to the amount of wages paid to the staff. In what are undoubtedly oversimplified terms, treatment systems provide an opportunity for the ecosystem to support both staff and clients for an amount no greater than that required to support either staff or clients alone. The distribution of decision-making, power, and competence demands is similarly disproportionate. In an ecosystems frame of reference, the term *human resources* has a double meaning: human resources are those utilized by human beings, but they may also be human themselves. In an ecosystem that lacks natural predators of another species, it becomes necessary for the population to implement its own regulatory system.

The Basis of Individual Dysfunction

The energy resources of a community are typically distributed through pyramidal structures. That is, a typical organizational chart is small at the top and becomes larger at the bottom. This scheme allows organizations to become extremely complex, extremely effective, and extremely powerful; it allows the size of organizations to extend in an almost limitless fashion. But with increased size comes increased disparity in decision making. The effect may very well be that the role occupied by many inhabitants of the particular system—that is, the "normal" role—may be one that is extremely stressful for the individual if not for the system. Further, the efficiency of the system demands that persons who cannot perform competently be excluded. It is in the interest of the larger pyramidal ecosystem to exclude as many people as possible when a large population base exists. The system then retains only those who are most competent. Those excluded must occupy either the deviant or the sick role.

When viewed from this perspective, many drug treatment efforts emerge as an ecological disaster. First, the patient may occupy only one setting: the treatment unit and its adjacent areas. Most of us are inhabitants of many settings: family, work, recreation, and others, which provide us some resources and which make specific demands for conventional behavior. But we have options in many areas, the possibility of movement from one setting to another, and escape (at least intermittently) from settings that coerce, frustrate, bore, or otherwise make life unpleasant. Not so for some of our traditional "rehabilitation" systems: there is one place, one set of expectations, and one source of reward and punishment.

Second, the setting is pyramidal, with the client as base. The organizational chart that is a map of power in the setting shows room at the top for a single leader, a niche or *zone* in the setting that will be occupied by a chief or director with full ultimate authority, regardless of the individual's personal capacity to make decisions or provide leadership. Below this point on the pyramid is the specialist or supervisor zone, occupied by a few individuals who impose management functions over a specific part of the setting: chiefs of a service, counselors, etc. Then there is a staff zone, a larger group that carries out the routine functions of the setting. At the bottom is the client, an involuntary guest who owns and decides almost nothing in the setting and whose behavior is evaluated and coerced by others. The client zone, by definition, involves a lack of responsibility for self and others. This is not to say that the client is free of demands; on the contrary, he is bound to be irresponsible and must be incapable of decisions, for there is no other zone and no other setting.

A similar relationship between person and system can exist at a total community level. Clinical settings that deal with populations at the lower end of the socioeconomic scale have long posed a substantial dilemma. The clinician is trained to treat pathology. But the individual may be discharged free of pathology and still return to other patterns simply because there are few realistic alternatives. The person who is "cured" but unable to compete in the community confronts the clinician with a simple fact of life: the absence of psychopathology is relevant only to tertiary prevention. Health is in the hands of the community, not the therapist.

In the case of drug abuse, the discrepancies between health on the one hand and the absence of pathology as defined by typical outcome measures can be enormous. It is not unusual to see program evaluations in which the mean usage of selected illegal drugs is lower following discharge, but where the frequency and amount of either prescribed or legal substances (e.g., alcohol) is increased.

Our confusion around definitions of personal and system dysfunction leads many professions to attempt to include all behavior within a single professional sphere. In the mental health system, an individual who is essentially deviant—engaging in antisocial behavior—may be diagnosed as sociopathic. But sociopathy is not an illness; it is a disruption of community norms. The individual diagnosed as neurotic does in fact enter into an illness contract with the healer: such individuals suffer anxiety and guilt in relation to external demands and expectations of others; treatment may be effective and appropriate. But the diagnosis of depression is often applied to individuals who suffer basically from a lack of health: the inability to impact or change the surrounding environment in an energetic or active fashion. The essence of depression is a feeling of hopelessness and helplessness in which action is unwarranted because it cannot affect the current situation or the future course of events. And finally, when an individual fails to behave in accordance with the most basic norms of social behavior, the mental health context diagnoses psychosis. The psychotic is described as out of touch with reality, but the specific reality with which he is out of touch is not his own but that of others. The distinction between psychosis and eccentricity varies greatly from culture to culture and time to time.

The situation is even more chaotic with respect to drug abuse. Klassen (1977), for example, studied 484 substance abusers admitted to 16 programs in a major metropolitan area. Each client was asked to identify all settings entered by him or her during the specified time period, and the interaction between person and community was then categorized. Twenty-seven percent of the clients did not present substance abuse as a major problem but nonetheless found their way into the treatment system. They were involved in treatment essentially because they had been identified as deviant, most often because of accidental involvement in a legal offense such as possession of marijuana or driving while intoxicated. Other groups were found for whom drug usage appeared to be a major issue: heroin users, drug dealers, and an employed white male group with a high level of polydrug abuse. But these three groups differed on many measures. The heroin users, while they might be seen as having a specific illness, were often not engaged in criminal activity and in some cases were involved in a relatively normal life-style apart from their heroin usage. The dealers were involved in clearly deviant behavior but tended to be relatively energetic, healthy, young, male, and financially successful. The employed 20–29-year-old white males were most "normal" by all conventional standards but appeared to suffer in the extreme from a lack of health: in order to maintain their own functioning and their involvement in the community as a whole they had learned to use substantial amounts of chemical support.

If the population was quite diverse, the treatment system itself appeared to involve several different processes as well. Some programs implemented what might be described essentially as an *overt* therapeutic contract. That is, the bulk of the treatment was formal psychotherapeutic intervention around the formal diagnosis of substance abuse. The client, the therapist, and the community at large recognized these activities as directed toward the reduction of the specific symptoms of drug abuse as an illness.

A second type of treatment program implemented what might be described as a *strategic* intervention. That is, the bulk of the program was directed toward modifying the individual's patterns of social interaction and general life-style. The goal of the treatment system appeared to be a readjustment of the balance or the proportion of the activities that characterize the individual's interaction with the community: increased health.

A third treatment organization might be termed a general *ecosystem* intervention. Such programs were organized largely around vocational and educational activities, representing an attempt to redefine the individual's formal role and basic relationship to the community. For such individuals, the thrust of the treatment delivery system was to develop a new set of skills with which the total community might be engaged: increased normalcy.

The existence of three very different types of response to drug abuse implies three very different types of problems that have been thrown together under the drug abuse label. Each may be examined as potentially effective for the right client under the right conditions.

Overt Therapeutic Contracts: Illness and Treatment

When the healing process begins, an ecounit is formed that permits certain predictions. In conventional terms, the outcome of therapy depends to a large extent on the client's expectations of outcome and the extent to which the therapist can meet these expectations. This is expressed in the overt contract between therapist and client, but it is also reflected in a variety of subtle behaviors on the part of both client and therapist. As long as both do what is expected, the therapy is likely to be considered effective.

What prevents this simple transaction from taking place is ambivalence. A client may enter the treatment system with an awareness of problems and solutions, but he is also aware that any change in behavior is a risk in life-style terms. The client has, after all, established certain consistent patterns and relationships; to change one's life-style pattern and relationships requires significant support.

Under ordinary circumstances, the therapeutic contract itself allows the patient to reject dysfunctional behaviors, attitudes, and commitments. The contract exists not only between the therapist and the client but also between the client and the ecosystem surrounding both client and therapy. Voluntary psychotherapy is generally supported by a variety of individuals in the client's life space.

In the case of drug abusers, the situation may become more complex. First, treatment entry is frequently coerced; the client expects to "go to jail" if treatment is refused, but has few expectations of the process itself. Similarly, the treatment program may focus largely on the elimination of certain chemical usage patterns with little awareness of other life-style effects.

The client's reluctance to enter into unknown changes is often termed a lack of motivation, defensiveness, or resistance. The words themselves are revealing of the processes. A person defends against attack; the defenses of the client protect him from the destructive potential of an ecosystem in which personal needs are not likely to be supported by social context. The process becomes resistance when the treatment system seems to "take sides"—that is, begins to coerce the patient on behalf of the system or force the patient to act without recognizing a legitimate basis for his defenses. The frequency with which drug-abusing clients are described as unmotivated, dishonest, and generally resistive suggests that the treatment system itself may enter into the clash between person and setting that lies at the heart of drug-abuse process.

What must be recognized is that the symptomatic behavior of the client is not the essential focus of the therapeutic process. Any client could obtain expert suggestions or sensible alternatives from a number of sources, and the therapist rarely suggests solutions that could not be obtained equally well from persons already known to the client. The task of the therapist is generally to discover the client's potential solutions and create a treatment environment in which these can be developed. The therapist in a conventional psychotherapy does this by recognizing the patient's defenses as self-protective and supporting a slow process of change. The patient is then free to improve.

The Strategic Contract: Regaining Health

But, as has been noted thus far, drug abuse is often a function of the total imbalance of life-style and individual needs. Thus, simply facilitating a change on the part of the client is not always a sufficient therapeutic contract. In conventional psychotherapies, the therapist often conveys to the patient gradually the knowledge that the client's problem is embedded in a total ecosystem and that the client is experiencing distress related not only to drug abuse but also to what is *not* occurring in the total system. Problems with a marital partner, a lack of effective stress-reducing or stress-coping resources, difficulty in the employment situation, and a variety of other discrepancies in the client's relationship to the total community may require an adjustment of what occurs on a 24-hours-a-day and 7-days-a-week basis.

A lack of awareness of this process may well be related to the persistence of the substance abuse problem. With stringent law enforcement and consistent drug prevention efforts, the psychedelic drug use pattern of the 1960s has diminished among youth. What has occurred instead is the epidemic increase of use of substances such as PCP and alcohol. In point of fact, we have made drug abuse more difficult for the at-risk population. As a result, the population continues to be immersed in a life-style that requires chemical adjustment and offers few sensible alternatives. But with the risk of sophisticated detection systems and possible legal consequences, drug abuse has become not so much a social rebellion to support a new life-style as it has become an attempt to utilize cheaply and quietly any substance that may be personally destructive but allow short-term survival. In our original efforts to combat drug abuse, we supported our cultural pathology by excluding alcohol; we were successful, for the youngest and most impressionable segment of the society no longer "drop;" they drink.

Where strategic healing interventions are effective in other cultures, there appears to be a congruence between the goals of the community as a whole and the problems experienced by the client. In Mayan communities, for example, the shaman will initially obtain a detailed history of the patient's activities either from the patient or from the head of the household.

He will then diagnose the malady and give some details as to how it may have occurred. The diagnosis is generally consistent with the perception of family and community members. The ceremonial phase of curing has much in common with Western group and family psychotherapy. It breaks the patient's preoccupation with his complaints as his attention is fixed on goals outside of himself. Reassurance is given the patient by his kinsmen, who assist him in the ceremony. The patient becomes the center of group attention. The group reasserts the importance of his continued participation, and a pattern is offered for the reestablishment of social contacts.

The Ecosystem Contract: Redefining Normalcy

The third type of contract is related to the broader sociocultural process. On a formal level, this contract is often expressed as prognosis, a prediction of outcome based on symptoms. What the prognosis indicates, in essence, is the extent to which the society at large will allow and support changes in behavior for a person of a particular age, sex, socioeconomic level, symptom complex, and set of circumstances. At the most basic level, the total ecosystem expects only a certain amount of change for a given individual. For the therapist to attempt to modify the effects of this prognostic contract requires manipulation not of the client but of the external ecosystem.

Many programs focus heavily on the client's involvement in different social networks, different modes of dress, different organizations, and a variety of other behaviors that clearly send a message about the client's "place" in the ecosystem: the therapist is attempting to reclassify the client in the eyes of the community. On occasion, the therapist may do this by literally changing the client's demographic characteristics, for example, by including further education as a major component of the treatment system. Treatment systems that deal primarily with disadvantaged persons are likely to have an outcome that is determined largely by the treatment system's access to restructuring resources in the community—job training, living arrangements, legal services, employment agencies, and social networks.

Examples of effective ecosystem intervention can be found in relation to other types of personal dysfunction and other cultural settings. For many cultures, the healer's role involves not only modification of the behavior of individuals but also sanctioned intervention into the process of the community as a whole. Within contemporary health delivery systems, examples of this process may be seen: the prevention of epidemic physical illness through vaccinations is considered an acceptable role for the medical practitioner in addition to the treatment of those illnesses as they occur on an individual basis. But it still maintains a distinction between intervention in the health/illness process and the separate function of social control (the normative/deviance process). In the case of drug abuse, such a comprehensive and well-coordinated role definition on the part of those given responsibility for control has largely been lacking. At best, control mechanisms are invested in the legal system whereas treatment functions have been isolated within the health professions. The emergence of paraprofessional programs and service delivery models may well suggest that the system as a whole is lacking a comprehensive role that includes both prevention and treatment; many paraprofessional programs have attempted to intervene not only at the level of support for individual drug abusers but at the level of community networking and educational efforts to modify epidemic patterns of specific substance abuse.

Conclusions

It is evident that drug abuse can be defined in a variety of ways. But the inconsistency of its definition as a quasi-illness, a behavior that requires treatment because it is illegal, makes effective response unlikely.

Drug abuse is an illness only when two conditions are present: the problem is specific and the treatment is voluntary. Addiction or dependence on a specific substance, for example, may be recognized by the community as an illness for which known treatment can be obtained by agreement between client and therapist.

Drug abuse is a deviant behavior only when two different conditions are present: the behavior is prohibited under specific conditions and in specific settings. The deviant behavior is fully the responsibility of the individual and penalties are based on the act alone, as in the case of driving while intoxicated. The penalties may be legal or they may be social or economic—being asked to leave a party or being fired from a job.

Drug abuse is unhealthy under different conditions: unhealthy behavior is not labeled as either deviant or sick and requires a community-level intervention. That is, more positive alternatives are made available (e.g., safer foods through FDA standards). Where an individual seeks support, the intervention is strategic, as in the case of community multiservice centers or personal growth "therapies" or public education programs. Where social controls are implemented, it is the environment that is modified, as in the case of safety standards or pollution control.

Drug abuse is abnormal only by group consensus: the norms of a society are not legislated and the individual participates by choice. The reduction of abnormal behaviors is impacted only by increasing resources to the total population and demanding performance that can be implemented.

In the final analysis, drug abuse is a mirror of the total psychosocial process. It has been labeled and projected on the few, but it is more accurately a reflection of the difficulty we have in making what is normal for most of us also healthy for all of us.

References

Holland, W. R., & Tharp, G. Highland Maya psychotherapy. *American Anthropologist*, 1964, *66*, 41–52.

Kennedy, J. G. Nubian Zar ceremonies as psychotherapy. *Human Organization*, 1967, *26*(4), 185–194.

Klassen, D. Person, setting and outcome in a drug abuse treatment program. *Psychiatric Annals*, 1977, *7*(8), 80–104.

Newman, P. L. Wild man behavior in a New Guinea highlands community. *American Anthropologist*, 1964, *66*, 1–19.

O'Connor, W. A. Ecosystems theory and clinical mental health. *Psychiatric Annals*, 1977, *7* (7), 63–77.

Wallace, A. F. C. The institutionalization of cathartic and control strategies in Iroquois religious psychotherapy. In M. K. Opler (Ed.), *Culture and mental health*. New York: Macmillan, 1959, pp. 63–96.

Wilkinson, C. B., & O'Connor, W. A. An ecologic approach to mental health. *Psychiatric Annals*, 1977, *7* (7), 10–15.

9

Views on the Psychosocial Dimensions of Cancer and Cancer Treatment

Stephen P. Hersh

> They cannot scare me with their empty spaces
> Between stars—on stars where no human race is.
> I have it in me so much nearer home
> To scare myself with my own desert places.[1]
> —Robert Frost

My work with children, adolescents, and young adults who have various forms of cancer provides the source materials for this chapter. Their families and those responsible for their medical care receive more of my time as a psychiatrist than do the patients themselves. This distribution of my professional time developed in response to my understanding of the psychological and social effects of cancer as well as to a decision concerning the most potent forces for therapeutic change.

The Dreaded Disease

Cancer, actually a word referring to a group of diseases, symbolizes to the public mind loss of control. It presents one's own body destroying one's

---

[1]From Desert Places. In Edward Connery Lathem (Ed.), *Poetry of Robert Frost.* New York: Holt, Rhinehart & Winston, 1969. Copyright by Holt, Rhinehart & Winston. Reprinted by permission.

Stephen P. Hersh • Director, Division of Children and Adolescent Services, St. Elizabeth's Hospital, Washington, D.C. 20032.

self. Appearing to come from nowhere, it strikes without warning. Cancer potentially can show itself anywhere within the individual at any time.

It affects the entire age range but increases in frequency with advancing age. Current information indicates that 1 in 4 persons will eventually develop a cancer (American Cancer Society, 1975). That means that of every 100 persons reading this article, 25 will eventually develop cancer. Indeed, barring major new improvements in therapeutics, 15 of those 100 will die from cancer or its related effects.

No wonder the word produces anxiety and fear. No wonder in a culture that teaches that one can assert control over existence through technology, as long as one marshals resources to attain that technology, we spend vast sums and significant scientific manpower on conquering "the disease" rather than on prevention of it.

Cancer represents *the* abnormal condition of physical self that symbolizes both our tenuous hold on life and the fragile reality of our control. The war on cancer is psychologically bigger than the mortality produced by it. (If mortality by itself so frightened us, we would declare a war on accidents.) It is a crusade involving our search for control, knowledge, and power against an enemy that is within ourselves.

Metamorphosis of the Cancer Crusade

A metamorphosis is in process. The cancer crusade recently has begun to assume a new, more mature form. It is no longer so in need of stimulating fear, righteous rage, and the determination to overcome distant enemies, and is settling down for a more reflective and long-term campaign.

Five things account for this ongoing change. First, there are the successes produced by the crusade—an increase in survival and some cures especially with skin cancers, choriocarcinoma, Hodgkin's disease, and a few of the childhood forms of cancer. Second, derivative of the efforts of, at first, Elizabeth Kübler-Ross (1969), but many others since, our culture slowly is looking again at life as a cycle and death as part of that cycle. Third, in medicine we are learning to see the limits of technology simultaneously with the true complexity of the history of disease states within each individual (DeVita, 1978). Fourth, modern treatments confront us with significant iatrogenic effects (Leventhal & Hersh, 1974). Indeed, sometimes the morbidity from treatment may not give a quality of life worth preserving. Fifth, our culture has begun to rediscover the ancient—i.e., life rhythms, nutrition, and family now seem "scientifically" related to the quality of life; health maintenance takes on an increasing attractiveness despite our continuing romance with disease treatment.

We hope that this metamorphosis of the cancer crusade will continue.

We will cease trying to exorcise an imaginary devil within our bodies and we will come to terms with both the intimacy of the body–mind interface and the power of the individual in group–social system interfaces. Increased interest in quality of life will lead eventually to a better balance between health maintenance and the technologies of disease treatment. What is euphemistically called "death education" moves us toward this better balancing as it attempts to decrease the fear of death and to increase an understanding of death through a better understanding of ourselves. Who knows, perhaps even the churches and synagogues will rediscover themselves over such issues!

Illness, Even Death, Are Living Things: Patient Self-Awareness

Visualize children and adolescents living under what to outsiders appear as death sentences—sentences deferred for unknown spans of time. Either these young people will not attain adulthood or they will proceed merely a short way beyond its threshold. Picture robust children, carrying on with their worlds as best they can while they lose their muscle mass, their hair, their skin color and tone; sclerose their veins; tolerate repeated painful procedures, violent emesis, and sometimes loss of body parts. Add to this image the pain, disruption, helplessness, and anxiety of their parents and their siblings. This sketch portrays a pediatric oncology service.

We often treat both children and chronically sick older people in similar ways by self-protectively failing to associate with them the possession of a conscious, potentially reflective awareness of self, others, and events. Such behavior, especially exaggerated toward the seriously ill, is not a new issue as is illustrated in the following excerpt from Leo Tolstoy (1886/1967):

> What tormented Ivan Ilych most was the deception, the lie, which for some reason they all accepted, that he was not dying but was simply ill, and that he only need keep quiet and undergo a treatment and then something very good would result. He however knew that do what they would nothing would come of it, only still more agonizing suffering and death. This deception tortured him— their not wishing to admit what they all knew and what he knew, but wanting to lie to him concerning his terrible condition, and wishing and forcing him to participate in that lie. Those lies—lies enacted over him on the eve of his death and destined to degrade this awful, solemn act to the level of their visitings, their curtains, their sturgeon for dinner—were all a terrible agony for Ivan Ilych. And strangely enough, many times when they were going through their antics over him he had been within a hairbreath of calling out to them: "Stop lying! You know and I know that I am dying. Then at least stop lying about it!" But he had never had the spirit to do it. The awful terrible act of his dying was, he could see, reduced by those about him to the level of the casual, unpleasant, and almost indecorous incident (as if someone entered a drawing room diffusing an unpleas-

ant odor) and this was done by that very decorum which he had served all his life
long. . . . This falsity around him and within him did more than anything else to
poison his last days.

Tolstoy's Ivan Ilych character illustrates how friends, families, medical teams all avoid their responsibilities when they fail to listen but engage
in the kind of deception described. The responsibility to not deceive in these
matters is part of our role in helping others under stress to cope. Denying
their reality to them undermines such coping.

Patient self-awareness has been written about most feelingly by a
variety of parent authors. Their writings convey with great insight the
broad spectrum of psychological as well as social challenges cancer patients
and their families must meet. Examples of such parent authors include John
Gunther (1949), Doris Lund (1974), Mickie Sherman (1976), and Nancy
Roach (1977).

Professional writings have also added greatly to our understanding the
awareness patients have of their struggles. Early writings concentrated on
behavior and intrapsychic phenomena (Bozeman, Orbach, & Sutherland,
1955; Chodoff, Friedman, & Hamburg, 1964; Green & Miller, 1958). Over
the past decade the literature has expanded greatly, emphasizing the emotional effects of cancer on patients, families, and even school systems (e.g.,
American Cancer Society, 1973; Binger, Ablin, Feuerstein, Kushner, Zoger, & Mikkelson, 1969; Kirten & Liverman, 1977). Unfortunately, with a
few exceptions (e.g., Korsch & Negrete, 1972), there has not been enough
emphasis on communicating with patients.

A basic element of communicating with patients (indeed, a major
"tool" in our therapeutic armamentarium) is listening. Listening to patients
is particularly instructive. By listening, one taps directly into their self-
awareness while simultaneously encouraging it. Listening serves as a high-
way that leads the clinician to insights concerning the psychosocial dimensions of living with cancer and its treatments. The best way to illustrate this
point is via the presentation of the following four life sketches. Each sketch
exhibits one communication of a different child or adolescent during various
stages of the disease process. All are cancer patients.

Life Sketch Number One

"Dear Friends and Relations:
    Well, it is almost a month now since I got out of the hospital and I
am assured by my doctors that I am on my way to a cure that rivals
anything yet achieved at Lourdes. Unfortunately, the drugs which produce the cure also produce side effects which could be classified under
the general heading of Instant Aging. I have developed incipient bald-
ness, dry skin rashes, irregularity, and the posture and gait of a retired

British Admiral with an old wound. . . . Although I have managed to qualify for Medicaid, I will still wind up well over a thousand dollars in the hole after paying off the diagnostitian, the surgeon, the hematologist and other fun-loving practitioners of the medical trade.

It certainly has been an Instructive Experience to Face Death Eyeball to Eyeball (when Death could get his Eyeball under the pillow which I kept firmly pressed over my head the whole time.) . . . I have learned much, and, yes, suffered much . . . perhaps some good can come out of it all if I can pass along some of what I have learned to you, in case, God forbid, you should ever have to undergo a similar experience.

. . . Having cut you open, seen what is wrong with you, stripped you of everything they can, checked the points, the plugs, rotated the magneto and dialed 800 toll-free, they actually are going to set about curing the disease. . . .

Well, friends . . . I am living much the same life I have always lived, counting the dreams that flee from my grasp and when I run out of these, I can now count the hairs that are falling from my head. . . ."

Life Sketch Number Two

". . . A girl . . . who had to . . . understand her own thoughts and make her own decisions.

The decision and thoughts were about going into a room, in which she couldn't touch her mother and family. . . . I had never explored the Air-Flow Room very well and so I didn't know what to expect. It was just like looking into a mirror for something that wasn't there. . . .

The nurses cleaned my body as if I were going into a new world of my own. . . . I was really scared and frightened . . . especially when they began rolling me down the hall in a wheelchair with a sterile sheet over the chair and over me. It was just like being blindfolded and dropped at the end of the world. . . .

When they stopped pushing, I knew this was it. . . . They pulled the sheet down and asked me to walk across the red line. . . . I felt all alone—no one to even talk to or hold in my arms."

Life Sketch Number Three

Nurses Note: I sat down by the head of her bed—held her hand and she started to talk. . . . She talked and cried until she fell asleep.

". . . Why does all this have to happen to me. . . . I missed out on a lot. . . . The other kids went . . . I can't go anywhere without NIH and the doctors bothering me. I just want to be normal. Be like other kids. . . . I don't have any control over anything. I can't plan anything. Everything centers around this place. . . . Look at what the drugs have done to me. . . . My equilibrium . . . a brace and a cane for a while . . . I

can't play the piano anymore . . . my eyes aren't right either . . . a wig
. . . all the needle marks on my arms—I look like a drug addict. All the
kids at school look at my arms and avoid me. I know what they're
thinking. They think I'm an addict. Everyone treats me different when
they see my arms. . . . I have to have some control over my life. I have to
be able to plan. I am so discouraged."

Life Sketch Number Four

An early grade school child makes a drawing several days before
his death. That drawing shows in it the figure of a woman in a loose-
fitting dress. The woman has long hair and a smile. Her arms are
upraised, with the hands and fingers very huge compared to her body.
She seems to be standing next to or leaning over an elipse. Within the
elipse is a tall cross. Next to the cross is a bouquet of flowers and a
headstone with a small cross on it and written within a rectangle in the
elipse is the name "Jeff." In the upper left-hand corner of the picture is
a sun with its rays coming out. The sun has two eyes and a mouth. The
mouth is open as if crying and out of the corner of one of the eyes is
drawn a tear. To the right of the sun is a cloud.

In words, this child communicated very little to his parents and the
staff. He said nothing about his awareness of the seriousness of his
illness. He said nothing about his thoughts concerning the present or
future. Yet, he told everyone through his drawing a great deal. He
showed his awareness of his impending death. He told some of what it
meant to him: separation from mother and her large, embracing arms;
separation from the flowers and sky and sun; the sadness he projects
(the sun's tear) that will be felt over this separation.

The life sketches presented are written, oral, and pictorial communications from children. As highlighted, they illustrate the expressed self-
awareness of children and adolescents. The age, sex, experiences, neurological intactness, and intelligence of the individual will determine, along
with the immediate opportunities of the environment, the form such expression takes. A conscious, reflective awareness of self, events, and others
does indeed exist.

In the first life sketch, a late adolescent uses a form letter with ingra-
tiating humor and clever satire to share his experience and cope with his
isolation and fear. The second life sketch was one of several attempts by
another midadolescent to communicate her experience, perpetuate herself,
reduce her loneliness through formal, schoollike essays. The third sketch
represents the capturing of spoken words by an observer and caregiver.
This sketch presents selected excerpts from a sobbing adolescent overwhelmed in the late night quietness of the hospital by her difference, her
aloneness, and her loss of control. Her psychological pain is poignantly

displayed, as are indications of her dramatic struggles with the physical and social changes in her self-image. Finally, how can one see drawings like that described in Life Sketch Number Four and then talk about the noncommunicative child? Words are only a small part of our communications, and the younger we are the more obvious this is. The use of few words or no words does not equal stupidity, lack of self-awareness, or lack of understanding. This drawing told us that a child knows he is dying, knows that dying means separation. It told us something about his mother and her arms. It told us about sadness—perhaps both his own and his desire for the world to feel sad. All children, preschoolers and older children, are continually communicating such awareness and insights to us through their drawing and play. We need only to "attend."

The Price Paid for Survival: Secrets and Separation

The wise man . . . lives as long as he should not as long as he can.
                                                          —Seneca

The quote from Seneca raises issues for discussion, and that is the purpose of this section. Again, I turn to patients as the sources of insight.

1. Diana at age 5 years (2 years after her diagnosis as having acute lymphocytic leukemia) is at home chatting with her mother in the kitchen. She asks: "Mommy, when you had leukemia as a little girl, did you get so many needles and bone marrows?"

This sketch is a humbling reminder that what we think we communicate to children and what they understand are often dramatically different. Misperceptions, as in this case, can be, in part, a function of the patient's developmental level.

2. Ginger, aged 8 years, has had acute lymphocytic leukemia since the age of 6 years. Since she has had a series of relapses, the medical staff believe she is on her last protocol (last attempt at medical control of her disease). The staff finds her frequently in the chapel and then observes her getting other children to go up to the chapel with her. While in the chapel, she leads the other children in bargaining with God for improvements in her white blood cell count and platelet levels.

In this sketch, we see an example of attempting to gain control through bargaining and through magic ritual.

3. Billy, an 11-year-old boy, arrives newly diagnosed with osteogenic sarcoma of the femur (long bone of the leg). His parents accompany him. Siblings and other family members and friends are left in their home community, which is far away. It is 3 days prior to surgery and Billy remains ignorant of his diagnosis or the nature of the surgery he will undergo. He

wonders to his doctor what bad he had done to deserve surgery and if he will wake up.

With Billy's situation, we see highlighted some issues of communication within families and among family, patient, and physician. In addition, the sense of stigma and sin in association with a dread disease fosters in such situations a holding of secrets and enhances the fears of both separation and death.

4. Zeke is 16 years old. A pain started during the summer in his left knee. Several months later he saw a doctor, and osteogenic sarcoma was diagnosed. The family is very resistant to Zeke's receiving any form of treatment. The father says to his son while the physician is present, "No matter whether you get treatment or not, you're going to die, you're dead!" The mother says that what is happening is God's will.

In situations such as described, one sees highlighted issues of fear, lack of trust, superstition, misinformation, and problems in communication, particularly between a family and the medical community.

5. Jim, at age 18 years, developed aplastic anemia. He had a bone marrow transplant. After 4 months, Graft versus Host disease developed (his body reacting to the foreign bone marrow and the foreign bone marrow reacting to his body). He is tall, skeletal, with sunken cheeks, prominent facial muscles, and prominent green eyes; his teeth look too big for his face, and his skin, sparsely covered with hair, has red dots, scabs, and a basic yellow green tone. He takes exquisite care of his hands, soaking them for long periods, manicuring them carefully. (His hands are the only healthy looking part of him). He shows little motivation for anything. His family finds him repulsive. When he is able to get a nurse's attention, he will recount macabre stories of hatchet killing and other gruesome murders to the nurse. He is depressed.

This sketch is an example of the situation in which some of our patients find themselves. They suffer dramatic physical changes secondary to their treatments and disease. For such patients, the sense of being grotesque is reinforced by the reactions, in this case ostracism, of others. Anger and depression soon follow.

6. Eleanor, at age 20 years, has a rare and out-of-control neoplasm. Only storing her bone marrow and administering a very aggressive course of chemotherapy in a laminar airflow room (one kind of germ-free environment) will give her any chance of survival. This means a 1- to 2-month period of isolation from her husband and her 3-year-old daughter. She agrees to this heroic treatment, entering the laminar airflow room with enthusiasm. After 3 weeks, she stops keeping her diary, becomes disinterested in all things, is lethargic and withdrawn.

Submitting oneself to the "high" medical technology of ablative chemotherapy in a laminar airflow room represents a surrender of one's self to modern medicine in exchange for a promise of potential survival. For both the patient and the family, the loss of control is significant. Depression often develops rapidly as those involved (particularly the patient) experience the dramatic limitations their situation has placed upon them. Such depression can be ameliorated through appropriate interventions. These consist of encouraging the ventilation of feelings while simultaneously working out ways in which one can return to the patient some degree of control over his daily existence.

The above cluster of vignettes present dilemmas created by cancer and by the treatments used to combat it. No matter what the age or developmental stage of the involved individual, a heightened awareness of self is forced upon them by their situation. The dilemmas with which they are faced, as presented in the vignettes include:

1. Loss of control—both an objective reality and a feeling state.
2. Finding ways to regain control—bargaining, wishing, magic, rituals, rationalization.
3. Coping with periods during which one has an overwhelming sense of isolation from others, isolation in part based on having thoughts and experiences (hence, secrets) one cannot share with others.
4. Recognizing and learning to deal with misinformation and misperceptions.
5. Learning to trust one's own feelings (anger, depression) and those of others (their fear and rejection).
6. Learning to live with one's own feelings (particularly anger and depression) as well as the feelings of others (e.g., fear, ambivalence).

Returning to the quotation from Seneca, one recognizes the greatest dilemma of all: When, if ever, should an individual refuse further treatment? At what point has one pursued far enough elusive survival or even more elusive cure? At what point can one say that the physical pain from disease and treatment, as well as the isolation and loss of control, exceed a threshold of tolerance? And does such a threshold exist? Clinical experience suggests that no objective, describable tolerance threshold exists. Human tensile strength, hunger for life, and influencing variables (family, religion, job, etc.) differ and change too much. If any generalization can be reasonably made, it is that few individuals ever state unequivocally that they have reached or passed their level of tolerance for further treatment or existence.

Comments on Coping

As medical professionals, we must deal simultaneously with many factors in individuals who, from the disease, the treatments, and the reactions to both, physically and psychologically suffer changes in their social environment, their energy levels, their sensorium, and their physical selves. Morbidity, perhaps even mortality, are to some extent related to coping. (Medical scientists studying such relationships include Robert S. Brown of the University of Virginia, George F. Solomon of Stanford University, and Dr. R. W. Bartrop of St. Vincent's Hospital, Sydney, Australia. The number of individuals engaged in such studies is increasing.) Coping itself is related to an intact nervous system, temperament (e.g., inward- versus outward-directedness), sex, intelligence, the premorbid personality, the capacity to tolerate anxiety, the ability to rehearse in fantasy for the purpose of problem solving, the family structure and experience, the peer group, the community, and the involved health care professionals (Anthony, 1974). Those particularly able to cope seem to have a great, stubborn capacity to avoid being overwhelmed or engulfed by their symptoms. They also seem to come from home environments where there was a consistency of signals. Finally, they use selectively but intensely the coping mechanism of denial.

Among the most neglected topics important to coping is that of sexuality. The scope of sexuality includes "not only manifest sexual behavior but such concepts as body image, object relations, self-esteem, ego ideal. . . . [It] is expressed not only in sexual acts per se but also in one's capacity for human relationships. . . ." (Blos & Finch, 1974). (It should be noted that this broad definition of sexuality creates some confusion, given the context of our current society, a society that aggressively, continuously promotes the sex act and its "accoutrements." In addition, some distinguished psychoanalysts and psychiatric educators define sexuality more narrowly than do Blos and Finch, specifically referring to "manifest sexual behavior." They reject those related behaviors and feeling states when the goals are different—i.e., touching, holding, cuddling for the sake of feeling secure, protected, and comforted (M. Hollender, personal communication, 1977). In the text that follows, I use the broader Blos and Finch definition.)

Only during the past 7 years has meaningful attention been paid by the medical community to the sexuality of handicapped individuals. For those with chronic diseases and fatal illnesses, the limited literature about sexuality naturally tends to be problem-oriented (Levy, 1974; Siris, Leventhal, & Vaitukaitis, 1976; Watts, 1976). Indeed, Blos and Finch (1974) clearly summarized our knowledge base in clinical practice regarding the sexuality of patients with chronic disease and conditions: "Most startling was the paucity of data when the need for such knowledge seems so obvious. It is our speculation that this neglect is analogous to the neglect accorded, until recently, the phenomenon of death and dying. Both topics are difficult, threatening, and painful for all to discuss. . . . What must often happen . . . is an unspoken collusion between doctor, patient, family, and peers to avoid references to sexuality or, if the question is raised, to 'reassure' with generalities."

Our culture's "collusions" to avoid the most basic issues, death and sexuality, are amazing, yet understandable in the context of our striving for control and our fear of noncontrol. Death and sexuality imply both mysteries and loss of control. Profoundly important yet simple equivalencies can be ignored less and less as we gain more control over our biological selves and generate more questions about the meaning of existence.

In hospitals (and unfortunately this washes over to outpatient care situations, too) the norm for staff, patients, and friends is to pretend sexuality does not exist. The little homage paid to its importance is disguised by "safe" rituals—the back rub, the application of body lotion, occasionally sitting and holding hands. In continuing to embrace this "norm" we all minimize or deny a basic range of communication while suppressing a significant part of our human selves. The relative elimination of an important realm of communication and comfort, as well as the nurturant source of "body image, object relations, self-esteem," produces in the patient emotional-physiological stress. Coping with this stress creates another demand on an already stressed (ill) individual. Such a situation cannot help the patient deal with the disease. Indeed, some of us, based on clinical impressions, believe it to be harmful. At the least, the medical care system's relative denial of sexuality in its broadest sense creates an avoidable stress. And, perhaps, more is involved—there are scattered clinical impressions, combined with recognition of sexuality's role in physical, psychological, and social development from conception onward, that raise the question as to whether acknowledging a patient's sexuality within the treatment setting helps us approach treating the whole person and thereby dramatically improving the quality of life for that person. Meeting the needs of some patients through nonverbal comforting, physical boundary setting, and contact may indeed positively influence both morbidity and mortality.

I have listened to staff discussions about conjugal visits in the hospital, echoing similar discussions by penal experts concerning prisoners. I have learned from some teenage cancer patients how their dramatic, painful feelings of being isolated, alone from everyone (moments of existential terror) are helped only by being held in someone else's arms. I have worked with nursing staff confused as to how they should respond to a male or female patient's apparent indifference to nudity or openness of masturbation or grasping, fondling hands. I have listened to the fears of young people (as in Life Sketch Number Two) about aloneness and "no one to hold in my arms." I have seen the drawings of school-age children (as in Life Sketch Number Four) with the adults portrayed as having huge, outreaching hands and arms.

Sexuality is reproductive behavior and all those psychological and socially determined differences that distinguish males from females. Its purpose is not only species-specific survival through reproduction, but also contact, relatedness, and serving as a vehicle for reducing anxiety and aloneness. Its expressions and purposes are different at different developmental stages, but it is just as real an issue for the 2-year-old as for the 20- or 40- or 70-year-old.

Important new contributions to our understanding of sexuality and the cancer patient are found in a recent article (Lieber, Plumb, Gerstenzang, & Holland, 1976). More such contributions to our understanding of sexuality and the cancer patient are needed. Although further studies are in progress, I suggest that sexuality as defined become an ongoing topic of discussion for the staffs of inpatient and outpatient services with oncology patients. I further suggest that—just as they did with the issue of death and dying— patient care advocates, self-help groups, and counseling groups thoughtfully assist in opening up this area for discussion. (A conference on this subject sponsored by the D.C. Division of the American Cancer Society and the National Association of Social Workers was held on October 19, 1977, at the National Presbyterian Church and Center in Washington, D.C.)

Behavioral Science Research

Cancers and their treatments produce observable changes in the patient, subjective changes, and changes in the individual patient's manner of relating to others. Observable changes may include alterations in hair, features, skin, stature, and strength, loss of body parts, and scarring. Subjective changes involve body image, sense of autonomy, disaffection, panic states, rage, hopelessness, self-destructive wishes, and depression. Changes that involve the patient's relating to others include the trade-offs made by accepting treatment, dependency, and stigma.

Our goals for the diseases called cancer are prevention and, when that has failed, cure. When cure is not likely, we seek health maintenance and prolonged survival while protecting the patient's autonomy as much as possible. Hence, enhancing quality of life presents itself as a significant challenge to health care providers.

This challenge is greatest when one deals with a rapidly developing individual such as a child or adolescent. Despite this fact, there have been few basic developmental inquiries concerning the effects of loss or absence of physical well-being on child development (Moss, Yarrow, Jacobs, Nannis, Hersh, & Levine, 1976). Knowledge concerning the needs and coping mechanisms of such children is far from sufficient. Parents and the medical community are still programmed by their own fears rather than by understanding. They continue to debate whether or not a child or adolescent should be told his diagnosis, whether or not to mobilize cooperation, whether or not to encourage the asking of questions (Hersh, 1978).

Treatments involving the disease, as well as the disease itself, exact a price (Hersh, 1976). As investigations into these issues proceed, we are uncovering often unpredicted effects, effects that assume special importance in the light of both the cures obtained and the chronicity of many cancers. One example of such effects involves those on the intellectual development of children treated for acute lymphoblastic leukemia (Eiser & Lansdown, 1977) and on brain tissue postcentral nervous system irradiation (Peylan-Ramu, Poplack, Pizzo, Adornato, & Dichiro, 1978). Expanded behavioral science investigations into all spheres of coping with cancer and its treatments are unquestionably called for. Studies should include not only the more obvious issues involving the patients but also the psychophysiological and social responses of their families and those who provide their medical care.

Toward a New Definition of Health for the Cancer Patient

Somehow the population's image of cancer must change. Cancer, "the dreaded disease," must become more more what it objectively is—a group of related diseases, chronic in their course, usually of unknown etiology, which currently effect someone in every family.

Through obtaining greater control over diseases, we demythologize them. Smallpox and bubonic plague were, in their time, dreaded diseases. Control has removed the fear, leaving echoes of the mythology. The diseases, however, still can be found. For cancer, control will come also, most probably through preventive measures (Boyce & Max, 1976; Strickland, 1978).

Today, the mythology concerning cancer and its symbolic meanings still rides high. Maintenance of autonomy, control (ability to choose), the ability to pursue the hope of continued existence, and the freedom to balance morbidity against death, all color the quality of the individual patient's coping with cancer. In such a struggle, the support systems of family, medical personnel, and the community are critical. These often go awry. In part, this occurs because of the impact the mythology of cancer has on these systems. For example, we discover heinous bits of behavior stimulated by fear, such as neighbors organizing to prevent the purchase of a home by a family with a leukemic child. We note the stresses on marriages and on individual patients—chronic diseases have a wearing-away effect not only on the bodies but on the psychology and social structure of those suffering from such disease. Parents and spouses recount in a guilty, confessional fashion how they arrive at a point where they do not want to know more; they do not want to give more; they wish it was over. And siblings, be they children or adults, are also affected profoundly. Their anxiety and fears of loss of control as well as guilt manifest themselves in increased irritability, sleep problems, and psychosomatic fears. Child siblings show school and behavioral problems, not infrequently more dramatic than those found in the cancer patients themselves.

One group not usually talked about in terms of the patient's coping includes the medical staff (Artiss & Levine, 1973; Heinemann, 1976). We forget that we are cut out of the same cloth as the patients and their families. Indeed, part of our armor is to forget this reality.

The modern physician in cancer therapeutics, while having a grasp of the technology, should have equal sophistication in the psychosocial area. Unfortunately, this is not always so. Such relative lack of sophistication is illustrated by the existing misuses in which patients and physicians engage, with Elizabeth Kübler-Ross's *On Death and Dying:* "The five stages [of reactions to, and adjustments to, having a fatal disease] . . . have been perceived by some in a mechanical fashion as providing a sure-fire progession to a happy ending . . . and dying persons who do not follow the script run the risk of being considered failures or even forfeiting the compassion of those caring for them . . ." (Steinfels, 1975).

Besides seeking a new definition of health for cancer patients through demythologizing the disease itself, one must also promote changes in both the process and the role of being sick. This process and role have been described in the following way: They involve exemptions from responsibility for having fallen ill and from normal social obligations/expectations combined with acceptance *both* of sickness as a socially undesirable state and of a doctor's (or medical system's) authority (Cole, 1976). Once an individual has accepted the role of being ill and the label, the patient and the social system see that individual as marginal. This brings a process of partial extrusion from the family and the social system (Cole, 1976). With all chronic diseases, including cancer, the need is for a buffering, even a reversal, of this partial extrusion phenomenon.

Methods to resist extrusion are most obvious when the patient is a child or an adolescent. One can insist on attendance at school if it is at all feasible. One can work with their families to help parents maintain discipline and limit-setting as close to the way it existed before the illness (assuming "normal" limit-setting) as possible.

For the adult, approaches include emphasis on maintaining family, work, and other social roles as much as possible. In addition, for adolescents, adults, and family members, group meetings are dramatically helpful. Groups not only allow for ventilation and sharing of coping strategies but also powerfully assist in resisting social extrusion while reinforcing both the autonomy and the interdependency with others of the individual with cancer.

Discovering those behaviors and attitudes that resist partial extrusion of the cancer patient from the family and the social system has already resulted in new group behaviors. These include the development of organizations such as The Candlelighters and Make Today Count. The Hospice Movement is also included. Together, they represent three living examples of movement toward demythologizing cancer, redefining the sick role, re-evaluating physicians' authority, and hence, creating a new definition of health for the cancer patient.

References

American Cancer Society. The child with cancer. In *Proceedings of the American Cancer Society's National Conference on Human Values and Cancer* (Atlanta, 1972), 1973, 118–149.

American Cancer Society. *Cancer facts and figures 1975*. Publication # 5008 LE. 3.

Anthony, E. J. The syndrome of the psychologically invulnerable child. In *The child in his family: Children at risk*. New York: Wiley, 1974, pp. 529–544.

Artiss, K. L., & Levine, A. S. Doctor–patient relationship in severe illness. *New England Journal of Medicine*, 1973, *288*, 1210.

Binger, C. M., Ablin, A. R., Feuerstein, R. C., Kushner, J. H., Zoger, S., & Mikkelson, C. Special article: Childhood leukemia: Emotional impact on patient and family. *New England Journal of Medicine*, 1969, *280*, 414–418.

Blos, P., Jr., & Finch, S. M. Sexuality and the handicapped adolescent. In J. A. Downey & N. L. Low (Eds.), *The child with disabling illness: Principles of rehabilitation*. Philadelphia: Saunders, 1974, pp. 537–538.

Boyce, T., & Michael, M., III. Nine assumptions of Western medicine. *Man and Medicine*, 1976, *1*, 319–320.

Bozeman, M. F., Orbach, C. E., & Sutherland, A. M. Psychological impact of cancer and its treatment, III. The adaptation of mothers to the threatened loss of their children through leukemia: Part I. *Cancer*, 1955, *8*, 1–33.

Chodoff, P., Friedman, S. B., & Hamburg, D. A. Stress, defenses and coping behavior: Observations in parents of children with malignant disease. *American Journal of Psychiatry*, 1964, *120*, 743–749.

Cole, S. A. Liminality and the sick role. *Man and Medicine*, 1976, *2*, 41–53.

DeVita, V. T. The evolution of therapeutic research in cancer. *New England Journal of Medicine*, 1978, *298*, 907–910.

Eiser, C., & Lansdown R. Retrospective study of intellectual development in children treated for acute lymphoblastic leukemia. *Archives of Disease in Childhood*, 1977, *52*, 525–529.

Green, W. A., Jr., & Miller, G. Psychological factors and reticuloendothelial disease: IV. Observations on a group of children and adolescents with leukemia: An interpretation of disease development in terms of the mother–child unit. *Psychosomatic Medicine*, 1958, *20*, 124.

Gunther, J. *Death be not proud*. New York: Harper & Row, 1949.

Heinemann, H. O. Incurable illness and the hospital in the twentieth century. *Man and Medicine*, 1976, *1*, 281–285.

Hersh, S. P. Psychosocial aspects of chronic yet fatal illness in children. In D. V. Siva Sankar (Ed.), *Mental health in children* (Vol. 2). New York: PJD Publications, 1976.

Hersh, S. P. Meeting the psychosocial needs of children and adolescents with cancer. In *Proceedings of the Second National American Cancer Society Conference on Human Values and Cancer*. Philadelphia: G. Stickney, 1978.

Kirten, C., & Liverman, M. Special educational needs of the child with cancer. *Journal of School Health,* 1977, *47,* 170–173.

Korsch, B. M., & Negrete, V. F. Doctor–patient communication. *Scientific American,* 1972, *227*(2), 66–75.

Kübler-Ross, E. *On death and dying.* New York: Macmillan, 1969.

Leventhal, B. G., & Hersh, S. P. Modern treatment of childhood leukemia: The patient and his family. *Children Today,* 1974, *3,* 2–6, 36.

Levy, N. B. Sexual adjustment to maintenance hemodialysis and renal transplantation: National survey questionnaire: Preliminary report. In N. B. Levy (Ed.), *Living or dying: Adaptation to hemodialysis.* Springfield, Ill: Charles C Thomas, 1974, pp. 127–140.

Lieber, L., Plumb, M. M., Gerstenzang, M. L., & Holland, J. The communication of affection between cancer patients and their spouses. *Psychosomatic Medicine,* 1976, *38,* 379–389.

Lund, D. *Eric.* New York: Lippincott, 1974.

Moss, H. A., Yarrow, M. R., Jacobs, B., Nannis, E., Hersh, S. P., & Levine, A. Behavioral studies of seriously ill children. A protocol submitted to the NIH Clinical Research Committee, February 18, 1976.

Peylan-Ramu, N., Poplack, D. G., Pizzo, P. A., Adornato, B. T., & DiChiro, G. Abnormal CT scans of the brain in asymptomatic children with acute lymphocytic leukemia after prophylactic treatment of the central nervous system with radiation and intrathecal chemotherapy. *New England Journal of Medicine,* 1978, *298*(15), 815–818.

Roach, N. The last day of April. New York: American Cancer Society, 1977.

Seneca. Letter 70: [Suicide] (M. Hadas, Trans.). In *The stoic philosophy of Seneca.* New York: Norton, 1958, p. 202.

Sherman, M. *The leukemic child.* DHEW Publication No. (NIH)76–863, 1976.

Siris, E. S., Leventhal, B. G., & Vaitukaitis, J. L. Effects of childhood leukemia and chemotherapy on puberty and reproductive function in girls. *New England Journal of Medicine,* 1976, *294,* 1143–1146.

Steinfels, P. Introduction. In P. Steinfels & R. M. Veatch (Eds.), *Death inside out: A Hastings Center report.* New York: Harper & Row, 1975, pp. 3–4.

Strickland, S. P. *Research and the health of Americans: Priorities, process and strategies.* New York: Aspen Institute for Humanistic Studies, 1978, pp. 7–8.

Tolstoy, L. The death of Ivan Ilych. In *Great short works of Leo Tostoy.* New York: Harper & Row, 1967, pp. 285–286. (Originally published, 1886.)

Watts, R. J. Sexuality in the middle aged cardiac patient. *Nursing Clinics of North America,* 1976, *11,* 349–359.

10

Labeling and Discrimination in Mental Health

Jonas Robitscher

When the label of "mental illness" is placed on an individual, a number of consequences follow. Some of these consequences are beneficent. Those who have been labeled mentally ill are given special protections and helps; they have the advantage—if it is an advantage—of stays of unlimited duration at state hospitals and of disability income provided by the state; they have a host of social work programs for their care and rehabilitation; and they have such special legal benefits as an excuse for criminal action and protection against disadvantageous contracts. (Some of these advantages are illusory. The theoretical entitlement to unlimited stays in government-supported hospitals, for example, may in real life be a series of short stays in a revolving-door system of commitment and discharge. The principle of special helps and benefits for the mentally disabled, however, is firmly entrenched in our legal and political systems.)

Many more of these consequences of the label are not beneficent. The mentally ill are kept from some jobs, and if they have been hired, they can be separated from the jobs after an evaluation of their competency. They are also kept out of some professions: attempts are made to screen out the mentally disabled from graduate and professional education and from professions that require licensure. Those who have been licensed may be subject to revocation of the license. At the extreme end of the loss-of-equal-

Jonas Robitscher • Emory University Schools of Law and Medicine, Atlanta, Georgia 30322.

status spectrum, the "mentally ill" can be held in mental hospitals for long periods of time against their will or, if they break certain laws, they can be diverted from the criminal justice system and held indefinitely in a mental hospital—usually the most unhuman kind of mental hospital, the hospital for the criminally insane—until a hospital superintendent cetifies them as "cured."

But usually the label of mental illness causes less dramatic losses— altered family and social relationships, and altered vocational adjustment. One common result of the label is the embarkation on a downward spiral of worsened interpersonal and vocational relationships that starts with job discrimination and the relegation to less important jobs or to no jobs at all; it continues with loss of earning power (and with it loss of the ability to purchase private psychiatric help); and continues further with relegation to the community mental health center system where chronic patients are often overlooked—a descending spiral of discrimination, loss of status and power, increasing inability to secure effective help leading to further pressures and symptoms, that in turn lead to further discrimination.

The neurotic, the psychotic, those labeled mentally ill may be victims of the "wallflower syndrome"—they are the least popular partners at the ball and the more rejected they feel the more symptoms they display. In contrast to the healthy and popular ball-goer who does not need partners to bolster her (or his) identity and confirm a sense of self-worth, but with whom everyone wants to dance, the "mentally ill" desperately need support and assurance but this need drives off prospective partners.

One of the ironies of the mental health care system is that the most "mentally healthy" who are employed and are often affluent have the benefits of earning power and often of mental health care insurance (this insurance can sometimes pay up to 80% of the cost of outpatient visits); the struggling, less affluent, mentally disabled person does not have earning power, does not have access to such insurance, and must seek psychiatric support from the community mental health system, which notoriously depends on short-term treatment ("crisis intervention"), chemotherapy, and inadequate follow-ups. An example of this irony, which indicates the difference in power of the mentally ill and the mentally well, is demonstrated by the insurance benefits to which mental health workers in my own state, Georgia, are entitled. The mental health workers are largely involved in the community mental health care system, where they provide treatment for the mentally ill. When the workers feel the need of psychiatric care—and a very large percentage do at one time or another—they take their problems to a private psychiatrist, escape the label of "mentally ill," and pay only 20% of the $45 or $50 an hour that their therapist charges; they do not take their problems to the community mental health care system; they do not receive the same kind of care they dispense. They can purchase for themselves an entirely different kind of mental health treatment—psychoanalysis—rather than the kind they provide for their clients.

A host of sociologists have centered in on diagnosing and labeling, and the resulting stigmatization as the core of the problem of the psychiatric patient. Psychiatrists see the problem differently: they see the diagnosing and labeling as a necessary part of treatment and they think patients are stigmatized not because they have been labeled "mentally ill" but because they have shown the lack of competent self-management that mental patients demonstrate.

Shakespeare has told us that "some are born great, some achieve greatness, and some have greatness thrust upon them."[1] In the same way, there are various methods of achieving the diminished status that results from the label of mental disability. The label can be conferred at birth, as in the case of congenital conditions; it can be secured through the seeking of help and the self-labeling that goes with this; or it can be imposed on an unwilling subject, an involuntary patient who denies mental illness but nevertheless is so labeled.

Thomas Szasz, the psychiatrist–psychoanalyst who is so suspicious of modern psychiatry and who denies the validity of the concept of mental illness, says that when psychiatrists put the label of mental illness or mentally disabled on people, they acquire power over them, that labeling is in fact the source of psychiatric power. The purpose of the power is not ostensibly to hurt the patient, but once the label has been placed on the patient there comes with it the authority to prescribe and treat and to hold involuntarily if the patient meets certain standards of dangerousness (which is also a psychiatric decision). An extraordinary variety of therapeutic modalities become available to the doctor; in the case of voluntary patients he can treat, prescribe, suggest, direct, and influence; in the case of the patient who meets the dangerousness criteria he has the authority to commit, inject, invade, subdue, shock, and impose any number of strange and novel treatment modalities.

Physicians, since they are authorities, are in the enviable position of setting up classifications that are accepted as classifications because they have set them up, of having recognized as diseases whatever they declare to be diseases. With diseases caused by organisms, wounds and breaks, cancerous growths, or the alteration of physiological functions, it is easier to define disease, but when the causative agent is less obvious, when the connection between cause and disease is not certain, or when the entity called a "disease" is a behavioral disturbance, then the definition of disease is less certain. No one doubts that typhoid fever is a disease, but back pain or fatigue may or may not be considered evidence of an illness, and at the

[1]Shakespeare, W. *Twelfth Night,* II, V, 159.

purely psychological end of the disease spectrum, check-kiting or exhibitionism or homosexuality can or cannot be seen as a disease depending on the point of view and the desires of the diagnostician.

Sociologists have been critical of medicine for its overinclusive definitions of disease, and in turn, physicians have accused sociologists of being misleading and unfair in their accusations. But physicians readily admit that most patients waiting to see doctors in their waiting rooms are not sick, ill, or diseased—at the most, they have symptoms that they wish to have differentiated from disease, so physicians cannot easily deny that they often deal with nondisease and that they have an incentive for defining disease broadly. Elliot Krause, sociologist at Northeastern University, has described physicians generally (not psychiatrists in particular) in their attitude toward disease:

> Taking strict medical definitions of physical illness, we can see that, in the United States, physicians in private practice have a patient or can treat an illness only if they can define the patient as officially ill. The physician's economic advantage, in private fee-for-service practice, lies therefore in overdefining people as ill. (1977, p. 519)

But it is not only the money inducement and the private fee-for-service that influence doctors to overdefine illness; it is to a much larger extent their need to preserve their own authority, to bolster their professional identities. If general practitioners and internists were to admit what is probably the truth—that the majority of the people they serve as "ill" are the end products of years of poor health hygiene and have fatigue, headaches, muscle tension, back pain, insomnia, or obesity not because they are "diseased" or "ill" but because they have developed a life-style inconsistent with maximum physical well-being and, although they may be in the process of acquiring a disease, are not at present diseased—they would have to abandon their pill-dispensing, reassuring approach to medicine or hand over a large part of their practices to nutritionists, physical activity specialists, and psychologists and dynamic (but not chemotherapeutic) psychiatrists. These purely medical doctors maintain their patients by treating them either for diseases or for nondiseases, in any case within the disease context.

If the problem of the overdefinition of illness is serious for general medicine, it is crucial for psychiatry. In psychiatry the conferring of the sick label gives the physician the power to use great persuasive leverage on his rational patients—"I am well and you are sick. Your desire to leave therapy proves how much you really need therapy. Your unwillingness to do what I say you should do (and I am backed up in this completely by all the members of your family) shows how sick you really are"—and it gives him complete authority—to eugenically sterilize, to (in the past) lobotomize, to put into a physical or a chemical straitjacket—over his designated patients.

The authors of *Comprehensive Textbook of Psychiatry* (Freedman, Kaplan, & Sadock, 1976) have commented on problems in defining psychiatric entities and even the grander concept of psychiatric disease. They say:

> None of the standard textbooks of psychiatry and neither the first nor the second edition of the American Psychiatric Association's *Diagnostic and Statistical Manual of Mental Disorders* provide a definition of mental disorder. Mental disorders are manifested by deviations in behavior (which includes ideation and affect) from some normative concept. The problem in defining mental disorder is that the widespread consensus that exists regarding the undesirability of specific manifestations of nonpsychiatric medical disorder—pain, disability, death—does not always exist for behavioral manifestations of what have traditionally been regarded as mental disorders.
>
> The lack of consensus regarding the specific manifestations of psychiatric disorder may take three forms: controversy as to whether a given condition should be regarded as undesirable at all; how undesirable a condition should be to warrant its designation as an illness; and whether the condition, even if markedly undesirable, should be regarded as within the domain of psychiatry or some other discipline. An example of the first form is the controversy as to whether preferential homosexual behavior should be regarded as undesirable. An example of the second form is disagreement about whether certain mild personality patterns are sufficiently undesirable to warrant designation as a psychiatric disorder or whether they should be viewed purely as descriptive traits. An example of the third form is the controversy as to whether certain forms of serious antisocial behavior should be regarded as sick (manifestations of psychiatric disorders) or bad (the responsibility of the criminal justice system). (pp. 406–407)

The authors state that most psychoanalytically oriented United States psychiatrists take a broad approach to mental disease and define as mental disorder anything that seems to them to be a significant deviation from an ideal state of mental health. "Thus, sexual practices, value systems, and personality traits that are deemed less than optimal or a result of intrapsychic conflict are viewed as manifestations of mental disorder" (Freedman *et al.*, 1976, p. 407). Almost all European psychiatrists take a narrow approach and restrict the disease label to conditions that are associated clearly with suffering or disorder. United States studies show a much higher incidence of mental disorder than is generally reported in European studies.

Putting the diagnostic label on the psychiatric patient not only raises the doctor, who gains tremendous authority over the patient in the process, but also lowers the status of the person receiving the diagnosis, who thereby loses authority. The stigma that goes with psychiatric labels is not undeserved; psychiatric patients who are irrational possibly should be stigmatized. The hallmark of psychiatric illness is unreason and erratic and unpredictable behavior, and our society is not only made uncomfortable by such behavior (as Thomas Szasz emphasizes) but it is often forced into a position where it has no alternative except to treat the person as different, often to impose controls or involve the criminal justice process. But even though I see as unremarkable the stigma that accompanies deviant behavior —usually leading to condemnation of the person who is different, although sometimes attributing the difference to superior or remarkable abilities or divine favor—I do not accept the lack of rigor with which the labels are applied, labels that to some extent are causal factors in the stigmatization. (Even if we do not put specific labels denoting disease entities on psychiatric patients, we would still designate them as different and might want to deal with them differentially; usually the mental patient is not different because he is labeled but is labeled because he is different.)

Psychiatrists are at a great advantage when they move to pin their labels on their subjects. In the first place, the area of mental peculiarities and disabilities (if you prefer, mental disease) is relatively unknown territory where psychiatrists have had experience and others have not. Occasionally, someone challenges the authority of the psychiatrist, so we have had Thomas Szasz (1967); Erving Goffman (1961); Otto Friedrich, (1975), a journalist, who (correctly) points out that "going crazy" is a unique experience with a different meaning for everyone who has experienced it; D. L. Rosehan (1973), a psychologist, who (incorrectly) equates psychiatrists' tendency to respect the history given by the patient (in a situation in which there is no apparent motive for deception or malingering) with an inability to diagnose. But, for the most part, the psychiatrist's assertion that he is an expert in the diagnosis of mental illness remains without challenge. Families, the police, judges, juries, insurance companies need someone to tell them whether or not someone is sick, and the psychiatrist fills that need.

Second, under the peculiar rules that psychiatrists have worked out, a patient cannot challenge his diagnosis. If he does, he is labeled as negativistic or paranoid or a troublemarker or litigious. Joseph Heller (1955) has helped us define one of the many variations of Catch-22—if the patient admits he is sick he can eventually be certified as well, but as long as he denies he is sick he can never be diagnosed as well.

Third, the psychiatrist can manipulate the symbols and labels so that someone is sick for differential purposes, and as a result he can be of great service to his patient. A man is so sick that his treatment should be paid for by his medical insurance, but at the same time he is so little sick that his employer should not fill his job but should keep it open for him. A man is so dangerous that he should be committed, but if he commits suicide in the hospital a label can be put on him posthumously of "not so dangerous that this could have been anticipated" to spare the hospital any financial liability for negligent care (or, alternatively, the psychiatrist can claim that he should never have been expected to have been able to predict dangerousness, since diagnostic skill does not extend *that* far). There are always data and a point of view that will justify any position—and this applies to the diagnostic process, too. There are always indications that can be used to emphasize ability and indications that can be used to emphasize disability. The psychiatrist treating an adolescent will label him as neurotically depressed and so qualify him for insurance coverage, but when this patient is applying for college admission he is seen as without mental illness or, at the worst, having suffered from "an adjustment reaction of adolescence." The psychiatrist can play with the label so it confers only benefits and no penalties on the patient, but he also has the authority to play with the labels so they apply only penalties and no benefits. He can change labels or he can apply one label for varying purposes. The sexual offender at the hospital for the criminally insane is seen as not sick from the point of view of insurance coverage for medical treatment—he is labeled a sociopath, which does not qualify for insurance benefits—but the fact that he does not have a curable or any other kind of medical condition does not prevent the label of sexual psychopath from subjecting him to the risk of an indefinite (perhaps lifetime) "therapeutic" commitment to last until he is "cured."

Fourth, the concepts that underlie the psychiatric labels are so vague and ambiguous that even a well-meaning and concerned psychiatrist will have trouble differentiating the well from the sick in many cases. Even if this psychiatrist does not go along with Szasz and deny the existence of mental disease, he has trouble, as a patient recovers from a psychotic episode, in saying when the patient has passed the dividing line between sickness and health and he may or may not see the "recovered" patient as still "sick," depending on his training, orientation, need to retain control, and other factors. The symptoms that are seen in acute or persistent form in "sick" patients are ubiquitous; they can be seen in all of us. The hypnogogic delusions that "normal" people have when they are falling asleep are not very different from the pathological delusions that "schizophrenics" have when they are awake; the primary process material that "normal" people express in dreams is not very different from the primary process material that "psychotics" express more directly. We have the concept of the normal individual, but perhaps he is always an abnormal person with the ability to control his public face. Perhaps the "normal" sublimates and, instead of going through life as a Peeping Tom, becomes a psychiatrist; instead of going through life as a paranoid, becomes a public interest lawyer; perhaps he merely hides pathology, as did such notables as Florence Nightingale, William Gladstone, T. E. Lawrence, and Woodrow Wilson—all in their times and afterward seen as great heroes and all shown by modern muckraking biographers to have had severe psychopathology. (The list could be extended indefinitely.) Then there is the question of the relation of psychopathology to unusual accomplishment—could it have been accomplished without the pressures of what, to some, would appear to be psychopathology? And should it always be considered "illness"?

The dividing lines separating normality, supernormality, and subnormality are tenuous, and they are sometimes related to the bias of the observer. Perhaps the psychiatric diagnosis is not objective except in acute, classical, or extreme cases.

Ronald Leifer, a psychiatrist and psychoanalyst who has adopted the Szaszian position and explicated this point of view in a well-thought-out and precise way, has stressed the fact that mental disease is diagnosed in a social context—the person is labeled mentally ill because he has deviated from some social norm and has strayed into ways so that his behavior is seen as "undesirable behavior." Leifer, who has been described as a disciple and systematic expounder of Szaszian doctrine with a much more sophisticated use of sociological theory (Sedgwick, 1973, p. 27, fn. 5), has given us a simple and logical approach to differentiating medical and nonmedical conditions that would cause chagrin to psychiatrists if they were knowledgeable about the attacks on psychiatric legitimacy, because it places psychiatric conditions squarely in a nonmedical, nondisease category. Leifer says that the term *disease* in physical diagnosis and treatment "refers to phenomena that are not regulated by social custom, morality and law, namely bodily structure and function," but that "in psychiatry the term 'disease' refers to behavior, which is subject to the regulation of custom, morality and law" (Leifer, 1969, p. 35). One of the consequences of labeling behavior a disease is that it gives psychiatrists control of behavior:

> Because the term "mental illness" refers to social conduct, it may be used to label any behavior as undesirable and the person exhibiting such behavior as in need of corrective action. Similarly, any behavior deemed disirable may be designated as "health." The interventions for transforming the undesirable to the desirable, "disease" to "health," may be described as "psychiatric technology." The rhetoric of health and disease is thus flexible enough to encompass all human activities. Psychiatric rhetoric may be used to justify social interventions in the name of the unimpeachable (and often unintelligible) authority of scientific (or medical) technology, rather than in the name of explicit social values and interests.
>
> The medical disguise of psychiatry makes it easy to smuggle in a number of social functions under the guise of medical treatment. In the guise of a physician, the psychiatrist may function as a policeman, a warden, a parent, a minister, an educator, a personnel manager, and a scientific expert on human behavior. Each of these activities is based on inexplicit social values and social purposes, which must be understood in the context of our social rather than our medical institutions. (Leifer, 1969, pp. 76–77)

The facility that the psychiatrist has to diagnose pathology is based on the fact that everyone has behavior that deviates from the norm, and if that test is used, everyone can be labeled as having pathology. Psychiatrists once diagnosed sociopathy as a disease and then, later, for legal reasons moved it back into a nondisease category. Homosexuality was diagnosed as a disease until social pressure from civil libertarian groups caused the classification to be reexamined; the decision was then made to call it nonpathological. Promiscuity and use of marijuana have been reasons for psychiatric hospitalizations, as has deviant political thought. Delusions concerning governmental interference into American life (not that all beliefs concerning being watched and harassed or adherence to conspiracy theories are delusional) are permissible if they come from certain sources—writers, intellectuals, political liberals, but they are unacceptable if they come from other sources—little old ladies in tennis shoes. Not everybody has demonstrable physical symptoms but everyone has psychiatric symptoms that may be revealed and that may subject them to psychiatric authority.

We are continually forced back to the basic question of the definition of mental health and mental illness and the differentiation of the two.

Psychiatrists could base their legitimacy on a long list of abilities—the psychiatrist is legitimate if he is able to empathize, if he is able to be helpful, if he understands and can communicate his understanding, if he does not intervene to be directive but lets the patient work through and reach his own solutions, if he understands and can make allowances for the countertransference. They can be judged on their ability to diagnose and bring into control acute psychosis. These are the kinds of criteria on which psychiatrists should be judged. Above all, is the psychiatrist able to be helpful? But all these are too imprecise and they are only relevant in the context of a therapeutic or treating relationship. When the state or other third parties are concerned, when legal issues are raised, when the psychiatrist is employed not to treat but merely to evaluate, then his legitimacy is judged on his ability to apply formal—statutory, regulatory, and contractual—definitions. Can the patient be classified so that he comes within the scope of the statute or the insurance policy? Is such a definition accurate? Is it accurate only in a majority of cases or in all cases? Are psychiatric patients dangerous? Can psychiatrists predict dangerousness? Are there effective therapies that psychiatrists can use with patients they are detaining because they have decided they are dangerous? These are the kinds of questions lawyers and sociologists and legislatures ask when they try to decide if psychiatry has legitimacy, if psychiatric intervention should be funded, if it should be countenanced or encouraged by the state. In the terms set by three of its most severe critics (all of whom are psychiatrists themselves), psychiatrists must show that there is such a thing as mental disease, although Thomas Szasz has said that there is not; they must show that psychosis is destructive, although R. D. Laing has seen it as constructive; and they have to justify psychiatric treatment as something more than witchcraft and mumbo jumbo, although these are how E. Fuller Torrey has described psychiatric treatment.

In the terms of less all-out critics, they have to prove that their diagnostic categories are sound and useful, that they have discriminating ability, that they are good predictors. Because mental diseases are strange and because mental patients are the special charges of those who specialize in their care, because mental disease is a medical subspecialty and psychiatrists carry the authority of doctors, because mental patients are potentially destructive or self-destructive and psychiatrists have been willing to try to impose control upon them, it has been unusual—until very recently—to challenge the ability of the psychiatrists to classify and to predict. The emphasis on scientism has put psychiatry above criticism.

Emil Kraepelin started it all when he constructed a psychiatric nosology that everyone agreed was modern, complete, and scientific. Kraepelin (1904/1968, p.v) stated three-quarters of a century ago that he tried at all times to keep the diagnostic point of view in the foreground because he was convinced of its fundamental importance, not only to the scientific advancement of psychiatry but also so the patient would receive the proper advice and be given the proper treatment. An intimate knowledge of psychiatric illnesses and their diagnoses was important for all physicians, he said, not for the variously branching scientific relations to so many other phases of human existence but rather for the extraordinary practical importance of the understanding:

> Insanity, even in its mildest forms, involves the greatest suffering that physicians have to meet. Only a comparatively small percentage of the mental cases are permanently and completely cured in the strictest sense of the word. And the number of the insane, which will hardly be exaggerated if we estimate it as amounting at the present moment to 200,000 in Germany alone, is apparently increasing with the most unfortunate rapidity. . . .
>
> All the insane are dangerous, in some degree, to their neighbors, and even more so to themselves. Mental derangement is the cause of at least a third of the total number of suicides, while sexual crimes and arson, and to a less extent, dangerous assaults, thefts, and impostures are often committed by those whose minds are diseased. Numberless families are ruined by their affected members, either by the senseless squandering of their means, or because long illness and inability to work have generally sapped the power of caring for a household. . . .
>
> For all these reasons, it is one of the physician's most important duties to make himself, as far as possible, acquainted with the nature and phenomena of insanity. Even though the limits of his power against this mighty adversary are very narrow, opportunity enough is afforded to every practical physician to contribute his share to the prevention and alleviation of the endless misery annually engendered by mental disease. Alcoholism and syphilis undoubtedly offer the most profitable points of attack, together with the abuse of morphia and cocaine, which so clearly owes its fatal significance to the action of medical men. Family physicians, again, can often help to prevent the marriage of the insane, or of those who are seriously threatened with insanity, and to secure a proper education and choice of occupation for children predisposed to disease. But it will be their special province to recognise dangerous symptoms in time, and, by their prompt action, to prevent suicides and accidents, and obviate the short-sighted procrastination which so often keeps patients from coming under the care of an expert alienist until the time for practically useful treatment has long been past. Even in those numerous cases which never become insane in the narrower sense,

the physician who has been trained in alienism will have such an understanding of the recognition and treatment of physical disturbances as will amply repay him for the trouble of his years of study. Even in my own experience it has happened very often that older physicians have regretted their defective knowledge of alienism, and complained that it was only in practical life that they learned how great a part is played, in the daily round of ordinary medical practice, by the correct diagnosis of more or less morbid mental incidents. I need hardly mention that, for various reasons, such a diagnosis is in constant demand by public authorities, courts of law, and trade societies. (Kraepelin, 1904/1968, pp. 3–5)

Kraepelin, in devising his grand scheme of nomenclature for psychiatric conditions, was synthesizing earlier approaches. The clinical descriptive approach dates back to the dawn of recorded history, but it is Hippocrates in the 5th century before Christ who is credited with formally introducing the concept of psychiatric illness into medicine. The English physician Thomas Sydenham in the 17th century, introduced a somatic approach stating that each kind of psychiatric illness had a specific cause. Philippe Pinel at the end of the 18th century simplified a disorganized diagnostic system by grouping psychiatric cases into four fundamental classes— mania, melancholy, dementia, and idiotism. Although Pinel did not accept Sydenham's specific etiology theory, most early 19th-century psychiatrists —including Isaac Ray—believed that mental disease was the manifestation of physical pathology, even if the pathology was reversible and so not discoverable at the time of autopsy or if the pathology could only be discovered by as yet undiscovered scientific techniques and instruments. Benedict-Augustin Morel in the 18th century, describing *dementia preaecox,* was the first to use the course or outcome of the illness as the basis for a classification. Karl Kahlbaum introduced the concept of organic and nonorganic mental disease. Kraepelin synthesized all these approaches into a grand nosological scheme, searching for the combination of clinical features that would best predict outcome, bringing together the manic and depressive conditions, distinguishing this affective condition from schizophrenia (which was still known as dementia praecox), differentiating paranoid and many other subtypes of dementia praecox, distinguishing the acute organic conditions or the deliria from the chronic brain syndromes or the dementias, and incorporating into the scheme such concepts as psychogenic neuroses and psychopathic personalities. Eugen Bleuler (1857–1939) refined the concept of dementia praecox and gave it the name of schizophrenia. Sigmund Freud expanded the boundaries of psychiatric disgnosis by dignifying the minor mental illnesses, the neuroses, and "raising" them to the status of medical entities. (Freedman *et al.,* 1976, pp. 408–409).

The tendency has always been to use an ever-expanding concept of psychiatric illness, and in this century psychosomatic disorders, chronic personality states that are not characterized by symptoms, and many kinds of criminal behavior have been included in the American Psychiatric Association Diagnostic and Statistical Manual, psychiatry's official nosological scheme. Transitory disturbances have also been included—adjustment reactions and brief situational disturbances.

Starting in 1917, the American Medico-Psychological Association, which later became the American Psychiatric Association, adopted a system of nomenclature that in 1934 was used in a revised form as the first official Standard Classified Nomenclature of Disease. In 1952, motivated by dissatisfaction with the classification by psychiatrists in World War II, a revision that depended heavily on a scheme in use by the Veterans Administration was published as the *Diagnostic and Statistical Manual of Mental Disorders*. It is known as DSM–I, and its revision of 1968, DSM–II, is in current use. The chairman of the committee that prepared the 1968 revision acknowledged in his foreword some of the biasing factors involved in giving names to conditions and also some of the controversy that existed about disease entities:

> Rationalists may be prone to believe the old saying that "a rose by any other name would smell as sweet"; but psychiatrists know full well that irrational factors belie its validity and that labels of themselves condition our perceptions. The Committee accepted the fact that different names for the same thing imply different attitudes and concepts. . . .
>
> In the case of diagnostic categories about which there is current controversy concerning the disorder's nature or cause, the Committee has attempted to select terms which it thought would least bind the judgment of the user. The Committee itself included representatives of many views. It did not try to reconcile those views but rather to find terms which could be used to label the disorders about which they wished to be able to debate. . . .
>
> Consider, for example, the mental disorder labeled in this Manual as "schizophrenia," which, in the first edition, was labeled "schizophrenic reaction." The change of label has not changed the nature of the disorder, nor will it discourage continuing debate about its nature or causes. Even if it had tried, the Committee could not establish agreement about what this disorder is; it could only agree on what to call it. (American Psychiatric Association, 1968, pp. viii–ix)

Commenting on the use of DSM–II, *Science News* has said: "[A]s in no other medically related discipline, psychiatry has spawned an avalanche of symptom labels that not only mystify the public but also, to a large degree, confuse and frustrate behavioral experts themselves. A recent study of diagnosis reliability revealed that when presented identical sets of cases, psychistrists rarely agree on the specific nature of the illness. (Greenberg, 1977).

I am not in agreement with Szasz and Leifer, although I think we owe them a debt of gratitude for forcing us to think about the way we are used as agents of social control. I think that some patients are suffering, if not from a disease, at least from some severe aberration that causes them to feel that they are going out of control, which makes their thoughts unmanageable, and which often makes them feel toxic and physically ill. I am persuaded by historical accounts that show that there has been a consistent pattern through time of seeing some people as being out of control and strange, and I would not be willing to side with Szasz and Leifer and say that we should not try to control them. When I look at the photographs Hugh Welch Diamond, superintendent of the Female Department of the Surrey County Lunatic Asylum, showed to London audiences on "the types of insanity" in 1852, which have been reprinted as *The Face of Madness* (Gilman, 1976), I see the faces of people who are distraught, disturbed, apathetic, withdrawn, or otherwise far from "normal," and they remind me of patients I have seen in my residency and in my brief excursions behind the walls of state hospitals. But, although I have no doubt that mental illness is more than a myth, I find the dividing line of disease and health very hard to place, the objectivity of my diagnostic impressions I find very hard to justify, and I would in many cases be uncomfortable in insisting that my diagnosis is correct or scientific.

The argument that psychiatric diagnoses are culturally and socially determined has some merit. Hallucinating mystics can be seen as holy men or psychotics depending on time, place, social context, relationship to the designator, and attitude of the designator. But cross-cultural studies show that cultures as different from Western society's as the Eskimo and the Yoruba have explicit labels for insanity referring to beliefs, feelings, and actions thought to emanate from the mind or inner state of an individual and to be essentially beyond control, and that people afflicted with these states seek the aid of healers. Jane Murphy (1976), anthropologist at the Harvard School of Public Health, says: "Almost everywhere a pattern composed of hallucinations, delusions, disorientations, and behavioral aberrations appears to identify the idea of 'losing one's mind' even though the content of these manifestations is colored by cultural beliefs."

Although I am not happy about the system of nomenclature used now, I have no suggestions for improving it. I would see as a better avenue to improvement an insistence that the labels be applied carefully, not be used in ways that are harmful to patients, and not be taken too seriously. Labels are used to denigrate people, to give the labeler control, to deprive the person labeled of legal rights; but labeling seems to be a necessary process, part of the job of differentiating the sane from the insane, the "sick" from the "well." All labelers are faced with the knowledge, although many do not always allow it to be felt deeply, that they are operating in an ambiguous area where a wrong decision can have powerful effects. John Spiegel (1975), in his presidential address to the American Psychiatric Association, called psychiatry a "high-risk profession." Psychiatrists "may never come up with the testable theory and replicated findings of the hard sciences," he says. "Because of the large number of variables underlying any type of human behavior, our therapeutic decisions are always taken in the context of a certain amount of ambiguity. Since the data available are never sufficient, we have to learn to live with uncertanty. Clinical judgment, based on training and experience, makes the uncertainty manageable, but *every decision we make is a risky decision.*"

The psychiatrist would be a more acceptable person and a more useful person if he could bring himself to admit that there is the possibility that he is wrong. The infuriating quality of psychiatrists is their insistence that they are scientific and correct and that their detractors, therefore, must be wrong.

In my own practice I do not use diagnostic labels except (usually kept to myself) as helpful in my own working hypotheses—and subject to change—or when they are necessary for purposes of (rare) hospital admissions and discharge or (frequent) insurance processing to secure third-party payments. But institutional psychiatrists, psychiatrists doing clinical forensic work for courts or prisons, psychiatrists testifying in personal injury cases, and psychiatrists working in community mental health centers spend a great deal of time and energy deciding on the right diagnosis.

Like most psychiatrists in private practice, I am not scrupulously honest about my diagnostic labels. When they are required by some outside party as a prerequisite to payment or in order to certify that an employee is able to return to his job, I feel this as an unwarranted intrusion into the doctor–patient relationship and I feel I am not obligated to transmit information that would not be in the best interest of my patient. What I see as a "schizophrenic reaction," which in the nomenclature is found under "Psychoses Not Attributed to Physical Conditions Listed Previously" as "Acute Schizophrenic Episode" (295.4), I will be happier calling "Adjustment Reaction of Adult Life" (307.3) or (grounding only one leg of a multiple diagnostic label in the official terminology and exercising a creative approach to the filling out of forms), for added labeling, "Anxiety Neurosis" (300.0) "with hysterical features in an immature personality." As long as I give one classification that corresponds with a number in the DSM–II, I can pile diagnosis on diagnosis. Most of the reports I send out to other doctors show my uncertainty about the true classification by their reliance on two or three diagnostic categories—e.g., depressive neurosis in a schizoid personality. This is a common practice, perhaps a usual practice, in psychiatry. A case vignette in a journal article, for example, describes a patient as having "an obsessive character neurosis with hysterical, depressive, and narcissistic trends" (Lax, 1977). Advantages of such a loose diagnostic labeling system are that it is flexible and it can be used very descriptively; it also can be used to protect the patient and minimize the severity of the psychopathology. The disadvantage is that it is unscientific—it is not only imprecise but it is sometimes used deliberately to becloud the issue—and under its broad scope almost any human attribute can be described as having something pathological about it. In particular, the altering of diagnoses to help the patient or to fit the exigencies of a social or political situation (like the manipulation of the term *sociopath* so as to selectively include or not include some criminals as "mentally ill") can be criticized.

Loren Roth, psychiatrist at the University of Pittsburgh, has deplored my willingness to manipulate and fudge diagnoses; because psychiatrists do this, Roth says, the basis of the collection of scientific data is imperiled. My thought is that it is better to imperil the basis of the collection of scientific data than to imperil the future of my patient's job or his educational progress. He is hiring my services to help him, not to hurt him, and he is not primarily interested in scientific progress. But I would not justify other uses of mislabeling and loose labeling, and I would want to point out the danger that any diagnostic scheme with this much flexibility carries with it by giving the labeler excessive power. A great variety of human activities can be labeled as pathological. For example, in Russia, political dissidence is seen as pathological, and in Pennsylvania, Paul Reese was committed in 1973, after he addressed a letter to the local planning commission, "My dear blood sucking parasitic bureaucrat," as an "immediate threat to society."[2]

Because some of the patients they saw did not seem to fit into any of the accepted categories, psychiatrists have been adding new disease entities not found in DSM–I or DSM–II. At one time schizophrenia was characterized by an absence of affect of feeling, but when it became apparent that many schizophrenic patients were elated or depressed, a category was added to the official nomenclature, "schizophrenia, schizo-affective type" (295.7).

Another group of patients who displeased their doctors because they presented with the typical neurotic symptoms of anxiety, depression, compulsions, obsessions, and episodic emotional outbursts but did not show the expected improvement were diagnosed as "pseudoneurotic schizophrenics." The term has never been officially adopted. These patients were sometimes called "borderline" cases; the criteria for the diagnosis were multiple neurotic symptoms in addition to pervasive chronic and severe anxiety that did not seem to be attached to any specific situation (Hoch & Polatin, 1949).

In 1953, Robert Knight published a paper on "Borderline States." He noted that up to that time the term, which had received no official recognition, had been used to label persons who were "quite sick but not frankly psychotic," who had not "broken with reality" but who were too disturbed to be included in with run-of-the-mill neurotics (Knight, 1953).

[2]*Reese v. Nelson*, C.A 74-1653 (D.C.E.D. Pa. 1973), commented on by Von Hoffman, N., *Chicago Tribune*, July 12, 1977, sec. 3, p. 3.

The borderline category is a part of the spectrum concept in which mental illness runs a range from the normal to the severely psychotic; the term fills a gap between psychotic and neurotic. But researchers who do not conceptualize mental conditions as fitting along a spectrum, who see them instead as existing separately (although each separate condition can have its own spectrum), find the concept difficult to integrate into their system. Melitta Schmideberg (1959, pp. 398–418) conceptualized these borderline states as representing a clinical entity that stood on the border not only between the neuroses and the psychoses but also between normality and psychopathy.

At a meeting of the American Academy of Clinical Psychiatrists, Charles Rich (1977), psychiatrist at the University of Pittsburgh, suggested that the term *borderline* should be eliminated from the psychiatric vocabulary because of its multiple meanings. In a study of 20 charts of patients with the diagnosis, Rich reported that the patient history was insufficient for the diagnosis in 7 of the cases and that each patient of the 20 had received an average of three other, nonborderline diagnoses. Rich suggested that even if there is such a syndrome, the diagnosis is usually misapplied. The term is frequently used, he said, to cover up the lack of a clear-cut diagnosis, to avoid the admission that the case is in reality "undiagnosed," to satisfy the insurance companies that require a recognized psychiatric diagnosis, and to give something concrete to patients and their relatives.

But the term has attained popularity in a very few years and it will not be abandoned. The American Psychiatry Association Task Force of Nomenclature in 1977 sent questionnaires to all association members asking for help in developing criteria for a category of Borderline Personality Disorder for the next DSM edition (Spitzer, 1977). The request said:

> As you know, although there is considerable interest in this diagnostic category, there is as yet no consensus as to how it could be defined. Superstition, clairvoyance, poor school achievement, unstable interpersonal relationships, extreme sensitivity to personal rejection, problems tolerating being alone, and undue social anxiety were some of the items which this Committee wanted considered in attempting to come to a clearer definition of borderline, or borderline personality, or borderline personality organization or borderline schizophrenia, synonymous terms.

The purpose of some of the newer classifications is to distinguish more serious conditions from the neuroses, but according to a standard text, the classification of neuroses from which the newer designations are being differentiated is itself in need of clarification:

> It is difficult to classify neuroses. At one time, anyone who evidenced some psychological imbalance was presumed to have a neurosis. . . .
> In the process of civilization, the drives can never be fully or directly expressed, always leading to some internal conflict and to conflict among total

personalities of others. Therefore, the neurotic process is ubiquitous. Its quantitative degree and its fit for special life situations determine whether the neurosis is healthy or an illness. This discrimination depends not only on the degree of conflict but also on the method of defense used by the ego and the life situation in which the bearer of a lifestyle finds himself. . . .

The classification of neuroses is based on the mode of psychological defense and the degree to which one aspect of the personality dominates internal or external conflict. Since the situational component and the phase of development are important determinations of neuroses, the course is variable, and the degrees of crippling in the end are determined by nonpsychological external elements. . . .

Since everyone is, to some degree, neurotic, the definition of normality or health is indeed difficult. The estimation of mental health is based on a combination of descriptive and psychogenetic studies concerned with development, anecdotal incidents about reactions to life situations, stress, and critical periods of growth. (Freedman *et al.*, 1976, pp. 415–416)

One of the most common psychiatric diagnoses is neurotic depression. Gerald Klerman, then a Harvard psychiatrist (now administrator, Alcohol, Drug Abuse and Mental Health Administration), after a study of 150 patients, said that the term is used to designate five conditions that may overlap but that are distinct. It can mean a reaction to life stress, a preexisting personality disorder, depression with less social incapacitation than is found in psychotic depression, the absence of the symptoms of endogenous depression (or, to express this in another way, the concordance of external predisposing events), and, finally, depression that has less severe psychiatric symptoms than psychotic depression. The five meanings of neurotic depression are not mutually exclusive—they overlap in many cases—but Klerman's complaint is that the term is used in clinical practice for all five conditions without clarification (Diagnosis of Neurotic Depression, 1977). Other authorities say that the distinction between psychotic and neurotic depression, formerly a major issue in psychiatry, has lost its importance as the frequency of psychotic depression diminishes in the population (Freedman *et al.*, 1976, p. 496).

DSM–II had one large section entitled "Personality Disorders and Certain Other Non-Psychotic Mental Disorders." These were described as conditions characterized by "deeply ingrained maladaptive patterns of behavior that are perceptibly different in quality from psychotic and neurotic symptoms." The list of conditions that follows includes various kinds of personalities (paranoid, cyclothymic, schizoid, explosive, obsessive compulsive, hysterical, asthenic, antisocial, passive-aggressive, inadequate, and immature), various kinds of sexual deviations (homosexuality, fetishism, pedophilia, transvestitism, exhibitionism, voyeurism, sadism, masochism, other sexual deviation), alcoholism (episodic, habitual, and addictive), drug dependence (with nine conditions in this category depending on the substance to which the person is addicted, opium, analgesics, barbiturates, tranquilizers, cocaine, marijuana, and hallucinogens). Richard Schwartz and Ilze Schwartz (1976), of the Department of Psychiatry of the Cleveland Clinic Foundation, have said that to call personality disorders diseases imperils the integrity of psychiatry as a part of medicine.

They state that in general medicine, the hallmark of disease is the impaired structure or function of some organ system of the body leading to pain or some other reduction in the sense of well-being. Organic psychiatric conditions meet these criteria and can easily be considered diseases; they say functional psychiatric conditions are associated with malfunctioning of the central nervous system manifested by abnormal emotional states, clouded or confused thoughts processes, and abnormal physical functioning, and so also meet the criteria. (The point is arguable.):

> The personality disorders on the other hand lack these attributes of disease. They are characterized mainly by maladaptive patterns of behavior learned in childhood without any apparent abnormality of functioning in the central nervous system or other organ system and without any associated pain or discomfort. . . .
>
> Symptomatic relief can be achieved in patients suffering from classical psychiatric disorders by means of tranquilizers and antidepressant medication. . . . In the personality disorders, since there is no somatic dysfunction, medication plays no role in the treatment, which consists largely of attempts to reeducate the person's basic attitudinal and behavior patterns.
>
> In the case of a classical psychiatric disorder, medically oriented criteria enable one to differentiate the disease state from normality. . . . With respect to personality disorders, there are no good criteria for separating illness from health, and the criteria used are more sociological than medical in nature. How passive or inadequate does a person have to be to be "diagnosed" as a passive or inadequate personality, or how antisocial to be classified as an antisocial personality. (Schwartz & Schwartz, 1976)

These authors see four detriments resulting or that will result from this inclusion of personality disorders in the disease category.

First, there is an excessive demand for psychiatry to perform nonmedical functions. When psychiatric illness is so broadly defined that it includes "all kinds of personality problems, problems in living and maladaptive behavior," large numbers of psychiatrists are forced to occupy their time in activities other than the direct care of patients with bona fide psychiatric illnesses, performing duties that could be carried out quite well by nonpsychiatrists; the definition of this category of mental illness means that a "high proportion" of the population is mentally sick and in need of services. It results in the drift of psychiatrists away from direct patient contact into such roles as administrators, supervisors, and consultants, since the sheer number of patients to be treated is so enormous.

Second, the expansion of the concept of psychiatric illness has required that nonmedical mental health professions be called into service—clinical psychologists, psychiatric social workers, other mental health professionals, and mental health nonprofessionals. These nonphysician mental health workers have redefined people seeking psychiatric service as "clients" rather than "patients" and as "people with problems" rather than "people with illness." The authors feel this undermines the credibility of psychiatrists and—perhaps just as important in their view—that the morale of medical psychiatry is hurt "if a person interested in psychiatric work can become eligible to carry out the functions of a psychiatrist with status and pay equal to a psychiatrist without having to undergo the rigorous and expensive educational process required to become a physician." Another adverse effect as they see it is that patients seen by nonphysicians and needing chemotherapy will receive only psychotherapy.

Third, psychiatrists are forced to become agents of social control, with responsibility for producing conformance to society's norms for the antisocial personality, the alcoholic, the drug addict, the sexual offender, and the violence-prone and explosive person, all of whom are regarded as mentally ill solely because their behavior is socially deviant. "The police and courts in most jurisdictions are allowed to commit any person who exhibits any of the above behavior patterns to a mental hospital for an indefinite period. The psychiatric profession is required to accept and treat these persons, against their will if necessary, and may be held responsible for subsequent misconduct perpetrated by these offenders." The role of the psychiatrist is not the traditional healing role but "has more in common with a jailer, subjecting involuntary subjects to enforced confinement and treatment."

Fourth—here the authors stress the materialistic motive—the broadened concept of psychiatric illness makes it less likely that coverage of psychiatric treatment on a basis equal with medical and surgical coverage will be included in any future national health insurance program. "Such exclusion would of course have the effect of reversing decades of progress in the upgrading of psychiatric treatment and in gaining the public's acceptance of psychiatric illness as no different in principle from any other illness."

Of course, many of the arguments made by Schwartz and Schwartz could lead to conclusions far different from those they reach. If psychiatrists drift away from direct patient contact and end up as administrators and consultants, that may not show that too many people have been defined as patients; it might show—although this is doubtful—that psychiatrists can be effective in their roles as administrators and consultants; it might show—and this is more plausible—that many psychiatrists are not interested in people, in their needs and their dynamics, and prefer to insulate themselves so that they will not be in touch with patients. The Schwartzes are incorrect when they state that nonphysicians can secure pay and status equal to a psychiatrist's unless they are referring only to the institutional superintendent or administrator who may be paid at a roughly similar rate whether or not he has a medical degree. They do not consider an important possibility, that if some psychiatric conditions are not illnesses and so should be excluded from health insurance coverage, then perhaps other psychiatric conditions are equally nonillnesses and should also be excluded. Their arguments are heuristic, their point of view materialistic; they do not protest the role of psychiatry as an agent of social control because it causes unnecessary pain to individuals or because civil liberties are trampled upon, but because it is burdensome and opens the way for possible malpractice suits. But their main point is valid—the inclusion of personality disorders as psychiatric disease entities has been a matter of psychiatric discretion. No physician could sit down and debate whether to include smallpox as a disease, but psychiatrists do debate whether to include immature personality functioning or voyeurism as diseases. The labeling is much more arbitrary. What the authors fail to see is if they cede to psychologists and social workers this vast domain of psychiatry, they may find they have given away their defensible borders and that many other psychiatric conditions will also be seen as equally nonmedical.

One of the most effective attacks on psychiatric diagnosis has come from sociologists who consider some of the ultimate ramifications of being given a special status as "mentally ill." A large but inconclusive literature has developed on the sociological theory concerning the uses of labeling in social deviancy and in psychiatry. Labeling theory, also called societal reaction theory, has been effective in its criticism of psychiatry because it is a sociological approach and therefore "scientific" (although anyone with any degree of sophistication knows that sociology is no more scientific than psychiatry). Thomas J. Scheff, a lawyer-sociologist, has stated that the purpose of labeling theory is "*not* to reject psychiatric and psychological formulations in their totality." He says, "It is obvious that such formulations have served, and will continue to serve, useful functions in theory and practice concerning mental illness." The labeling theory model of insanity —that insanity is a culture-based concept imposed on some individuals in order to maintain a societal status quo—is described by Scheff as more of a sensitizing theory—directed to the recognition of new data, the development of new ways to perceive old data, the challenging of "taken-for-granted assumptions," and the shattering of "the attitude of everyday life" —than it is a step in the development of a scientific alternative to medical labeling (Scheff, 1975a, pp. 22–23).

Scheff gives some of the presuppositions underlying the labeling theory criticism of psychiatric practice. Many behaviors in society deviate from the accepted but are not necessarily criminal; these deviations may have such very different sources as the organic, psychological situations of stress, and volitional acts; this kind of deviance is very common in society but most of the behavior is rationalized and in any case has only transitory significance; when stereotypes learned in early childhood are applied to deviant behavior, the stereotypes are continually reaffirmed in ordinary social interactions; there are rewards for the person labeled in accepting the label and penalties when he tries to return to a conventional role (Scheff, 1975b, p. 9).

Murphy (1976, p. 1019) has a similar but not identical list of salient features of the labeling theory as applied to mental illness: there are deviations from what is believed to be normal in the sociocultural group; the norms are different in different groups; the deviation from the norms leads to stigmatization and disapproval; a label of mental illness becomes fixed; the person so labeled is encouraged to accept that role identity; powerless individuals are more vulnerable to this process than individuals with power; social agencies by contributing to the labeling process, are part of the problem rather than part of the solution.

Sarbin (1969, pp. 9–31), upholding labeling theory, rejects the concept of "internal states of mind" as unobservable and as a diversion from a consideration of causal factors in the social world; he sees what we call disordered conduct or mental illness as following from or concurrent with "attempts to solve certain problems generated in social systems." He sees the best metaphor for mental illness as a "transformation of social identity." Becker (1969, pp. 488–499) has said, "[D]eviance is not a quality of the act a person commits, but rather a consequence of the application by others of rules and sanctions to an 'offender.' The deviant is one to whom that label has successfully been applied; deviant behavior is behavior that people so label."

The literature on labeling theory is a debate, although most of the contributions have come from antipsychiatrists rather than from defenders of current practice. Some of the defenses have been by Walter Gove, Jack Gibbs, Nanette Davis, and most recently by Loren Roth (1975, for reference to this literature, see Scheff, 1975c, pp. 31–34). Roth, who teaches legal psychiatry at the University of Pittsburgh and is also a practicing psychiatrist, does not deny that the labeling perspective has some validity. He does not wish to discourage this perspective in research into the nature of mental disorder. He calls attention to the possibility for useful research in the field of transient stress, which occurs more frequently in the lower social class as it relates to mental life; the study of when and how mental disorders begin; the relationship of the prevalence of mental illness and social structure. However, he gives important arguments against the position of the labeling theorists:

1. Labeling theory does not try to explain why a deviance from the group norm occurs in the first place.
2. Empirical data do not support the contention that people enter into the hospital system only after brief or "ritual" screening.

3. Labels can act to deter deviance just as they can act to reinforce continuing careers of deviance.
4. The labeling position ignores the severity of illness; impairment is one method of providing a cutoff point between disorder and nondisorder.
5. Labeling theory does not give cognizance to the evidence that those whom we label mentally ill may not only have problems in their relationship to the mental health establishment but often have childhood, school, marital, family, job, drug and alcohol, and other problems, indicating that more than labeling has produced the phenomenon.

At the same time that psychiatry is subject to criticisms for its labeling methods and its lack of accurate predictive skills, the labeling process continues to extend itself by application to uses other than medical diagnoses—and many psychiatric determinations have to do with such subjects as ability to return to employment, ability to continue with employment, suitability of patients for discharge, suitability of dangerous prisoners for release, and many other kinds of pigeonholing and classifying that are not entirely diagnostic but are predictive. All these classifying activities—performed by psychiatrists, clinical psychologists, industrial psychologists, corrections personnel, and many others in modern society—are usually less scientific than they appear, but they serve to put the classified person in a category where he may easily feel discrimination and loss of status.

Hans Toch (1970), professor of psychology, has said:

> To me, the point of concern rests in any labels that lead to sorting or dispositions. Categorization that is used privately, as an aid to thinking, seems harmless. True, it can produce communication gaps (one man's crutch may be another man's confusion), but such a consequence is remediable and even self-correcting.
>
> Unfortunately, man is an influencing animal, not a communicating one. We seek to convince and are eager to adopt. Categories that start as private tools tend, ultimately, to become guides for action. At this point they acquire life—and results—of their own. Mao Tse-Tung once classed conversation as "propaganda." This makes sense, presuming that eventually one of the conversational parties is a decision-maker.
>
> A seminar on diagnosis in social work creates no problems for me. But when a graduate of this seminar, in his capacity of probation officer, submits a presentence report, I would argue that he may become a propagandist, and must cope with this danger.

The main point to be made about labels that go on record, says Toch, is "that they stick." "Even if we can forget to use labels—or pretend to—we cannot depend on our colleague down the assembly line. He may be more desperate or have less time, or he may be under pressure to produce." But since Toch told this to a panel at the American Psychological Association in

1969, the methods of labeling have become more standardized, and the labels have been fed into computers to ensure that the typologies will stick.

About fifteen years ago a popular but well-researched study of the industry that assesses personality and fits individuals into categories, "brain watching," became a best-seller, but all the misuses of behavioral science that it cites still flourish and the industry is now far larger than the $50,000,000-a-year affair at which it was then estimated. Some of the abuses described in *The Brain Watchers* (Gross, 1962) at that time were (1) the imputation of homosexuality by responses on a masculinity-feminity scale that indicated the subject liked art galleries and would not enjoy being in a posse pursuing a bandit; (2) the estimation of executive abilities to subjects who showed a greater interest in Henry Ford than in Florence Nightingale; (3) the evaluation of a school child by his or her agreement or disagreement with such statements as, "the things that some of my family have done have embarrassed me."

At the time *The Brain Watchers* was published, 15 medical schools were using personality tests in processing applicants and 11 others indicated that they were interested in using such testing. For 6 years the State University of New York College of Medicine in Brooklyn had asked applicants to draw a figure, and on the basis of the drawing a psychologist answered the question: Are there indications that he has sufficient resources to stand up under the inevitable stresses of medical school, or would his sensitiveness and human insecurities be too heavily taxed? (The medical school had abandoned the test as not helpful, but no amends were made to the applicants who had been rejected in part because they had not drawn the right figure.)

Candidates for theological schools and Catholic seminaries have been tested and categorized as acceptable or nonacceptable as students; in many localities candidates for police and fire jobs are routinely psychologically assessed.

In the years since *The Brain Watchers* appeared, the marketing of easy pencil tests of personality and pathology has continued and grown, the commerical potential has received even more exploitation, and use has extended into areas further and further removed from professional scrutiny. Schools and correctional institutions particularly rely on testing instruments of doubtful validity and bypass psychiatrists, psychologists, and social workers in the process. An advertising brochure comes across my desk; it is directed to users in "both clinic and nonclinic settings." "Do you need to measure differences among antisocial individuals? Do you need a test that makes sense to everyone? Do you need help in diagnosis, counseling or research with criminals or youth offenders? If you do, they you need the Bipolar Psychological Inventory, a 45-minute, 300-item test that will give the testee's "bipolar dimensions" in regard to lie/honest, defense/open, psychic pain/psychic comfort, depression/optimism, self-degradation/self esteem, dependence/self-sufficiency, unmotivated/achieving; socially withdrawn/gregariousness, family discord/family harmony, sexual immaturity/sexual maturity, social deviancy/social conformity, impulsiveness/self-control, hostility/kindness, and insensitivity/empathy. One version of the test also gives a problem index for the subject. It is easy to administer, score, and interpret; machine scoring is possible; it has proven useful "as an aid in counseling, diagnosis, and as a research tool." The Bipolar Psychological Inventory Booklets are $.50, the answer sheets $.10, the adminstration manual $2.00, the keys of hand scoring $5.00, the profile sheets $.05 and $.07, and the individual scale items $1.00 (Psychological Resources, 1977). What is not described in the brochure is how many criminals and youthful offenders have been diagnosed, classified, assigned, granted parole, or refused parole on the basis of their penciled-in responses.

The determination of "illness" status—the so-called stigmatization of the mental patient—leads, as I have noted, to difficulties in securing a job, pursuing interpersonal relationships, and securing competent psychiatric help—and that in turn leads to alienation, more symptoms, and further discrimination. Mental health professionals and ex-mental patients feel bitter about discrimination against those who have been labeled "mentally ill" or who have been labeled "recovered from mental illness." These who may need a job most find the most impediments placed in their way. In the report of the Joint Commission on Mental Illness and Health (1961), the disadvantages that stigmatization usually brings are stressed:

> The nonconformist—whether he be foreigner or "odd ball," intellectual or idiot, genius or jester, individualist or hobo, physically or mentally abnormal—pays a penalty for "being different," unless his peculiarity is considered acceptable for his particular group, or unless he lives in a place or period of particularly high tolerance or enlightenment. The socially visible characteristic of the psychotic person is that he becomes a stranger among his own people. . . .
>
> The principle of *sameness* as applied to the mentally sick versus the physically sick and the mentally sick versus the mentally well has become a cardinal tenet of mental health education. But this principle has largely fallen on deaf ears. . . . The "deaf ears" of society translate in less anatomical terms as the "stigma of insantiy." It has been observed countless times that the sight or thought of major mental illness, as our culture has come to understand it, stimulates fear—fear of what an irrational person might do, fear of what we ourselves might do if we acted out our impulses in a similar manner, fear arising from the power of suggestion that we, too, might suffer a similar fate. (pp. 59–60)

The report says that the social stigma of mental illness is a real and persistent problem, that evidence of this includes the fact that although mental institutions are called "hospitals," the patients who are released are regarded very differently from "ordinary" convalescents.

The answer to the problem of rejection and stigmatization, according to *Action for Mental Health,* is to admit that mental patients are different and to try to come to terms with this difference in a rational way. The report states that it is not so much that the mental patient has strange symptoms—many other people in society have equally strange symptoms—but that his behavior has reached a point where "people can no longer stand it:"

> It is not so much that he physically endangers them (though they may fear this); violence is more the exception than the rule among psychotic patients, popular misconceptions to the contrary. Basically, normal people are disturbed by his refusal to comply with expectations of time and place. . . . The mentally ill tend to require other people to adjust to them at every point in their illness from onset to recovery.

However, stigmatization and the effects of stigmatization do not disappear as easily as this indicates. Other workers on the problem of stigma see it as a more entrenched phenomenon and they would see the solution to the problem as related to defining fewer people as mentally ill. Since stigma is a real phenomenon and since it affects people permanently, then it becomes more important to be sure that the diagnoses, the labeling, and the profiles have validity and are being applied properly, and it becomes important that confidentiality should be observed so that mental patients, if they wish, can preserve their anonymity and masquerade as nonpatients rather than revealing their status.

Edward Sagarin (1976), sociologist, has said we do people a disservice when we ask them to accept their labels without shame because the labels give only an imputed identity—an alcoholic, a schizophrenic, a drug addict, a homosexual, a sadomasochist, a pedophile, a juvenile delinquent—which he calls a "special kind of mistaken identity." According to this argument, when we label someone a thief we do it on the basis of his actions and we do not see his total identity as thief but only a part of his identity, but when we label someone schizophrenic or homosexual and then convince the person that he has this identity, we are locking him into an at least partially—or very incomplete—false category and we are giving it a changeless character.

Phillips (1963) has pointed out that the utilization of certain kinds of psychiatric help involves not only the possible reward of securing help but the possible cost of rejection by others and a negative self-image. In his study of attitudes in a southern New England town, townspeople rejected other members of the community in direct relationship to the professionalism and specialization of the source of help—someone consulting a clergyman would be least rejected, with more rejection for those consulting physicians and still more for those consulting psychiatrists and the most rejection reserved for those who sought help in mental hospitals. Such stigmatization may be unfortunate in some ways, but to change it would mean changing established attitudes that are not entirely irrational and that act to serve the patient as well as to harm him. A study conducted among 127 supervisors in Philadelphia showed that almost 6 out of 10 felt that even if an employee had a good rating, the knowledge that he was seeing a psychiatrist would be a hindrance and would be likely to rule out a promotion. The supervisors included 55 government supervisors. The responses were more negative toward mental illness than if the employee was obese; had a major limp, a heart ailment, a facial twitch, or a history of asthma attacks; was under treatment for a noticeable skin cancer; was half of a racially mixed marriage; was an atheist; wore a long beard; was 60 years old; had a foreign accent; or smoked marijuana on weekends. The mentally ill and homosexuals were seen as equally unlikely to be recommended for a promotion. Half of the supervisors would make a note of the mental illness problem in the employee's record (Snider, 1975). To study a hierarchy of prejudices, John L. Tringo (1970) of the University of Kentucky tested 455 people—including rehabilitation workers—to find which disabilities they found to be most and least acceptable. Those with ulcers, arthritis, asthma, diabetes, or heart disease, as well as amputees, the blind and the deaf, and stroke and cancer victims were the most acceptably disabled. Those with old age, paraplegia, epilepsy, or cerebral palsy, and those who were dwarfs or hunchbacks ranged from the middle downward on the list. The five least acceptable of the 21 kinds of disabled were the tubercular, ex-convicts, the mentally retarded, alcoholics, and at the very bottom of the list, those with mental illness.

Unless patients are stigmatized as being different, they have no claim to the benefits of their status as mental patients—free or low-cost psychiatric services, special job protections, freedom from responsibility for some criminal actions, vocational and rehabilitation programs. There is no way to consider mental patients and former mental patients as just like everyone else for the purpose of public acceptance but also as unlike everyone else so they can receive special benefits.

Patients feel the conflict between stigma and reward when they are asked to allow insurance companies to have information about them so they can be reimbursed for treatment expenses. Releasing the information may lead to stigma, but the financial reward makes the risk tolerable.

In many situations there is little reward, and often the stigmas create great harm. Studies done on the effect of brief psychiatric hospitalization on poor patients who do not have resources of family and friends show that often only a few days' absence from job and lodging place will mean the job has been given to another, the room has been rented to another, personal possessions have disappeared, life has been completely disrupted. At all socioeconomic levels, the effect of having been labeled mentally ill can be crippling or catastrophic. Says Goffman (1963), "Ex-mental patients . . .

are sometimes afraid to engage in sharp interchanges with spouse or employer because of what a show of emotion might be taken as a sign of" (p. 15). He tells us of former mental patients securing jobs through the help of a rehabilitation service but leaving these jobs when they have a little money saved up so they can find work in a situation where their former status will not be known (p. 94).

The bitterness that mental patients and former mental patients feel concerning their rejection is not only confined to those who have had serious "illness"—who have been hospitalized or who have had to interrupt carreers or schooling. Psychiatrists know that many people who consult them are much less "sick" than many or most of the general population. If these patients had decided not to be "patients" but "clients" or "parishioners" and had taken their problems to a social worker, a pastoral counselor, or a faith healer, they would not have incurred appreciable stigma. Their problems in living would not have been defined as medical and there would be no "illness" on their record. Some patients who want the services of a psychiatrist or a psychoanalyst pass up medical insurance benefits to which they are entitled—in the case of one of my psychoanalytic patients a matter of thousands of dollars yearly over a number of years—so that their status as patient would not be on any public or corporation record. The ubiquitous questionnaires that ask, "Have you ever consulted a physician for a physical or emotional or mental condition?" do not take account of those who should have and haven't, or those who are able to answer "no" because they have taken their problems to an encounter group, a sensitivity-training session, an ert seminar, or a consciousness-raising group—and so have escaped the discriminatory effect of seeking "help."

Goffman (1963) has written about the difference between the discredited person, who is seen when he presents himself as obviously abnormal, and the discreditable person, whose differentness is not immediately apparent and is not known beforehand. The discredited individual has the task of managing the tensions caused by the reaction of others to his differentness; the discreditable individual has a completely different kind of task—that of managing information about his failing:

> To display or not to display; to tell or not to tell; to let on or not to let on; to lie or not to lie; and in each case, to whom, how, when, and where. . . . [I]t is not that he must face prejudice against himself, but rather that he must face unwitting acceptance of himself by individuals who are prejudiced against persons of the kind he can be revealed to be. (p. 42)

So the mental patient or the ex-mental patient often "passes," or at least he tries to. Some patients or ex-patients want to be accepted with full knowledge of their status—sometimes to the point of volunteering information that will surely cost them the job, the acceptance of their school application, or their entrance into a licensed or regulated profession. Some would have liked to "pass" but had a failure of nerve when they thought of the penalties they could incur by lying on an application for federal employment and the less severe penalties that can occur for giving false information to less official questioners. (Applicants for the State of Georgia Bar examination, like applicants in many other states, are required to answer such questions as "Have you within the past ten years undergone treatment or consulted any doctor about the use of drugs, narcotics, or intoxicating liquors? If so, please state the approximate dates, details, circumstances and names and addresses of the doctors so consulted. Have you ever received diagnosis of amnesia, or any form of insanity, emotional disturbance, nervous or mental disorder? Have you ever received regular treatment for any of these conditions? If so, please state the names and addresses of the psychologists, psychiatrists, or other medical practitioners who treated you." Law students applying to take the bar who have had treatment for some emotional problem—very common in our therapeutically oriented society—consider it an invasion of the privacy of their relationship with their therapist, although there is no known instance of this information having been used to keep an applicant from taking the examination or from being admitted to the bar. (There are instances of barring of applicants in other jurisdictions.) The applicant does not like to have this information on record, he does not know what the precise use of the information will be, and he suspects that if he says he has been in treatment he will be asked to sign a release of information that will authorize his therapist to share details about his treatment with the State Board of Bar Examiners of Georgia.

(A year ago some students consulted me about this, and I wrote a letter asking the Emory Student Bar Association to consider initiating action or securing support to have these questions eliminated. The Student Bar Association has not taken any action, so the inequity is allowed to persist.

(There are many good arguments against this intrusive practice. I outlined some of them in my letter to the Student Bar Association. It penalizes those who have sought help, even though those who have not sought help may be more severe "psychological risks." It penalizes those who seek help from psychologists or psychiatrists or other physicians in contrast to those who seek help from other less professional sources. It puts the treating therapist who receives the release of information form in an extremely difficult situation; he does not feel he has the right not to release information after the patient has authorized the release, but he feels he is being forced into an unprofessional stance in retailing confidences. It places the therapist at times in a position where he has to divulge information harmful to the patient—a violation of the Hippocratic injunction to "do no harm"—or alternatively has to give a false picture of the patient to the inquirer. It raises a complicated informed consent question—if the patient had not been coerced or if he knew what was going to be divulged, would he have signed the release of information form? It blackmails the therapist into giving information because if he refuses to give information he may be blocking the professional progress of his patient or at least he may be giving the impression that there is something to hide.)

Most patients and ex-patients, if they feel they are not incurring the possibility of too great a penalty for lying, will not give truthful answers to questions about psychiatric treatment. Psychiatric hospitalization is more difficult to dodge; this is often a matter of public record. By concealing any or all of his mental health background, the person escapes being discredited, but he is in the uneasy position of living a lie and knowing that he is in danger of having this information discovered. Dr. Jerome Biegler, chairman of the committees on confidentiality of both the American Psychiatric Association and the American Psychoanalytic Association, testifying before a government commission on the protection of privacy, has said that people who have been treated for emotional problems should try to keep this information out of the their job records. "It is common knowledge," Biegler (1976) has said, "that promising young corporate executives dare not take advantage of insurance coverage for psychotherapy lest their employers stigmatize them for having a disorder of mental health and arrest their careers." If the former patient fails to reveal his psychiatric history he can have his career arrested, and if he reveals it he can have his career arrested.

Here are some of the discriminations that have been practiced against mental patients, some with justifiable rationales, some without:

1. There has been discrimination against addicts and alcoholics in the job market.

2. The history of mental illness has kept many patients and former patients from getting jobs and from being able to rent housing.

3. There has been widespread zoning discrimination against halfway houses and addict rehabilitation centers.

4. There is job discrimination against homosexuals.

5. Parents, particularly mothers, who have had a history of mental illness are often deprived of their children in custody disputes.

6. In 1972 the regulations of the Commissioned Corps of the Public Health Service denied appointments for individuals in psychotherapy. (This ruling under a full disclosure policy would have disqualified 15 to 20% of the students at some medical schools and an even higher percentage of medical students planning to become psychiatrists.)

7. State regulations promulgated in 1971 for all licensed and practical nurses in Pennsylvania required that all those admitted to a hospital for psychiatric treatment were to be reported so that licenses would be suspended and all nurses in outpatient treatment were to be reported with a statement to describe the level at which they could function. Because of opposition to these regulations, the outpatient regulation was modified so

outpatients who were not incapacitated in the performance of their nursing duties would not have to be reported but those who were incapacitated would have to be reported.

8. Until very recently the government pursued a policy of discrimination against job applicants who had received psychiatric help—although contradictorily it allowed jobholders great liberty in securing psychiatric therapy on office time and great assistance in paying for the therapy; a liberal government policy pays 80% of the cost of psychiatric treatment.

In questions having to do with job applications and qualifying for professional licensure, there is a gray area where one can surmise that the stigma of the psychiatric diagnosis or history has been the reason for rejection, but the applicant cannot be sure since the rejection is justified on some other ground. The most interesting case on discrimination against former mental patients is *Glassman* v. *New York Medical College*.[3] Myra Lee Glassman graduated from college Phi Beta Kappa and magna cuma laude and was in the 99th perentile in the Medical Aptitude Test. But she was even smarter and more qualified for medical school than this indicates. Her lawyer, Bruce Ennis, in courtroom testimony obtained the admissions from the Medical College that Myra Lee was quite possibly the only member of Phi Beta Kappa among its 2,870 applicants that year, and that she had placed 12th in a statewide New York test for college graduates who demonstrated exceptional promise for medical school, an award shared by less than 8% of the successful applicants; Dr. Benjamin Sadock admitted on the witness stand that her Medical College Admission Test score placed her within the upper 8% of those applicants who had been accepted for the class and that she may have had the highest score—neither he nor anyone he had talked with knew of any other applicant with as high a score or higher. She gave the truthful answer in her application to New York Medical College that she had been in a mental hospital. She had spent a year between her sophomore and junior years as a voluntary patient at Hillside Hospital. The Medical College claimed that she had made two suicide attempts—although Myra Lee described them not as attempts but as gestures—and established that she had interrupted her undergraduate studies for 14 months while she was an undergraduate; during this time she was in psychiatric treatment. New York Medical College was one of the 13 schools she applied to that rejected her.

Three psychiatrists and a clinical psychologist who had been one of her college professors, all of whom were aware of her psychiatric history, recommended her for medical school without reservations. Their recommendations had been glowing. (Dr. Richard Green, clinical director of the adult inpatient services at Hillside, submitted an affidavit for the later trial point-

[3]*Glassman* v. *New York Medical College*, 64 Misc. 2d 466, 315 N.Y.S. 1 (1970).

ing out that Myra Lee was "better equipped to deal with the rigors of medical school than most other applicants" because she had succeeded in recovering from the effects of emotional stress that are likely to affect everyone at some point in life. Nicholas Papouchia, a clinical psychologist who had been a professor of Myra Lee's at City College, told the court in his affidavit that he found "no evidence in her behavior that would indicate any difficulty handling the rigors of medical school training or the professional demands of medical practice. Her capacity to work independently, as indicated in the course of the semester, suggested, rather, that she would be an asset to any medical school." Other professors saw her as an "unusually mature, well-adjusted student" and saw no reason "to question her emotional stability." Two independent psychiatrists who examined Myra Lee for purposes of the trial found her completely qualified for medical school. They minimized her past illness by describing her condition as "an adjustment reaction of adolescence" and by stating that the suicide "attempts" had been to manipulate the situation but had not been veritable attempts because they had not been designed to put her life in danger. They found no evidence of any psychiatric condition that would impair her current or future functioning). For purposes of her trial Myra Lee submitted to an examination by two independent psychiatrists and one psychologist, who gave as their opinions that her past history of mental illness would not have an adverse effect on her future in medical school or in the medical profession. Court testimony brought out that she had been interviewed by two members of the New York Medical College faculty, one of whom, Dr. Raymond McBride, had found her a "most impressive person" and had "strongly" recommended her acceptance but who had also recommended a psychiatric interview. That interview was conducted by the psychiatric consultant to the admissions committee, Dr. Benjamin Sadock. Dr. Sadock is one of the co-authors of the widely used *Comprehensive Textbook of Psychiatry* (with Alfred Freedman and Harold Kaplan), which decries the use of labeling as a method of social control. It was on his recommendation that she was rejected.

New York had a statute, unlike any statute in any other state at the time. It provided that a mental hospital admission should not be the reason for the deprivation of any civil right including "civil service ranking and appointment or rights relating to the granting, forfeiture or denial of a license, permit, privilege or benefit pursuant to any law." Myra Glassman sued the New York Medical College. (Dr. Sadock was one of the named defendants in the case.) Myra Lee's position was not that her past condition was irrelevant—she felt that the Medical College had a right to consider it—but that her present condition should be the determinant of her admission application and that the Medical College had not considered her current condition. The court held that New York Medical College had not denied

Myra Glassman admission because of her mental hospitalization but because she had interrupted her academic career for 14 months and made two suicide attempts. "If the plaintiff never had been admitted to a mental hospital but had indicated that she had interrupted her career for over 14 months and that she had made two attempts at suicide, she would have been rejected by the Admissions Committee as a risk to a successful completion of her medical courses and as a practicing physician."[4] Not past medical history but an "aggregate of factors" was behind the rejection, said the court, and "the determination as to what factors should enter into the standards set for college admission was within the exclusive province of the college authorities. The judicial task ends when it is found that the applicant has received from the college authorities uniform treatment under reasonable regulations fairly administered."[5]

The court decision does not mention some other pertinent factors in Myra Lee Glassman's background, which Bruce Ennis, her lawyer, relates in his *Prisoners of Psychiatry* (Ennis, 1972, pp. 162–176). (The chapter is entitled "Stigma.") Her parents had been Orthodox Jews and she had attended the Yeshiva of Flatbush, a Hebrew parochial high school. Much of her conflict with her parents while she was in college was about her deviation from Orthodox Judaism. Ennis quotes one psychiatrist who saw her as attributing her difficulties to "a sadistic, guilt-provoking, and dependent mother," and although I am skeptical of the validity of dynamic formulations without considerable evidence, it seems plausible that, as Myra Lee herself would testify, her emotional problems had been related to her movement toward independence and her conflicts about separation from her parents. She would testify that her hospitalization was the result of a psychiatrist's recommendation that she should live away from home and her inability to follow the recommendation by less drastic alternatives. She denied the seriousness of the suicide "attempts" and pointed out that both times that she took an overdose of medication her condition was not seen as sufficiently risky to warrant pumping her stomach. Her estrangement from her parents went so deep that during the year she was at Hillside they visited her only three times, although they lived near the hospital. Following her hospitalization she had completed the last 2 years of college with highest scholastic honors.

(The New York Medical College did not have the benefit of later research, but a study done of 116 students from the University of Michigan who in the period from 1958 to 1967 were hospitalized in acute treatment centers in Ann Arbor because of profound emotional disturbances showed that compared to a control group of students without an interruption in their

[4]*Glassman v. New York Medical College*, p. 4.
[5]*Glassman v. New York Medical College*, pp. 4–5.

studies, the effect of hospitalization was minimal. The study speaks of such "prejudicial policies of not admitting or readmitting students who have had or are undergoing psychotherapy, of requiring dropouts to remain away from scholastic pursuits for prescribed periods of time, or of requiring them to obtain and maintain jobs for a definite duration." The research indicated that emotional problems, even those serious enough to require hospitalization, have essentially no effect upon academic success; similar conclusions were reached in a study at Harvard [Nicholi, 1967; Reinhard, Lohr, Schaefer, Burlinger, & Huddleston, 1972]).

Before she brought suit, Ennis had asked the college to reconsider her application taking only present mental condition into consideration. The Medical College had refused.

On the witness stand Myra Lee told of a remarkable hospital and posthospital history. After several months in the hospital, while still an inpatient, she had begun to work 20 hours a week as a biochemistry research assistant for a Hillside doctor who had a grant to study drug metabolics and hormones. While still in the hospital she had resumed classes at City College and earned A's in two 4-credit-hour courses—comparative anatomy and honors economics. In the summer of 1967 she had left Hillside, found an apartment, found a job in a federal poverty program as a counselor for disturbed children, and earned two more A's in summer school. In the fall of 1967 she returned to full-time studies at City College while supporting herself with a job at the Jewish Guild for the Blind.

The story that Dr. Sadock told on the witness stand was equally remarkable. Although the official minutes of the admissions committee said that Myra Lee had been rejected because of an "ongoing" psychiatric illness, he denied telling the admissions committee that she had an ongoing illness. (He had conducted the only psychiatric examination for the school.) He conceded that he had not performed a mental status examination or made any current diagnosis. His report to the admissions committee had concluded, on the basis of the history of hospitalization, "probable diagnosis of latent schizophrenia," although the DSM–II clearly limits the diagnosis to people who have "clear symptoms of schizophrenia." Dr. Sadock admitted on the witness stand that in Myra Lee's interview with him she had appeared perfectly normal and did not exhibit "any withdrawn, regressive, or bizarre behavior." Asked to explain his diagnosis, he said on the stand:

> As I said, I did not do a history and mental status. I am not prepared to say that Miss Glassman is schizophrenic. What I am prepared to report to you is this fact, that most hospital admissions carry a diagnosis for schizophrenia. The majority of people who have been in mental hospitals in a particular age group, her age group, have a diagnosis of schizophrenia, and it was on that, sir, that I made that comment. . . . I did not make that comment on the basis of a history

and a mental status. I am not prepared at this point to defend a diagnosis of
schizophrenia in Miss Glassman. . . . I trust she does not have that illness.

He testified that she was an academic and emotional risk because
people who have interrupted their college careers are less likely to graduate
from college than those who have not (but she had already graduated from
college) and that persons who had attempted suicide were more likely to
commit suicide than persons who have not (although all the evidence indicated these were not real suicide attempts).

So the stigma of past psychiatric hospitalization was enough to cause
Myra Lee to be rejected by New York Medical College (as well as 12 other
medical schools) and the unsupported word of one psychiatrist was used to
label her as having an ongoing mental illness and to reject her on this basis.

By the time the decision against her was announced 6 months after the
court hearing, Myra Lee had been accepted by a midwestern school for an
unusual joint program in which she could receive medical and pharmacological degrees in 5 years of postgraduate study so her case was never
appealed. Bruce Ennis reported that after 2 years in the program she had
earned honors in most of her courses and superior grades in all the rest.

Myra Lee Glassman was luckier than most people who are rejected on
the basis of past psychiatric histories. Usually they do not have the legal
resources or the willingness to be in the limelight to pursue legal remedies,
and they accordingly never find out the basis of their failure to be employed,
to get into school, or to receive some other kind of advancement.

There are a few signs that psychiatrists are becoming more aware of
the harm they can do to patients by furnishing stigmatizing information.
The Blue Cross in Washington, D.C., has had a policy of requiring much
detail from a therapist before it would pay for mental health benefits under
the Federal Employees Program. The therapist was required to answer
questions of the patient's family and social life, presence of suicidal tendencies, and degree of anxiety and depression. A therapist in Maryland wrote
to Blue Cross indicating he would not disclose the information for three of
his patients and sent a copy of his letter to his congressman. Blue Cross had
consistently maintained that the information it collected would in no circumstances be made available to outside sources. When Blue Cross answered the therapist, it sent a carbon of the letter—with the names of the
three patients neatly typed in the letter—to the same congressman. The
Blue Cross later announced a change in its policy; it withdrew the questions
from the insurance claims forms. The change in policy was made after the
Mental Health Law Project threatened a class action suit against Blue
Cross, citing the cases of a number of people who had not entered treatment
or had terminated treatment because of the threat of this intrusion into their
privacy. Paul Friedman, in this case, speaking for the Mental Health Law

Project, said he saw a serious inconsistency between the attitude of psychiatrists who were anxious to get insurance reimbursement for their patients' fees and the same psychiatrists' attitude when other kinds of threats to confidentiality were the issue (Blue Cross, 1977a,b,).

We have embarked on a new phase of our treatment of the mentally disabled and other handicapped people. Possibly the rejection that Myra Lee Glassman received could no longer occur under new government regulations that were announced in April 1977, when Joseph Califano, Jr., secretary of Health, Education and Welfare, promulgated a controversial set of regulations designed to implement the Rehabilitation Act of 1973, banning discrimination against the handicapped by those receiving federal funds.

Under the regulations all programs supported in whole or in part by federal funds—which include federally supported schools, colleges, graduate schools, health and welfare institutions—are not allowed to discriminate against the handicapped. The handicapped comprise an estimated 35 million Americans, many of whom have physical handicaps—and public buildings are being remodeled extensively to give them access to all parts—as well as the psychoneurotically disabled, the psychotically disabled, the retarded, alcoholics (10 million of these), and drug addicts (1.5 million of these). Programs or activities in existing facilities must be made available to the handicapped. Employers may not refuse to hire handicapped persons if reasonable accommodations can be made for them and if the handicap does not impair the ability of the job applicant or the employer. Employers may not require preemployment physical examinations and may not make preemployment inquiries about whether or not a person is handicapped. Colleges and universities must make reasonable modifications in academic requirements to ensure full opportunities for handicapped students. Doctors who treat Medicare or Medicaid patients must make their offices accessible to the handicapped or go to accessible facilities to treat them, even if that means making house calls. How all this applies to the mentally disabled, alcholic, and addict population is not clear and will have to be worked out through court cases.

The concept of continuing to differentiate the mentally disabled, the alcoholics, and the addicts by labeling them but refusing to let these labels be used to hurt the individual is humanitarian, but it disregards many aspects of mental illness and drug and alcohol abuse—that the prevention of discrimination may require individuals who do not want to hire the mentally ill, the alcoholic, and the addict to hire them, and they will feel that their autonomy is being taken away; that the definition of these conditions and the differentiation of the degree of handicap is hard to fix; that the freezing of these individuals into these disabled categories may work against the possibility of improvement; that the responsibility of the government to secure redress for the individual relieves him of the responsibility of doing for himself (Regulations, 1977).

It is easy to see how the new regulations will be implemented as far as paraplegics, the crippled, the deaf, the blind, those suffering from heart conditions, and other physically handicapped are concerned; in some cases special teaching programs or training programs and accommodations in physical structures designed to facilitate movement will be all that is necessary. It is much more difficult to know how alcoholics, drug addicts, and the mentally ill will be aided by the new regulations. The regulations prohibit discrimination by the covered institutions and agencies in hiring and promotions, but in order to benefit from the regulation the person must "qualify" for available employment. Probably it was in response to the controversy caused by the inclusion, after years of debate, of the mentally ill, drug addicts, and alcoholics that Attorney General Griffin Bell advised the Department of Health, Education and Welfare that the new regulations do not require that a person "be hired or permitted to participate in a Federally assisted program if the manifestations of his condition prevent him from effectively performing the job. . . ." Bell stated that behavior that was "unduly disruptive to others" would not be covered under the new rules (Hicks, 1977; Mosher, 1977).

The new regulations provide for a great government superstructure to ensure compliance and to investigate and hear complaints. Each recipient of federal funds must keep records and file compliance reports to show that it is not discriminating; HEW officials are given access to records so they can police the practices; information must be made available to the disabled; investigations are to be made periodically and also on the basis of complaints; a hearing procedure has been set up with such safeguards as timely notice and the right to counsel; provisions for hearing examiners and for review of their decisions have been set up. We know discrimination is an evil; we do not yet know whether the procedures to do away with the discrimination will be workable.

Before the new regulations, a number of actions concerning discrimination against the mentally ill, addicts, and alcoholics were brought under the civil rights law. *Beazer* v. *New York City Transit Authority* was a case that resulted in the hiring of a heroin addict by the New York City Transit Authority after attorneys from the Legal Action Center of New York and a Columbia law school professor had brought a suit on his behalf.[6] The New York City Transit Authority had had a blanket policy of not hiring former heroin addicts. The basis for the successful suit to force Beazer's hiring was the contention that such a policy had a discriminatory impact on blacks and Hispanics. After winning the case, the successful attorneys petitioned the court for an award from the New York City Transit Authority of the legal

[6]*Beazer* v. *New York City Transit Authority,* No. 72 Civ. 5307 (S.D.N.Y. Jan. 13, 1977).

fees Beazer had incurred in fighting for the job. The court, after taking into consideration the financial difficulties of the troubled New York Transit Authority, awarded the attorneys $375,000, which represented an incentive award of $75,000 for righting this civil wrong and $300,000 for approximately 4,500 hours of work on the basis of $60 an hour for lawyers with 2 to 4 years experience, $100 an hour for lawyers will 9 to 11 years of experience, and $110 an hour for a lawyer with 15 years of experience. One of the issues the court considered in setting the fee was whether there should be a reduction of the award because plaintiff's attorneys were salaried employees of a public interest law firm receiving outside funding; the decision was that there should not be. (Attorneys' Fees, 1977).

The field of discrimination against the mentally disabled will be a fruitful field of law, and lawyers will be favorable to this new policy. Psychiatrists who consider the matter may see it as another diversion of the mental health dollar, which is increasingly being diverted from patient care to patient protection. Psychiatric institutions and agencies will find the new policies irksome because they will have to hire many varieties of the disabled—the argument could be made that former patients and addicts and alcoholics have a special claim to jobs in hospitals, community mental health centers, and treatment programs.

Psychiatrists will be kept busy evaluating the degrees of disability, separating the handicapped from the nonhandicapped. The problem of stigma has been dealt with by increasing the benefits of the stigmatization; a more promising approach would have been to devise ways of keeping the condition of patients and former patients out of public records, by decreasing the numbers of people who were subject to stigma instead of by devising complicated ways of securing redress for the effects of stigmatization.

The new antidiscrimination regulations apply only to agencies and institutions that receive federal funds. Discrimination can continue in private employment. There may be good reasons for this discrimination; possibly an employer is within his rights in preferring to hire someone who has not been an addict rather than someone who has been an addict if two applicants have similar qualifications. Many recovered mental patients are fragile and they may be temperamental, touchy, and generally less desirable as employees than people who have been more stable. There are good economic reasons for not hiring the formerly mentally ill or those who are in psychotherapy. The health insurance costs of the employee may be raised and this creates an additional burden for the employer. We get into a vicious circle here: those who need employment most because they have suffered from a disability and have been stigmatized are selectively kept from employment, and as a result they do not have the health insurance, access to good living quarters, work relationships, job satisfactions, and other benefits of employment that help maintain their stability. (The same kind of discrimination keeps heart attack victims and other physically handicapped people from competing equally in the private sector of the job market.) There are few judicial precedents, statutes, regulations, or constitutional provisions that will help the disabled or formerly disabled. There are rehabilitation and vocational training programs and welfare benefits, but they involve emphasizing the status of handicapped.

Forcing private employees to employ the disabled would raise issues of invasion of privacy and problems of enforcement. It is often easy for the applicant to be turned down for another reason or an aggregate of reasons, not because of the psychiatric history. Stigmatization will continue to be a problem; discrimination will continue to exist. The need for psychiatrists to be more certain of their diagnoses and evaluation procedures and to preserve confidentiality will continue to be paramount. Most patients will want to continue to attempt to "pass." The best protection for the former patient will be not public acceptance of his patienthood but assurance that the fact that he was ever a patient will be kept secret. Even better would be to try narrowing and confining of the definition of mental illness so that the labels "patient" or "former patient" need never have been incurred at all.

References

American Psychiatric Association. *Diagnostic and statistical manual of mental disorders* (DSM-II). Washington: American Psychiatric Association, 1968.

Attorneys' fees of $375,000 awarded in suit against transit company for failure to employ former heroin addicts. *Clearinghouse Review,* June 1977, p. 159.

Becker, H. Becoming a marihuana user. In D. Creasy & D. Ard (Eds.), *Delinquency, crime, and social process.* New York: Harper & Row, 1969.

Biegler, J. Quoted in Keep a low emotional profile. *Business Week,* August 23, 1976, p. 73.

Blue Cross to withdraw sensitive queries from form. *Psychiatric News,* July 1, 1977, p. 1. (a)

Blue Cross/Blue Shield gives in on a privacy issue. *Behavior Today,* July 4, 1977, p. 5. (b)

Diagnosis of neurotic depression said to be vague, no longer of clinical value. *Clinical Psychiatry News,* June 1977, p. 1.

Ennis, B. *Prisoners of psychiatry.* New York: Harcourt, Brace, Jovanovich, 1972.

Freedman, A., Kaplan, H., & Sadock, B. *Modern synopsis of comprehensive textbook of psychiatry/II.* Baltimore: Williams & Wilkins, 1976.

Friedrich, O. *Going crazy.* New York: Simon & Schuster, 1975.

Gilman, S.D (Ed.). *The face of madness: Hugh W. Diamond and the Origin of Psychiatric Photography.* New York: Brunner/Mazel, 1976.

Goffman, E. *Asylums.* Garden City, N.Y.: Anchor Books, 1961.

Goffman, E. *Stigma.* Englewood Cliffs, N.J.: Prentice-Hall, 1963.

Greenberg, J. How accurate is psychiatry? *Science News,* July 9, 1977, pp. 28–29.

Gross, M. *The brain watchers.* New York: Random House, 1962.

Heller, J. *Catch-22.* New York: Simon & Schuster, 1955.

Hicks, N. Equity for disabled likely to be costly. *New York Times,* May 1, 1977, p. 29.

Hoch, P., & Polatin, P. Pseudoneurotic forms of schizophrenia. *Psychiatric Quarterly,* 1949, 23, 248–276.

Joint Commission on Mental Illness and Health. *Action for mental health.* New York: Basic Books, 1961.

Knight, R. Borderline states. *Bulletin of the Menninger Clinic*, 1953, *17*, 1–12.

Kraepelin, E. *Lectures on clinical psychiatry* (Thomas Johnstine, Rev. and Ed.). New York: Hafner, 1968. (Originally published, 1904.)

Krause, E. *Power and illness: The political sociology of medical care.* New York: Elsevier, 1977.

Lax, R. The role of internalization in the development of certain aspects of female masochism: Ego psychological considerations. *International Journal of Psycho-Analysis*, 1977, *58*, 289–300; 292.

Leifer, R. *In the name of mental health.* New York: Science House, 1969.

Mosher, L. The high cost of aiding the handicapped. *National Observer*, May 16, 1977, p. 3.

Murphy, J. Psychiatric labeling in cross-cultural perspective. *Science*, March 12, 1976, pp. 1019–1028; 1027.

Nicholi, A., Jr. The return of the dropout. *American Journal of Psychiatry*, 1967, *124*, 105–112.

Phillips, D. Rejection: A possible consequence of seeking help for mental disorders. *American Sociological Review*, 1963, *28*, 963–972.

Psychological Resources. Mailing. Grein, Utah, 1977.

Regulations of April 26, 1977, implementing § 504, Rehabilitation Act of 1973, 20 U.S.C. 706, 1 *Mental Health Disability Reporter*, No. 5, Part II, March–April 1977.

Reinhart, M., Lohr, N., Schaefer, D., Berlinger, N., & Huddleston, J. Evaluation of academic performance in a neuropsychiatric hospitalized population. *Archives of General Psychiatry*, 1972, *26*, 68–70.

Rich, C. Quoted in Wants "borderline" stricken as psychiatric term because it has multiple meanings. *Clinical Psychiatry News*, February 1977, p. 3.

Rosenhan, D. On being sane in insane places. *Science*. January 19, 1973, pp. 250–258.

Roth, L. Some comments on labeling. *Bulletin of the American Academy of Psychiatry and the Law*, 1975, *3*(3), 123–131.

Sagarin, E. The high personal cost of wearing a label. *Psychology Today*, March 1976, p. 25.

Sarbin, T. The scientific status of the mental illness metaphor. In S. Plog & R. Edgerton (Eds.), *Changing perspectives in mental illness.* New York: Holt, Rinehart & Winston, 1969.

Scheff, T. Learning theory as ideology and as science. In T. Scheff (Ed.), *Labeling madness.* Englewood Cliffs, N.J.: Prentice-Hall, 1975. (a)

Scheff, T. Schizophrenia as ideology. In T. Scheff (Ed.), *Labeling madness.* Englewood Cliffs, N.J.: Prentice-Hall, 1975. (b)

Scheff, T. *Labeling madness.* Englewood Cliffs, N.J.: Prentice-Hall, 1975. (c)

Schmideberg, M. The borderline patient. In S. Arieti (Ed.), *American handbook of psychiatry.* New York: Basic Books, 1959.

Schwartz, R., & Schwartz, I. Are personality disorders diseases? *Diseases of the Nervous System*, 1976, November, 613–617.

Sedgwick, P. Illness—Mental and otherwise. Hastings Center Studies, 1973, *1*(3), 19–40.

Snider, A. Report on a study by Gerald A. Melchiode, Hahnemann Medical College and Hospital: Seeing a shrink? Don't tell the boss. *Atlanta Journal and Constitution*, May 18, 1975, p. 19-C.

Spiegel, J. Psychiatry—A high risk profession (presidential paper). *American Journal of Psychiatry*, 1975, *132*, 693–697; 697.

Spitzer, R. Letter, American Psychiatric Association Task Force on Nomenclature and Statistics, January 3, 1977. (Mimeograph).

Szasz, T. *The myth of mental illness.* New York: Delta, 1967.

Toch, H. The care and feeding of typologies and labels. *Federal Probation*, 1970, September, 15–19.

Tringo, J. The hierarchy of preference towards disability groups. *Journal of Special Education*, 1970, *4*(3), 295–306.

III

Health Needs of Special Groups: Some Specific Examples

Introduction

Students of social epidemiology have long noted that health conditions differ systematically not only among societies but within each society along such demographic variables as age, sex, race, and social class. If different population groups possess distinct health needs, then health delivery systems must be especially adapted to the specialized needs of the group being served.

In this section we have presented several articles that address the unique health needs of special groups—the aged, minorities, traditional population groups possess distinct health needs, then health delivery systems must be especially adapted to the specialized needs of the group being served.

The first chapter, by Havighurst, deals with the special health problems of the aged. He points out that 12 to 15% of those aged 65 or over in North America and Western Europe are "very sick" in the sense that they need constant attention. In this age group chronic illness is more prevalent than acute illness. This condition calls for personally oriented, primary care that preserves the dignity and autonomy of the elderly rather than for high-technology, disease-oriented curative care. In particular, institutionalization tends to undermine the dignity and autonomy of the elderly and to aggravate existing conditions, whether purely physical or mental. Havighurst argues that institutionalization should be avoided as long as it is possible for the elderly to live in their own communities with proper medical care and with some household help.

The next chapter, by Weaver, highlights the racial and ethnic dimension of morbidity. It attempts to account for the higher incidence of such health problems as hypertension and heart disease among some ethnic minorities in the United States. Weaver offers an alternative to the hypothesis of the dysfunctional "health subculture" of some minority groups (e.g., they practice unhealthy dietary habits or avoid modern medicine because it is perceived to conflict with their cultural perceptions). Focusing on the social and economic causes of morbidity and mortality, he hypothesizes that the problems of poverty and discrimination both contribute to the initial onset of disease and restrict access to medical services. Thus, economic factors interact with cultural ones to produce poorer health conditions among minorities. For example, the relatively high incidence of hypertension and cardiovascular problems among Asian-Americans is noted. According to Weaver, this association derives from the interaction of several factors: poor dietary habits, outright discrimination, and a high level of stress responses. This stress is caused by the psychological pressures of acculturation and marginality and from the aberrations of lowered self-esteem to which minority group members are subjected.

Under such circumstances, the role of curative medicine in combating these problems is limited. What is needed, according to Weaver, is a "reordering of society's institutions, priorities, and values" that contribute to the health risks facing minorities.

Turning to an emphasis on the family as the relevant unit for health analysis and planning, Zivetz, in the next chapter, discusses some cultural factors affecting fertility in different societies. She asserts that fertility behavior is an outcome of both technological conditions (the availability of effective contraceptives) and cultural norms regarding optimal family size, the proper role of women, the meaning of family, etc. Reviewing a broad spectrum of contraceptive practices and policies, she emphasizes the importance of cultural attitudes and values—those of society and those of the individual—in motivating men and women to limit family sizes. Among the examples she cites are China's official policy of delayed marriages and the full participation of women in the labor force, and the United States' changing attitudes toward women's role and desired family size. She concludes that effective population control is possible only if both technological factors (the availability of contraception) and cultural factors (the motivation to limit family size) are taken into account.

In the next article David presents an extensive survey of the literature on healthy family functioning, together with a comprehensive bibliography. The survey is organized conceptually around the themes of life cycle phases, psychological stress, and communal coping.

This chapter represents a significant departure from traditional thinking in the field in several respects: First, most scholars and planners have focused on health as an attribute of individuals, whereas David addresses the family as a collective unit with its own dynamics rather than as an aggregate of discrete individuals. Second, most research has focused on mental and social illness in "problem families," while David attempts a positive conceptualization of mentally and socially healthy families.

Healthy family functioning is defined as a family unit that is "effectively coping with cultural-environmental, psychosocial, and socioeconomic stressors throughout the diverse phases of the family life cycle." It is recognized that considerable research is needed to develop satisfactory measures of family effectiveness. Nonetheless, enough is known, according to the author, to warn us against culturally biased definitions of "the family unit," and of complex concepts such as "health" and "unhealth," "functional" and "dysfunctional."

David proposes a cross-cultural approach to the development of a theory of healthy family functioning. This approach would focus on effective decision making in coping with different concerns, based on awareness of relevant contextual information and of available alternatives. Research should concentrate on family units in early stages of the life cycle, since "the basic unit of successful coping and healthy family functioning is likely to be the young family."

The last chapter in this section, by Ahmed and Davis, addresses the special health needs of urban populations in developing countries. The authors attribute the often deplorable health conditions of these populations to the dislocations of rapid urbanization, to the stresses of overcrowding, to environmental (air and water) pollution, and to the generally low standard of living. In addition, they consider several factors that contribute to the ineffectiveness of existing medical care. One such factor is the alienation of the recent rural migrant who is steeped in traditional forms of indigenous healing and is exposed to the unfamiliar processes and impersonal world of modern hospital medicine. Another factor is the prohibitive cost in time, money, travel, and professional specialization of modern medical services, which are more often than not ill-adapted to populations who are at risk and not in need of various services. Significant improvements in the health conditions of the cities of the third world, according to Ahmed and Davis, may result only from broad political, economic, and public health reforms. Political reform is needed in order to place higher priority on the health needs of the urban poor, economic reform in order to improve the standard of living and thereby reduce disease, and public health reform in order to make health services more accessible and more egalitarian. Regionalizing urban health systems, eradicating poverty, and ensuring community participation in health activities are necessary in order to attain health for all.

11

Coping with Health Problems in Aging

Robert J. Havighurst

A national poll made for the National Council on the Aging in 1974 disclosed the fact that poor health is regarded by 21% of people aged 65 and over as a "very serious" personal problem, and 10% report that "not enough medical care" is also a very serious problem for them.

Health Is a Social as Well as a Medical Problem

Elaine Brody, who is director of the Department of Human Services of the Philadelphia Geriatric Center, has written an important paper (1977), in which she says:

> One of the great philosophical thrusts of this century has been toward the concept of the "whole person"—understanding the relationship between psyche and soma, between the individual and the personal, social and physical environment—and that the homeostasis of the whole is affected by a disturbance in any of its parts. Practice approaches such as psychosomatic medicine, family therapy, network therapy (which may include the neighbors, the milkman and the family dog), and multi-disciplinary teams have been developed in order to implement the whole person concept. . . . Now, more than at any other time in history, there is a readiness to accept what might be called a psycho/social/somatic/environmental framework for health.

Robert J. Havighurst • Department of Behavioral Sciences, University of Chicago, Chicago, Illinois 60637.

Viewed from the perspective of older people, the inter-relationships stand out in bold relief because

- medical problems (disease and disability) increase with advancing age,
- those problems play more important roles as determinants of social functioning,
- the elderly are more dependent on and vulnerable to their physical and social environments,
- unlike children whose physical and social dependencies are transitional and are met primarily through the family, a proportionately larger share of the supportive and long-term health/social services needed by older people must be provided by the community.

During the past 30 years, research and experience in gerontology have resulted in the development of a considerable body of knowledge. There is still, of course, vast uncharted territory. But in sorting out where we are, some propositions are so well accepted that, though many subtleties and specific relationships remain to be determined, there is virtually no disagreement in principle.

Of the total body of knowledge, a significant portion concerns the reciprocal inter-dependence of the health of older people and social factors. Just as health has broad social implications, social factors in turn affect the health of the elderly, their families, and society as a whole. The role of social factors is accepted as being of major consequence, though there are no refined indicators of the precise proportions which they contribute to the health of older people, no more than such indicators are available for the contributions of medical conditions or the normal decrements of aging.

M. P. Lawton (1974) has summarized a host of studies that explore the relation of physical health to other types of well-being. "Nothing is more regular," he writes, "than the correlation between health and morale, health and social behavior, or health and leisure time activity."

Health Status of the Elderly

It is known that 12 to 15% of the people aged 65 and over in North America and Western Europe are "very sick" in the sense that they need attention from nurses or family members and cannot be left alone for more than short periods of time. The quantitative data come from surveys made by Ethel Shanas over a period of time from 1957 to 1975.

Shanas, (1962; Shanas et al., 1968; cited also in Anderson, 1976) estimated that among the older population not in institutions, 10% of all older persons interviewed (8% of all men and 12% of all women) were "very sick." As would be expected with advancing age, the proportion of the "very sick" increased from 9% for the age group 65 to 74, to 14% among persons 75 years and over.

Using 10% as the base figure for those interviewed in their homes, the older persons in institutions should also be added. This latter group is usually estimated at 4 to 5% of the persons 65 years of age and over. Thus, the total is roughly 14 to 15% of this age group.

From the age of 60, chronic rather than acute illness is characteristic of people. Chronic illness is incurable but requires treatment to alleviate pain and to help people cope with their condition. Anderson (1976) summarizes the situation in the United States as follows:

Of all discharges from short-stay hospitals reported for Medicare patients, 16% were discharged for diseases of the heart as the primary diagnosis, and 9% for malignancies—in all, one-fourth of all discharges. As is to be expected, hospital admissions increase with age. In the age group from 67 to 68 the discharge rate was 212 per 1,000 population compared with a rate of 370 for the age group 85 years of age and over. In 1973 the admission rate among Medicare patients was 320 per 1,000 population (the rate for the entire population is around 140); the admission rate to nursing homes was 19 per 1,000 population.

A survey by the National Center for Health Statistics estimated that in 1969 there were 815,000 residents 65 years of age and over in 18,000 nursing and personal care homes. More than one-half of nursing home patients were confined to the premises, the bed, or the chair. Further, in the week previous to the survey of all patients (of whom 89% were 65 years of age and over) 22% were given a full-bed bath, 29% were helped with eating, 12% had bowel and bladder retraining, and 19% were given enemas.

Anderson estimated that in 1975 in the United States health care for the population over 65 cost $1,200 per person, compared with $450 per capita for the entire American population. In other words, 10% of the population consumed 30% of the total expenditures for health services.

How do older persons utilize health services? In contrast to the under-65 population, senior citizens are admitted to hospitals about twice as often (in 1970, there were 220 admissions per 1,000 persons over 65 compared to 131 for younger persons); have hospital stays that are about twice as long (in 1970, 11.2 days per stay versus 6.2 days); visit a physician about 50% more often (in 1972, 6.9 visits per year versus 4.8 visits); and see a dentist only about one-half as often (in 1972, .9 visits per year versus 1.6 visits).

Another source of information on the extent of physical disability is found in a report from the National Center for Health Statistics (1975), which gave the data of Table I.

Mental Illness

Finding dependable statistics on the incidence and prevalence of mental illness is difficult. Admission rates to psychiatric services or facilities at best give us figures on utilization, not necessarily on the need for services. The most commonly used method of arriving at estimates of the incidence

Table I.   Persons with Limitations on Activity Caused by Selected
Chronic Conditions: 1972[a]

	All ages	65 Years and over
Persons with limitation (thousands)	25,868	8,613
Percentage limited by		
Heart condition	13.4	18.8
Arthritis and rheumatism	11.2	16.9
Visual impairments	2.3	3.0
Hypertension without heart involvement	2.9	4.0
Mental and nervous condition	3.7	1.7
All persons: percentage with		
No activity limitation	87.3	56.8
Activity limitation	12.7	43.2
Limitation in major activity	9.6	37.9

[a]Source: Library of Congress, Congressional Research Service, *Key Facts on the Handicapped.* Edward R.
Klebe, Education and Public Welfare Division, HD 7275 A. p. CRS4. Washington, D.C.: Government
Printing Office, 1975.

and prevalence of mental illness is the community survey. The National
Health Education Committe in 1957 estimated from four community surveys of mental illness among the general population that 16 million persons
have some sort of mental illness in the United States.

In 1970 it was estimated that 20 million persons, or 10% of the population, could benefit from mental health services (President's Task Force on
the Mentally Handicapped, 1970).

Federal government action on mental illness took a decisive turn in
1946 when Congress passed the Mental Health Act, creating the National
Institute of Mental Health, and in 1955, when Congress passed the Mental
Health Study Act of 1955, authorizing an appropriation to the Joint Commission on Mental Health and Illness "to study and make recommendations concerning various aspects of mental health policy." The report,
known as Action for Mental Health, recommended the establishment of
mental health clinics and attacked the state mental hospital. This report,
along with the advent of psychoactive drugs, led to the concept of community care where the emphasis is on outpatient care and short periods, if any,
of hospitalization.

In 1963, Congress passed the Community Mental Health Centers Act,
designed to reduce the discrepancy between the mental health care available
to the rich and that available to the poor.

The discharge from state mental institutions that followed (the population of patients in state mental institutions dropped from 505,000 in 1963 to

249,000 in 1973, more than 50%) has come under severe criticism since communities were, by and large, incapable of providing for the care of the chronically ill patients who were discharged. "Many of those patients have gone to live in boarding and nursing homes, most of whose operators have not had much experience with chronic mental patients . . . that such conditions are an improvement on the back wards of state hospitals is debatable" (Jones, 1975).

With the advent of psychoactive drugs and the concept of community care, there has been marked reduction in the median length of stay for hospitalization (from 6 months in 1948 to 41 days in 1972) and in the inpatient episodes of care (from 77% in 1955 to 43% in 1971) (Brown, 1973).

Thousands of mental patients who had resided in large state mental institutions were discharged to communities, where they have several options open to them: single rooms, halfway houses, foster care homes, nursing homes, and boarding homes—the latter since the enactment of the federally financed Supplementary Security Income program, which provides funds for the care of patients in private facilities rather than in public institutions.

Although single room occupancy in a low-cost rooming house has been criticized as approximating "living in a one-person chronic ward in a hospital," halfway houses have been more favorably regarded as promoting the return of the ex-mental patient to the community and as lowering the chances of residents being rehospitalized. Caution is advised, however, against socalled halfway houses that offer no more than low-quality custodial care (Rog & Raush, 1975).

Health Problems as Seen by the Elderly

To give some empirical information on the health status and health problems as perceived by various subgroups of the elderly population, we can use the results of a survey of people aged 60 and over made in Chicago in 1975, and reported by Bild and Havighurst (1976). Six hundred persons were selected by a sampling method and interviewed in their homes. They were asked a variety of questions, and their answers to questions about their health will be reported here. This sample of persons consisted of approximately one hundred of each of six subgroups that are visible in every large city and have different life-styles and probably have somewhat different needs.

We shall call these samples by characteristic names: homeowners, Polish-origin elders, low-income persons in residential hotels, a black population from a certain geographical area, a largely Jewish population from a certain geographical area, and a sample of elderly residents of subsidized public housing. We will report on these groups, knowing that each group is a sample of a clearly visible segment of the elderly population of a big city. We will also sometimes combine the data from the six subgroups to give a very crude picture of the total Chicago older population. In this case we will call our sample the "combined group," knowing that this is not a representative sample of Chicago seniors, but also knowing that the composite picture is not far off from representing the total Chicago senior population. We will generally call these groups by their characteristic names, and sometimes we will speak of them as groups of samples.

The elderly homeowners are the most stable and the most favorably situated in many respects, although some of them feel "tied down" to their property. They tend to congregate in the older residential areas that have maintained a stable ethnic composition.

Our Rogers Park and Polish subgroups have much in common with our homeowners, and they overlap in many respects. The Rogers Park group is largely Jewish middle and lower middle class in composition and can be seen as a stable ethnic group. They live in areas of relatively high elderly population.

The Washington Park group are the most stable black elderly; although their incomes are relatively low, they are fairly comfortable in other respects. The black elderly will increase rapidly in numbers over the next two decades.

The residential hotel groups (two of them) represent a growing proportion of the elderly—the "singles." Although half of them have adult children, their children are living in the suburbs or in other sections of the city, and they prefer to live independently. As we discovered, they have a wide range of incomes, and they tend to find residential quarters in areas that suit their particular economic level. Thus, the uptown area attracts people with lower incomes than those prevalent in the Hyde Park–Kenwood area. Women are greatly in the majority among residential hotel dwellers.

The public housing group represents a potentially large group of low-income people who have learned to accept poverty and live with it. The long waiting list for accommodation in public housing attests to this. These people, with resources generally limited to small Social Security benefits and Supplementary Security Income, may be found in small numbers wherever there are dwellings with low rents, but they are concentrated in the areas where public housing is located—generally in low-income areas. In some ways this group is the most secure, since it knows what to expect. It lacks property and gets little or no help from adult children, which sources are less reliable than the rock-bottom support level provided for the poor by the government.

All the information on the health of these people is subjective, inasmuch as it relies solely on the words of the respondents. Some questions capitalize on this subjectivity, as when the respondents were asked to characterize their health. Other questions, such as those asking for concrete information, are more objective, however. "During the past year did you ever have to stay overnight or longer in a hospital?" carries evidence of an evaluation external to the respondent.

A set of questions aimed at getting objective answers was used to arrive at the Physical Incapacity Index. These questions asked about ability to perform 11 usual daily activities: going on walks outside of the home, climbing stairs, walking in the house, bathing, dressing and putting on shoes, cutting toenails, eating without help, preparing meals, cleaning the house, shopping for groceries, and riding buses serving the city. For each of the 11 tasks a person was given a score from 0 to 2 or 3, depending on the degree of difficulty experienced by the person in performing the task. A low score indicated no difficulty; a score of 2 or 3 indicated that help was needed (a mechanical aide, such as a cane, a crutch, or a wheelchair) or that the task could not be done by the person. The total Physical Incapacity score for an individual varied from 0 to 33, with a 0 score indicating no physical incapacity, as measured by this index.

Analysis of Group Differences Concerning Health

Table II presents self-evaluations of their health by the Chicago seniors. The most favorable health conditions were reported by the homeowners, who have the highest incomes and the highest material standard of living. They evaluate their health positively. On the Physical Incapacity Index, they report the greatest physical competence and the least impairment.

Almost as consistent as the homeowners, but at the opposite extreme, are public housing and residential hotel residents. A high proportion cite health as a serious personal problem. They have the highest Physical Incapacity scores. A high proportion report visual problems.

People enter the retirement hotels when poor health, loneliness, or reduced income force them to acknowledge their need of some special facilities (communal dining for those who are no longer able to cook or who never knew how to cook and have been widowed, maid service for those in similar circumstances with regard to cleaning, subsidized rents to supplement a low and rather fixed income, a lobby and meeting rooms and some other residents willing to play cards and to chat, or staff whose duty it is to regularly check on the building's residents to make sure they have not had an accident or been stricken ill).

The residents of the low-cost retirement hotels are likely to be in worse health than their contemporaries who continue to live more independently in

Table II. Self-evaluation of Health, Chicago Senior Citizens[a]

| | | | | Subgroup | | Residential Hotels | | |
Self-evaluation	Home Owners	CNAS[b]	Rogers Park	Polish	Black	Uptown	Hyde Park	Public Housing
Very good	34	23	25	6	18	15	22	11
Good	29	21	24	16	22	23	32	22
Sometimes good, sometimes not	36	36	32	58	42	33	25	40
Poor	9	20	15	11	15	14	18	19
Very poor	2	—	3	9	2	15	2	7
Do you have health handicaps which limit your activities?								
Yes	42		48	42	40	65	52	58
No	58		52	58	60	35	48	42
Have you stayed in a hospital overnight during past year?								
Yes	16		22	19	21	35	22	38
No	84		78	81	79	65	78	62

Physical Incapacity Index (range 0–33)							
Score 0	66	45	46	55	34	36	19
1–6	16	33	32	22	38	38	52
7–27	18	22	22	23	28	26	29
By age group and sex (Y = 60–74, O = 75 and over)							
Men	Y O	Y O	Y O	Y O	Y O	Y O	Y O
Score: 0	90 56	65 43	71 25	68 59	44 44	56 30	50 20
Score: 7 and over	3 15	8 14	0 11	7 35	11 19	11 30	0 27
Women	Y O	Y O	Y O	Y O	Y O	Y O	Y O
Score: 0	67 45	62 21	68 18	61 38	27 26	33 27	25 0
Score: 7 and over	19 45	14 38	11 45	11 38	46 37	17 46	44 34

aSource: Bild and Havighurst (1976).
bCNAS is the Chicago Needs Assessment Survey made in 1972 on a random sample of the noninstitutionalized Chicago population aged 60 and over.

age-heterogeneous community situations. It is not clear whether the age-segregated, quasi-institutional setting aggravates the elderly person's health because of inadequate support systems, impersonal administration, or other reasons. But the health of the elderly people who live in these hotels is worse than the health of the elderly people in our community samples, even when age is controlled.

The Salience of Age. Although the several subgroups show differences in health status and physical capabilities, their advancing age seems to separate them from middle-aged adults. For example, in the least disabled subgroup, 40% admitted being restricted by disabilities. The comparable percentage of a younger group would undoubtedly be substantially lower. It was possible to compare the health self-reports of the younger segment of the old people (aged 60–74) with the older segment (aged 75 and over). There are some problems in drawing conclusions from such a comparison.

The older segment are not precise counterparts of the younger: they are self-selected in favor of greater physical strength or endurance, as they are composed of survivors of a diminishing cohort whose less hardy members have died. But these survivors are still in worse health than our younger groups, and they provide evidence for the decline of health with advancing years.

Splitting each sample into a younger and an older group yields 14 small subgroups, as seen in Table II. Because of the large number of comparisons involved, differences will be regarded as significant only when they recur throughout the samples. In at least six of our seven samples, the older subgroup said more frequently that poor health was a serious or a very serious problem; that they were restricted in some way by disabilities; that they do not go out daily in good weather or in winter; that getting sufficient medical care is a serious problem; that their eyesight is not adequate for reading, for distance, or for television; that they have difficulty or that they require help in bathing, going for walks outside, and cutting their toenails. The age subgroups show wide divergence on Physical Incapacity Index scores, the older subgroups having less total competence and autonomy and more frequent severe incapacity.

However, there are other health variables in which the influence of age is negligible or peculiar to a particular sample. There is no significant difference between the older and the younger subgroups in rating their health against their contemporaries, in evaluating their health positively or negatively, in attaching importance to the doctor, or in having been recently hospitalized.

Although the questions that clearly show age differences include both objective and subjective variables, the questions that show little or no difference by age are mostly subjective. An explanation will be offered. Since there is a direct relationship between old age and poor health, it is not surprising that this poor health is sometimes accurately evaluated by the old person and that there is sometimes agreement between the objective and subjective health variables. But neither is it surprising that as a person becomes very old, his subjective appraisal of his health alters to take into account the condition of being very old as well as his actual state of health, resulting in lack of agreement between objective and subjective standards.

The very old person, who is more likely than the less old to be physically restricted or incapacitated, is also more likely to have had contact with serious illness and death through his spouse or friends. He knows that his health is worse than it used to be, but he is less inclined to take good health for granted and is more grateful for the abilities he retains.

The differential significance of age to health variables is a result of the older person's accommodation to his and others' increasing frailty over time. He is more often exposed to serious illness and death in others (and so more aware of the threat they pose to himself), making his own physical problems seem less critical in comparison. One homeowner could perform only 4 of the 12 Physical Incapacity tasks independently without difficulty, could clean the house or shop for groceries only with help, and could not ride the bus at all, yet she rated her health as "good" and "about average" for her age. She said, "I'm going to be 77. I never thought I'd get that far." The old person's accommodation to declining health also acts on his conception of his own health as he becomes inured to it. As a constant or gradually deteriorating condition in his life, an incapacity becomes submerged into the norm from which sickness and other deviations constitute "poor health." One 93-year-old black woman listed arthritis and a pain in her chest as her disabilities and said that they hindered her in the performance of activities as elementary as walking. She had endured each of them for longer than 40 years. Of the 12 Physical Incapacity tasks, only eating was easy for her. She had very bad hearing and used a hearing aid. Her sight was not adequate and she had been hospitalized in the year previous to her interview. She said her health was "sometimes good and sometimes not," but "better than average" for her age.

Management of Mild Chronic Disease

A number of chronic conditions produce physical pain and discomfort, as well as depression. The latter condition may also be brought on by loneliness, or loss of a husband or wife. It now appears that this level of physical or mental distress can be alleviated by appropriate physiotherapy or by what may be termed *sociotherapy*.

At the mild physical level some headway is being made in treatment of arthritis and rheumatism that afflict people increasingly as they grow older. Physical education and recreation leaders are developing physical fitness programs for elders, which lead them to report that they feel better and are more active physically. This result may be due in part to the enjoyable associations they have with other people in these groups, since many of them have been lonely and depressed before joining the groups. However, physicians who are observing those programs carefully are inclined to believe that the mild exercises and the dietary advice they get in these groups have a physical as well as mental health value. Questionnaires filled out by members of these physical fitness groups report a general rise in morale and in life satisfaction as measured by a Life Satisfaction Inventory, and some indication that they go to a doctor less often.

Autonomy of the Elderly

Albert Jonsen, a Jesuit who is a professor of medical ethics in a medical school has written the following eloquent argument for making the autonomy of the elderly patient the primary goal of health treatment. He points out that a major distinction must be made between treatment for *acute illness*, around which American medical care is structured, and treatment for chronic disease.

> However, the elderly suffer largely from chronic disease. The preponderance of medical service which they seek is for the alleviation of chronic disease states. Such care would allow for the personal and the intimate. Not single-mindedly oriented toward cure, it would move at a measured pace to alleviate and sustain. Not dominated by the high technology of machines, it depends on the low technology of basically effective drugs. It is most often best provided, not by specialists, but by primary care practitioners who have ongoing, intimate knowledge of their patients.
>
> Nevertheless, care of chronic disease is a lost medical art. The characteristic needs of chronic patients are only vaguely comprehended. The elderly, who could best profit by chronic disease care, are bereft of it because, in the United States, it is poorly understood, poorly organized, neglected in medical training and badly financed. Thus, not only is the form of medical care largely unsuited to the medical needs of the elderly, but the form of medical care provided also compromises their profound moral need for the appreciation of individuality and diversity.
>
> Secondly, health care for the elderly must not only respect, but enhance their autonomy. Enhancement implies efforts to structure institutions and behavior in ways which make room for meaningful participation of the elderly. It is attentive to the problems of purpose and vocation, as well as effective employment of powers relative to age. In our current practices of retirement and institutionalization, those whose lives have been built on action and purpose are suddenly excluded. . . . Respect for persons requires openness in the social structure for purpose, vocation, engagement. Current patterns of institutionalization deny this openness.
>
> It is becoming clear that warehousing the elderly not only affronts their

dignity, but contributes to their deterioration and dependency. Indeed, it is likely that it is even economically inefficient. The growing awareness that the largest need of older persons is for services which will help them remain at home in familiar surroundings where risk of deterioration and disability is considerably less is prompting efforts for better, broader provision of home care. It would be a pleasant surprise if such a policy were not only more effective, more economical, but also most ethical!

Finally, respect for persons serves as a warning against that etymological oddity, paternalism toward the elderly. . . . The elderly, seen as persons in and for themselves, must be enabled, as far as possible, to be, as they were in their earlier years, deciders of their own ways and means. Our benevolence toward them must be respectful, that is, fully aware of their essential freedom in spite of their physical deficits. Concern for the protection and promotion of autonomy should serve as a basic constructive and critical principle in health care policy for the aged. Systematic departures from this ethical principle must be justified with cogent and equally ethical reasons. (1976)

Prevention of Heart Disease

The major cause of death in the population over 50 years of age—cardiovascular diseases—has decreased in several modern countries, including the United States, since about 1965, after a plateau that had persisted so long as to lead the medical profession and the demographers to expect no decrease unless new basic discoveries could be made, leading to further reductions around the close of the century.

In the United States and in Finland, to cite two rather different countries, there was a visible reduction of mortality from coronary heart disease in the 1960s and 1970s. In both countries, this is attributed to a decrease in cigarette smoking (inhalation of tobacco smoke), to a reduction in the consumption of saturated fats such as butter, and to more pervasive treatment of high blood pressure. The mortality decline was greater in men than in women, probably because women did not stop smoking in as large numbers as men. On the other hand, the theory that coronary heart disease is also related to mental stress for people in such occupations as those of surgeon, business executive, and others who must take responsibility for making decisions that may turn out badly is leading people to watch closely the cardiovascular mortality data for women since women are now moving into the more stressful occupations in larger numbers.

Home Health Services

For the protection of their autonomy, and for the maintenance of their mental and physical health, it is widely agreed that elderly people with mild levels of chronic disease or physical disability should remain in their own homes rather than be placed in a nursing home or a home for the aged. But this is difficult or impossible for those who live alone and have physical disability beyond a certain level, and even for those who live with an adult daughter or son, or with a spouse who has some physical disability.

To meet this situation, the 1972 Social Security Act Amendments included a Title XX, which provided $3 of Federal funds for every dollar of state or local money devoted to the provision of social services for needy people. Among the program goals of Title XX are preventing or reducing inappropriate institutional care by providing for community-based or home-based care, or other forms of less intensive care; and helping people achieve or maintain self-sufficiency.

The several states are given wide latitude in the creation of a Comprehensive Annual Services Program Plan, on the basis of which the federal money is awarded. Certain services can be provided to people with incomes up to the median family income, although persons with low incomes are generally favored. The amount of federal funding has been set at $2.5 billion annually, allocated to the various states in relation to their population.

The services that are primarily health-related for elderly persons are described as Home Health Services and include health care by a practical nurse, home-delivered meals, homemaker assistance, and physical therapy. These are described in a report by the National Council on the Aging (1976) entitled *Making Title XX Work.*

Mental Health Services for the Elderly

As people move past the ages of 75 and 80, some of them become confused about the life around them. They need someone to help keep them in touch with reality. This may be done by a husband or wife, or by adult children. But elderly people who are alone, without near relatives, often need some kind of attention. They may become near-senile.

In the early years of this century, such people were often sent to state or county mental hospitals. Kahn (1975) has described the situation and how it has changed in recent years. In 1904 there were 150,000 persons in mental hospitals in the United States, and this number increased to 633,000 in the peak year of 1955. The data on age of first admission show that people over 65 had much higher rates than any other age. In 1910 the rate for people 65 and over was 200 per 100,000 persons in this age group. This increased to 435 per 100,000 in 1950.

Kahn reports:

> After World War II there was a dramatic alteration in our conceptions and patterns of mental health care. With such milestones as the establishment of the National Institute of Mental Health in 1948, the organization of the Joint Commission on Mental Illness and Health in 1955, and the passage of the Commu-

nity Mental Health Centers Act of 1963, there was a more active and optimistic attitude toward mental illness, characterized by radically reducing the resident mental hospital population and developing such other services as psychiatric units in general hospitals, outpatient services of all kinds, and the vaunted community mental health centers.

These developments resulted in decreased admissions of older people, and increased admissions of younger people to state and county mental hospitals. Between 1946 and 1972 there was an 80% decrease in admissions of people aged 65 and over. Elderly patients were given tranquilizers, which helped them to get along in their own home quarters, and they were increasingly placed in nursing homes. There were 554,000 residents of nursing homes in 1963, and 1,099,000 ten years later.

Kahn says that nursing homes have replaced the state and county mental hospitals as "custodial warehouses" for elderly persons. Kahn reports: "In 1963 almost two-fifths of the aged who were diagnosed as mentally ill and who were in long-term care institutions were to be found in state and county mental hospitals, while 53 percent were in nursing homes and personal care homes. These proportions changed drastically in 1969, when 75 percent of the aged mentally ill were in nursing homes."

He goes on to say that "the patterns of psychiatric care of the aged can be better explained on the basis of a reciprocal aversiveness between the mental health establishment and older persons, based on the interaction of such factors as mental health ideology, social class characteristics, and considerations of age appropriateness."

It seems probable that the "old old" group—those over 75—will show more resistance to near-senility and to custodialism and custodial institutions such as nursing homes. They will be better educated and will have become accustomed to better comprehensive medical care. They will be better prepared for retirement, psychologically and financially. They may show fewer cases of disordered behavior than the elderly population of the 1970 decade.

We may anticipate that older people will expect to be more competent to care for themselves, and that the mental health experts will adopt a policy of "minimal intervention," which is least disruptive of usual functioning in the usual setting.

Elderly people who are in need of some care may be encouraged to stay with their families, who will receive some supportive help from staff of mental health centers.

Last Home for the Aged

For a number of unavoidable reasons, many people will come to the end of their lives in a home for the aged or a nursing home. Although approximately 5% of all people 65 and over reside in such institutions, this proportion rises with age, so that 16% of persons 85 and over are in institutions. The research by Tobin and Lieberman (1976) studied the entrants to three homes for the aged in Chicago, keeping in touch with them from the time they applied for admission until more than a year after they were admitted. These researchers also studied a group of 40 elderly people of the same age as the ones who entered the homes, but who continued to live in the community. This matched community sample consisted of 40 unattached elderly people, 34 women and 6 men, whose average age was 80 years and whose average educational level was eight grades. Half of this group lived alone; the others, in most cases, lived with their eldest daughter. These 40 people represented a wide range of personality types, a variety also exhibited in the primary study sample. Thus, no one particular type of person could be seen as more likely, on the one hand, to remain in the community or, on the other, to seek institutionalization. Rather, the data suggest that any type of older person may seek care in a home for the aged or may hold out against the forces of age and remain an independent community resident.

The psychological status of these very old community residents was impressively good, especially considering their physical status and the number of significant adverse changes they had experienced in the past 3 years. Two out of three, for example, reported the presence of two or more serious chronic diseases. Three out of five had lost some physical capacity in the past 3 years; two out of five had suffered the death of at least one significant other person; and an additional one out of five had experienced some other sort of decisive change in their relationship with significant others. One out of three had moved their place of residence, yet none had sought institutional care at this time. Many respondents in the community sample had discussed the possibility of institutional care with their families as a solution to the problems these losses had generated, but all had decided against giving up their independence. For all, institutional care was a feared or dreaded solution that would be taken only if necessary to assure survival. Although often physically impaired and having experienced many adverse changes, these community elderly were cognitively intact, in good rapport with themselves and the world outside them, and hopeful about the future. They recognized but were not preoccupied either with the losses they had already endured or with those that might lie not too far ahead, including the possibility of their own death.

A contrasting picture emerges in a description of the group who entered the homes for the aged, at the end of their first year. This group of 85 persons broke into two very different subgroups. Forty-four had deteriorated severally or had died. These people were characterized from the start by extreme passivity; they were less able to feed and care for themselves, and less hopeful of the future. Passivity seems to be a predictor of vulnerability to the stress of institutional life.

Those who suffered severe outcomes by the end of the first year gave signs of trouble after the first two months. It seems likely that the discontinuity of a move into an institution has adverse effects on practically all who enter, since those who displayed no marked negative effects nevertheless showed a lower level of feeling of well-being and some hostility to their staff members.

The group with more favorable outcomes after the first year had improved in life satisfaction after the first two months and exhibited lessened anxiety. Still, they were adversely affected by the change to institutional life. They became less hopeful, and perceived themselves as less capable of self-care. Even those who showed no marked negative effects nevertheless showed diminished feelings of well-being.

The conclusion of Tobin and Lieberman was that institutionalization should be avoided if possible. They say:

> It would appear from the data presented here that institutionalization, even in homes of the highest quality, should not be considered a first choice, but should follow only after serious efforts have been made to determine whether continued independent living might be possible if specific deficiencies were corrected through ancillary services. Stated another way, all efforts need to be made to prevent unnecessary or premature institutionalization. In practice, however, the distinction between unneccessary and necessary institutionalization is not easily made. Thus, it is essential that service providers become versed in the use of flexible service packages in order to help older people and their families understand and explore the available options.

Their conclusion about institutionalization for the elderly goes:

> By its very nature, institutional living is physically and socially discontinuous from autonomous community living. The best of long-term care institutions is still a foreign spatial environment inhabited by other old, sick, and needy people. While the caretakers may be able and loving, they are not one's own family. If the new resident is to receive the maximum benefits from this relocation, he or, more likely, she must become a part of the institutional fabric. In so doing, he or she experiences unavoidable negative effects such as a focal concern on mutilation and death that reflect an underlying experience of personal vulnerability and a deepening of hopelessness. Can we intervene to stop the development of such effects? Probably not. Even for the resident who is most successful in making the transition from preadmission to postadmission, as was the case for Mrs. A., there is an apparent unavoidable shift toward a focal concern of mutilation and death. Yet at the same time a sense of self was maintained, and the sought-after gains of care, people, and activities were achieved. Indeed, by the end of the first month or so, Mrs. A. was her old self in many ways. To be sure, individualized efforts were made to help her weather the impact of the relocation. Because a reaction was expected, she received help that reduced its intensity and foreshortened its expression. If appropriate help had not been available, the initial reaction might have crystallized into a permanent negative trend.
>
> The new resident must thus be helped through the transitional acute period with minimal negative effects. All people and objects from the former world that

are incorporated into the new institutional world become anchors for the new resident. Family and workers, as well as personal belongings that have special meanings, offer continuity. People and things that give continuity can offset some of initial sense of abrupt change, but the balance is tipped toward what the newcomer experiences as unpleasant because of having to learn new rules and to puzzle out the attitudes of a new environment when cognitive and perceptual functions may be weakened by age and anxiety. For some, the anxiety can be reduced by the assurance that strange or different behaviors during this period are expected as well as tolerated, and that there will be neither punishment nor explusion from the home for these behaviors.

Once the initial impact of entering and living in the institution has been weathered, the new resident can go beyond merely accommodating to the foreign world. A rewarding and life-enhancing adaptation can be achieved within the constraints of congregate living if the environment is sufficiently flexible and individuated. If a range of life-styles is actively encouraged, the heterogeneous population of residents play out the diversity of their idiosyncratic selves. Efficient operation obviously conflicts with maximum development of a flexible and individualizing environment. But if human losses are to be minimized, the struggle must be to help each individual express those aspects of self that yielded satisfaction in independent living. Self-continuity can be achieved and benefits can be accrued—as was generally the case for respondents in our study sample 1 year after admission to long-term care facilities.

Congregate Living Can Be Healthy

Older people can live in close proximity to each other without the disadvantages of institutionalization described by Tobin and Lieberman. They can maintain autonomy. Congregate living may have real advantages for the maintenance of health.

An example of such a health-promoting situation has been described by Frances Carp (1977) in her research on the experience of people in San

Table III.   Comparative Data on Tenants and Nontenants of Victoria Plaza

Condition (8 years later)	Percentage	
	Tenants	Nontenants
Self-rating on health		
"Good" or "excellent" decreased for	13	28
"Poor" or "very poor" increased for	6	18
Attitude toward health		
"Beginning to be a burden"	47	67
"Feel miserable most of the time"	6	17
"Bothered by" one or more health problems	59	75
Terminally ill or dead	26	37

Antonio who moved into Victoria Plaza, a high-rise low-cost apartment building for the elderly, around 1965. There were 352 legally qualified applicants, with an average age of 72. Of this number, 204 were accepted as tenants and 148 were not, since there was no more space for them. No one who was seriously ill or substantially handicapped was accepted as a tenant.

Eight years after this date, interviews were obtained with 127 tenants and 62 applicants who had not become residents. These interviews produced the comparative data shown in Table III.

A Comprehensive Health Care System

Tobin and Lieberman (1976) see that meaningful alternatives to total institutionalization of the frail elderly require a "Comprehensive Health Care System." They list general objectives of this kind of system:

1. Involving the elderly client in planning the regimen of care, thus combining client preference with professional judgment.
2. Provision of quality social care for all socioeconomic levels.
3. Coordination of preventive, rehabilitative and maintenance services under a comprehensive administration which employs a variety of professional and paraprofessional personnel.

A viable geriatric care system that fulfilled these objectives would care for a much larger number of older people than is typical today, especially of those 75 years of age and over. The future elderly will be better educated and have greater expectations of themselves and of service providers. They will make increasing demands on the social and health system. It is those above 75, however, who will most need a system that assures maintenance of functioning. For the coming group of "old old," whose children are themselves likely to be "young old"—in their 60s and 70s—a social and health system must be developed in which direct services are synchronized with emotional and practical supports that can be offered by the aging family. The long-term institution or facility would be an important component in a viable geriatric social and health system. Equally basic to the system would be a community social and health organization, under one auspice, that attempts to integrate a range of services. (p. 241)

References

Anderson, O. W. Reflections on the sick aged and helping systems. In B. L. Neugarten and R. J. Havighurst (Eds.), Social policy, social ethics, and the aging society. Washington, D.C.: U.S. Government Printing Office, 1976, pp. 89–96.

Bild, B. R., & Havighurst, R. J. Senior citizens in great cities: The case of Chicago. Gerontologist, 1976, 16(1), Part II.

Brody, E. M. *Health and its social implications.* Paper presented at the Institut de la Vie, World Conference—Aging: A Challenge to Science and Social Policy, Vichy, France, April 25, 1977.

Brown, B. S. A national view of mental health. *American Journal of Orthopsychiatry,* 1973, *43*(5), 702.

Carp, F. M. Impact of improved living environment on health and life expectancy. *Gerontologist,* 1977, 17, 242–249.

Jones, M. Community care for chronic mental patients: The need for a reassessment. *Hospital and Community Psychiatry,* 1975, *26*(2), 94–96.

Jonsen, A. R. Principles for an ethics of health services. In B. L. Neugarten & R. J. Havighurst (Eds.), *Social policy, social ethics, and the aging society.* Washington, D.C.: U.S. Government Printing Office, 1976, pp. 97–104.

Kahn, R. L. The mental health system and the future aged. In B. L. Neugarten (Ed.), *Aging in the year 2000: A look at the future.* p. 24–31. *Gerontologist,* 1975, *15*(1), Part II.

Lawton, M. P., & Cohen, J. The generality of housing impact in the well-being of older people. *Journal of Gerontology,* 1974, *29*, 194–204.

National Center for Health Statistics, Congressional Research Service. *Key facts on the handicapped.* Washington, D.C.: U.S. Government Printing Office, 1975.

National Council on the Aging. *Making Title XX work: A guide to funding social services for older people.* Washington, D.C.: National Council on the Aging, 1976.

National Council on the Aging. *The myth and reality of aging in America* (Harris Poll). Washington, D.C.: National Council on the Aging, 1975.

Neugarten, B. L., & Havighurst R. J. (Eds.). *Social policy, social ethics, and the aging society.* Washington, D.C.: U.S. Government Printing Office, 1976. (Stock Number 038-000-00299-6)

President's Task Force on the Mentally Handicapped. *Action against mental disability.* Washington, D.C.: U.S. Government Printing Office, 1970.

Rog, D. J., & Raush, H. L. The psychiatric halfway house: How is it measuring up? *Community Mental Health Journal,* 1975, *11*(2), 157–161.

Shanas, E. *The health of older people: A social survey.* Cambridge, Mass.: Harvard University Press, 1962.

Shanas, E., et al. *Old people in three industrial societies.* New York: Atherton, 1968.

Tobin, S. S., & Lieberman, M. A. *Last Home for the aged.* San Francisco: Jossey-Bass, 1976.

12

Toward a Definition of Health Risks for Ethnic Minorities: The Case of Hypertension and Heart Disease

Jerry L. Weaver

Recent epidemiologic studies have revealed that Asian Americans, Blacks, Chicanos, and native Americans have rates of heart disease, cancer, diabetes, mental illness, drug abuse, and other health problems well above the national norm. In seeking an explanation for these elevated risk levels, some analysts have pointed to the diet, living conditions, and health care behavior of members of the communities as the sources of many health problems (Suchman, 1964, 1965). For example, studies of the health care behavior of Chicanos in rural areas of the Southwest present a picture of belief in magical sources of many diseases and disabilities; a preference for seeking care from folk healers, family, friends and other "unscientific" providers; and an unwillingness to be hospitalized (Kiev, 1968; Sanders, 1954; also see Weaver, 1973). Similar behavior and attitudes are reported among traditional Japanese-Americans, Chinese-Americans, and other Asian populations. Blacks are said to avoid private physicians and dentists and to rely heavily on over-the-counter nostrums. Traditional diets of ethnic minorities are said to be deficient for promoting good health, especially for at-risk individuals such as babies and the elderly. Taken together, the patterns of behavior and beliefs about the causes and cures of illnesses that deviate from the "norms" of the larger (White) society have come to be labeled

Jerry L. Weaver • U.S. Agency for International Development, Washington, D.C. 20523.

health care subcultures. Thus, in explaining the high mortality rates of Chicano infants, for instance, some observers put much of the blame on the "Chicano subculture," which keeps sick children away from physicians and hospitals until it is too late (for an analysis of this literature, see Weaver, 1976).

There is no doubt that health care subcultures are *associated* with certain mortality and morbidity profiles. Avoiding physicians, hospitals, and modern medicines can and does kill people because such behavior delays or prevents timely and appropriate intervention. But looking at the particularities of communities and blaming their subculture for their health problems is simplistic. In the first place, not all members of a community practice the subculture: most Chicanos are urban-born and live in cities; unlike their rural grandparents or cousins, these urbanized Chicanos seek care from scientific providers and many are not even aware of *mal de ojo* (evil eye), *curanderos* (folk healers), and herbal remedies. Choice of provider is dictated by price, by availability, and sometimes by language. Similarly, research demonstrates that second- and third-generation Asian-Americans have few if any views on health and illness behavior in common with their traditional, pioneer-generation relatives. And if Blacks tend to use over-the-counter drugs and public health facilities more than Whites, it may be economics and racism rather than subculture that best explains these differences.

Examination of research reporting the prevalence of health subculture reveals that it is often based on isolated populations or is drawn from groups that are atypical of the overall community. Indeed, it is the uniqueness of the subjects that draws the attention of investigators. Moreover, most of the subculture research is now badly out of date because of the profound changes in the educational levels, residence, and availability of health care providers among minorities during the 1960s and 1970s. Both the Black and Chicano populations are now urban-dwelling, and Asian-American populations have educational attainment levels equal to or above the national levels.

Aside from failing the test of close empirical scrutiny, the subculture of health approach confuses primary and secondary causality. Disease and illness may be *caused* by poor sanitation, inadequate nutrition, and failure to respond to symptoms; but equally important to morbidity and mortality profiles are factors outside and beyond the control of the individual—price and availability of scientific providers; institutional restraints on accessing providers, such as racism, sexism, and agism; environmental pollution, and attitudes held in the dominant society that have pathological impacts on minorities. This latter set of secondary factors exacerbates and worsens diseases that they do not actually cause, often because they intervene between the patient and the receipt of professional care.

Indeed, there is considerable evidence that social and economic variables multiply the health risks of minorities. Studies show that as the cost of health services goes up, frequency of utilization decreases. Since disproportionately more ethnic minorities than Whites are poor, it follows that some of the minorities' avoidance of providers is economically, not culturally, based. Similarly, research in many different health care institutions confirms that minorities are treated differently (read: inferiorly). Hence, avoiding providers who are generally White may well reflect sociological and psychological factors that have nothing to do with the individual's culture. And levels of environmental pollution that are found in the living places of minorities (such as lead in the housepaint and in the air of inner-city ghettos, or the impure water of rural areas and small towns of the South and Southwest) are not caused by diets or beliefs about the origins of disease.

The basic inadequacy of the subculture model of minority health care problems is that it is too restrictive: it emphasizes only one—albeit an important—set of variables. In order to gain a more useful picture of the factors that shape the health care risks of minorities, equal attention must be given to factors outside the communities that impinge on the timeliness, appropriateness, and effectiveness of treatment and the severity of existing pathologies. In the jargon of social science, a useful model of risk factors must be additive and interactive. That is, it should combine subcultural factors with availability of providers, cost of care, institutional barriers to utilization, and sources of pathologies emanating from the institutions and practices of the dominant society.

Such a model must examine the combined weight of these variables to see how they affect individuals and minority communities. In addition, we must view the determinants of health risks interactively because health status is a dynamic, changing process in which a host of factors such as past experience, new knowledge, changing technology, and evolving institutional processes and procedures merge with biological and psychological elements. The environment in which diseases and illness occur changes; the attitudes and information of the individual change; and the nature of the health care delivery system changes. Only by seeing the individual, the environment, and the delivery system interacting simultaneously are we able to understand the comprehensive origins of health care problems.

A particularly good illustration of the pathological interaction of individuals, environment, and providers emerges from the study of the etiology of hypertension (high blood pressure) and heart disease. By framing the analysis of these maladies in the context of individual attitudes, values, and behavior (i.e., health care subculture), the impact on individuals of selected social institutions, and the response of providers to the problem, we see that controlling these health problems in the near term and reducing their frequency among minorities over the long haul requires the creative concatenation of technology, public education, and professional diagnosis with the modification of many basic American institutions. In other words, what is defined currently as constituting the source and remedy of hypertension and heart disease must be expanded considerably to incorporate factors that conventional health programs and treatments have hitherto ignored.

High Blood Pressure and Heart Disease among Minorities

A review of the prevalence and causes of high blood pressure, cardiovascular diseases, stroke, and related pathologies of the circulatory system among Asian-Americans, Blacks, and other ethnic minorities reveals how profoundly these communities are affected by the interplay of social and environmental forces that are little noticed by members of the dominant society—yet these same forces may very well be at the bottom of the high rates of similar diseases reported for Anglos. For instance, much is made, by students of heart disease among Asians, of the association between change in diet and changing frequency of disease. The same diet-related pattern of morbidity and mortality is cited by investigators of high blood pressure among Blacks. Other research points to the link between diet and heart problems for Anglos. Hence, by illuminating the problems of minorities, and thereby providing information for remedial action and further research, we will be casting light on problems common across the American society.

While hypertension and heart disease were once thought to be chiefly threats to high-pressure business executives and professionals, it is now clear that ethnicity rather than social class is the strongest predictor of risk. Although it has emerged slowly, the picture before us reveals that Black Americans, especially young Black males aged 18–35 and Black females, have the highest per capita rate of high blood pressure. As early as 1966, it was reported that "in any age group the likelihood of heart disease with hypertension is greater for Negroes than for white persons" (17 million Americans with Hypertension, 1966). Among Black adults in Harlem, 30–35% were shown to be affected by high blood pressure (Kilcoyne, 1973). Another study of over 11,000 residents of New Orleans showed that Black males exceeded Anglo males in the prevalence of hypertension in every cohort except the 30- to 39-year-old. Among females, however, the rate of Blacks exceeded the Anglos' rate in every age category: fully 71% of Black women over 50 years of age were found to have high blood pressure (McMahon, Cole, & Ryan, 1973).

A similar pattern of higher rates among Blacks was reported from Oakland, California: "Blacks had higher average diastolic and systolic blood pressures and a higher prevalence of hypertension than whites for both males and females and for all age groups. *When these distributions were examined by social class, Blacks in the lowest social classes had the highest blood pressures* (Syme, Oakes, Friedman, Feldman, Siegelaub, & Collen, 1974, emphasis added; see also Oakes, Syme, Feldman, Friedman, Siegelaub, & Collen, 1973).

Just as these recent studies have documented unexpectedly high rates of hypertension among Blacks, research comparing the frequency of disease between Asian-Americans and their heritage groups in Asia as well as between Asian-Americans and Anglos has pinpointed unexpected health problems. Specifically, there is mounting evidence that Asian and Pacific peoples living in the United States suffer from high rates of hypertension and circulatory problems. That this unfortunate condition is associated with residence in the United States is suggested by survey data showing that the frequencies of high blood pressure, stroke, and cardiovascular disease are greater for United States residents than for similar groups living elsewhere. For example, Kagan reports that for every heart attack suffered by a Japanese male in Japan, there are two for Hawaiian Japanese and 10 for California Japanese-Americans (Keys, 1966; see also Gordon, 1957, Kato, Tillotson, Nichaman, Rhoads, & Hamilton, 1973; Tillotson, Kato, Nichaman, Miller, Gay, Johnson, & Rhoads, 1973). Similar patterns of comparative disadvantages are seen in the lower rates of heart disease and hypertension among southeast Asian Chinese compared with American Chinese (Kleinman, Kunstadter, Alexander, & Gale, 1974). These cross-sectional or one-time survey data are augmented by longitudinal studies that suggest that the frequency of hypertension among Guamians and other Pacific island peoples has increased over the past two or three decades—a period that has seen the growing Americanization of island culture and increased contacts with Americans. Groups of islanders who have immigrated to the United States are found to have a dramatically higher percentage of hypertensive individuals than among island residents.

While the evidence of hypertension among Asian and Pacific communities is fragmentary and a great deal more research is needed to determine clearly the extent and nature of the hypertension risk they face, the present record indicates the need to explore systematically the roots of hypertension so that remedial actions can be undertaken. To date, those examining hypertension among Asian and Pacific peoples have emphasized the causal role of diet: it is widely reported that high blood pressure is associated with eating highly salty foods (which are commonly found in Chinese, Japanese, and other Asian traditional diets), refined flour and sugar, and animal fats, beef, and other foods high in cholesterol (Bennett, Tokuyama, & McBride, 1962; Gordon, 1967; Keys, Kimura, Kusukawa, Bronte-Stewart, Larsen, & Keys, 1958; Moellering & Bassett, 1967; Wenkan & Wolff, 1970). The greatest combination of these foods is found in the diets of second- and third-generation Japanese and Chinese and other peoples whose traditional diet has been augmented by dairy products, beef, and bakery products. The fact that these groups also have the highest frequency of hypertension is seen as proof that diet is the major determinant of high blood pressure.

Diet is also cited by students of high blood pressure as responsible for the inflated levels of hypertension among Blacks. The chief villain, according to many observers, is "soul food." Among the diverse elements of this diet are chitterlings, sweet potatoes swimming in butter or margarine, and collard greens with "fatback." On top of all this customarily floats the fat-rich juice from cooking, which covers the dish like an oil slick. Corn bread or hush puppies (corn bread batter fried in lard) usually complements the main plate.

Soul food is high in carbohydrates and calories, and may add pounds to regular practitioners. Since obesity is related to high blood pressure and heart disease, soul food may be linked indirectly to a number of health problems. But probably more important to high blood pressure than the calories is the high levels of salt contained in soul food. Salt tends to attract water and thereby increases the volume of water circulating in the body. This process is apt to accelerate blood pressure and aggravate circulatory problems.

Although there is good reason to suspect that diet is associated with a wide range of health problems, there is growing evidence showing that to blame a group's eating habits for its heart disease and hypertension rates is simplistic. For example, clinical research is now reporting that there is little association between the consumption of animal fats and one's level of serum cholesterol. (It is serum cholesterol that produces the "plating" of arteries and vessels that is thought to lead to hardening of the arteries and hence to heart disease.)

Moreover, it is unlikely that soul food is the chief villain in the Black high blood pressure drama since few individuals consume it as a steady diet. Rather, traditional dishes are eaten at holidays or special occasions with daily nutrition not significantly different from that of Whites of equivalent socioeconomic status. The same is true for the consumption of traditional foods by American-born Asians. Preparation, volume, and quality of *all* foods rather than emphasis on traditional dishes is the key to the diet/health puzzle.

If total diet is only one of several determinants of hypertension what other conditions might cause high blood pressure? Research points to a host of factors, including heredity, occupation, smoking and drinking, gender (in some populations, women have a greater—while in other populations, a lower—rate of hypertension), and obesity. But the fact that the frequency of hypertension among Asian and Pacific peoples is closely associated with their degree of acculturation into the dominant culture of the United States (as measured by the consumption of nontraditional "American" foods) points to the role of life-style as a factor worth considering. Looking so long at the association between westernized diet and hypertension may have hidden a more fundamental impact of American society on Asian and Pacific peoples.

For many individuals, being a part of American society generates high levels of stress (Chang, 1974; Henry & Cassell, 1969; Lamont & Tyler, 1973; Okano & Spika, 1971; Sue & Sue, 1971). "Stress" is the physical and emotional tension that makes it difficult or impossible to obtain the psychological comfort and reassurance that allows one to be at ease. Accommodation to this unsatisfactory situation may take many forms; commonly, however, stress results in poor mental and physical health: drinking and drug abuse, suicide, mental breakdown, psychosomatic complaints, ulcers, and, of course, heart disease have all been linked to high levels of stress. Of special interest to students of hypertension is the study of 3,500 tax accountants that shows that blood cholesterol levels shoot up radically around April 15 (income tax filing deadline) with no changes in diet or body weight, pointing to stress as a factor that cannot be ignored in the causality of heart disease. (Friedman and Rosenman, 1974; also see the discussion of the association between dietary cholesterol and level of serum cholesterol, Nutrition Newsletter, 1977).

As we shall see in a moment, stress and the coronary risks it entails comes from many sources: family, community, economic and social organizations—even from schools and the mass media. Sometimes it is blatant, such as racist discrimination. Often stress arises from subtle relationships, such as that between the characters in a television program or commercial and the minority community viewer. Sometimes stress results from something as apparently benign as teaching children how to arrange silverware at the dinner table. Yet explicit, subtle, or apparently benign, sources of stress must be identified because they pose potential health risks to millions of Americans. In the following paragraphs we shall illustrate a few of the many sources of stress.

Sources of Stress

Asian and Pacific peoples, along with all ethnic minorities in the United States, may suffer stress from being presented models of what constitutes a "successful" man and a "desirable" woman—models that they are physically and emotionally unprepared and unable to meet (Matsumoto, 1970). Remember also that the media present Asian and Pacific peoples with two views of themselves—the exotic female sex object and the maniacal practitioner of martial arts. Stereotypes of Asian and Pacific peoples, especially Japanese and Chinese, are permitted in the media that are now without parallel for Blacks, Jews, Italians, and other minorities.

The public school system offers scarcely a less distorted portrait of

Asian and Pacific peoples. Typically, the picture is one of quiet people dressed in "traditional" clothes—which may mean grass skirts— dancing, eating with chopsticks, or kite flying. All too often the "unit" on Asian and Pacific peoples consists of an Anglo teacher presenting slides of temples, dances, or art work. No attention is given the internment of the Japanese-Americans during World War II; the exploitation of Filipino, Chinese, Hawaiian, and Japanese agricultural workers during the 19th and 20th centuries is ignored; and the history of anti-Asian legislation is conveniently overlooked. Examples of successful Asian and Pacific individuals are sometimes used to show positive role models, but it is forgotten that Koreans, Indochinese, Indonesians, and Pacific islanders identify very little with Japanese senators, Samoan football players, and Chinese business leaders.

The criterion of measuring personal worth in terms of economic attainment that the media present is reinforced in many Asian and Pacific families by pressure on children to strive and achieve excellence in school and later in their careers. This pressure to succeed seems to weigh especially heavily on Japanese and Chinese men: the high rates of psychosomatic illnesses, alcoholism, suicide, mental breakdown, marital breakup, and heart disease among university-educated, professional, and semiprofessional Asian males are mute testimony of this emphasis on success and the terrible toll trying to be "successful" extracts.

While the typical Asian and Pacific family and community may generate pressures to be successful, individual members also are given a great deal of support and comfort from the complex network of social, economic, recreational, and cultural institutions within most communities. Here, traditional and familiar foods, games, languages, and styles of interpersonal relations are found and enjoyed. More and more, however, the children and grandchildren of the pioneer generation are leaving the "Little Tokyos" and "Little Manilas" and moving into the suburbs. Others are cut off from full participation in the traditional community by their lack of language fluency. Some have turned their backs on the traditional community in an attempt to become "good Americans" through assimilating into the dominant society and casting off as much of their uniqueness as possible.

Many individuals appear to have integrated successfully with the overall population, but countless individuals seem not to have made this transition. Psychologists speak of the "marginal man," the individual who has turned his back on his parents' culture or community but has not been accepted by (or become comfortable with) another group. Characteristically, the marginal individual is recognized by a host of psychological and even physical problems that have their origin in stress. While part of this stress is generated by pressures to be successful economically and socially, the person living on the fringe between the traditional community and the broader society is especially vulnerable to rejection and hostility coming from the latter.

Although most Anglos are ignorant of it, minorities are attuned to the melody of hostility that emanates from the dominant society. For Asian and Pacific peoples, the refrain is both familiar and clear. Examples of official hostility include anti-Asian legislation that forbids immigration, land ownership, citizenship, and entry into a wide range of occupations; the internment of tens of thousands of Japanese-Americans during World War II while German–Americans and Italian–Americans walked the streets; two wars during the past 25 years fought against Asian peoples—wars accompanied by atrocities against Asians that were widely reported but officially ignored. The negative reaction of many Americans, including spokespersons for other minority communities, to the resettlement of Indochinese refugees is seen as more proof of an underlying hostility to all Asians—or so many Asian and Pacific peoples believe.

This history of discrimination and persecution is a part of the legacy of every Asian and Pacific American and reminds even the most successful that they must be watchful for signs of renewed enmity. Is it possible to be fully at ease and without stress in a society that has so often in the past treated individual Asians as part of an undesirable collective?

The rising levels of hypertension among Japanese and Chinese who have entered the middle class should not be interpreted to mean that hypertension is a problem only of the well-to-do. Recent data from Hawaii demonstrate that low-income Filipinos, Pacific islanders, and other disadvantaged peoples also report a high incidence of hypertension. Moreover, although not all new arrivals are economically disadvantaged and not all poor Asian and Pacific peoples are recent immigrants, there is a very close association between poverty, recent arrival, and marginal assimilation and acculturation.

Female partners in international marriages (i.e., "war brides") form a distinctive group of high-risk Asian- and Pacific–Americans. Fragmentary reports from Los Angeles, Long Beach, Seattle, and elsewhere where there are outreach programs for these women suggest that many live in a particularly stressful environment. Language problems, the absence of community friends and family, being generally restricted in social and recreational contacts to their spouse's relatives and friends are widely reported conditions. Not surprisingly, these women also have high rates of alcoholism, drug abuse, nervous breakdown, child abuse, suicide and attempted suicide, and other indicators of severe stress. It would be unusual if hypertension were not also part of this syndrome of despair.

One of the starkest illustrations of the social origins of stress is reported in a recent Detroit study (Harburg, Erfurts, Hauenstein, Chape, Schull, & Schork, 1973; see also Harburg, Erfurts, Chape, Hauenstein, Schull, & Schork, 1973). A sample of Black males living in areas characterized by low socioeconomic status, high crime rates, high population density, high residential mobility, and high rates of marital breakup—that is, "high-stress environments"—contained higher frequencies of elevated blood pressure than a sample of Blacks living outside of the high stress areas. Here the association is clearly revealed between a group's physical environment and the life-style it creates (in this case, a life-style fraught with tension from the threat of physical abuse, from constant economic and psychological marginality, and from the inability to establish rewarding continuous relationships in one's living space).

Equally significant, however, is the finding that *color* is related to blood pressure. In the Detroit study, the highest aggregate blood pressure rates were reported for the element of the population with the darkest skin. That is, as the proportion of the study group with the darkest skin pigmentation increased, so did the percent of the group reported hypertensive. The significance of color to the etiology of hypertension has been reported elsewhere (cf. Boyle, 1970) and seems to confirm the hypothesis that there is a significantly greater prevalence of high blood pressure among dark compared with lighter Blacks.

Of course, the density of pigmentation *per se* has no bearing on blood pressure. Rising blood pressure levels are created by the irrationality and prejudice of the American society that has historically discriminated against individuals on the basis of their color. From slavery onward, White society has placed a premium on light skin. Those "Blacks" who could pass for White were able to escape the legal and social barriers that restricted their darker brothers and sisters. Within the Black community, light skin has been preferred traditionally by many community leaders and institutions—witness the cover girls of Black-oriented publications and the numerous advertisements for skin bleaches in these magazines. Consequently, dark-skinned individuals receive massive assaults on their sense of self-worth from such stereotyping.

Fortunately, the 1970s witnessed a change, at least publicly, in the image of what constitutes beauty in the Black community. The "Black Is Beautiful" movement, along with closer and wider recognition of African heritage and culture, has liberated many Blacks from racist stereotypes of personal worth. Yet we still do not know the extent to which self-hate and self-denial arise in the minds of Blacks and other minorities from their inability to appear "White." The psychological aberration caused by rejecting one's body can be corrected by publicizing authentic ethnic identities that are free of racist and sexist clichés.

Whether the origins of hypertension are traced to slavery, segregation, contemporary racism, diet, or heredity, it is certain that socially induced personal stress is a major determinant. Kramer (1970) points to both the psychological and physiological ramifications of being an ethnic minority in America when she links race to social acceptance:

> The psychological concomitant to racial visibility is personal invisibility. When a categorical status (being a "Negro") is internalized without another set of cul-

tural values even to cause conflict, there are no social alternatives available to serve as a source of identity . . . There is no positive response from within that can offer any psychological resolution. The resulting tension is all but intolerable. . . . (p. 18)

Limited Preventive Role of Health Care Providers

The emphasis that many scholars place on the role of traditional health care behavior—including diet, superstition, avoidance of scientific providers, reliance on ineffective patent medicines, and an unwillingness to be hospitalized—in fostering high mortality and morbidity rates among ethnic minorities offers an important set of insights for those concerned with promoting better health. Practitioners need to be aware of the idiosyncrasies of their patients in order to provide services. Also, people should be alerted to the risks involved in selected traditional practices.

Nevertheless, excessive concern with the subculture of health produces a distorted and potentially dangerous view of the health risks facing millions of individuals. There is arresting evidence that many health risks spring from institutions and forces outside the individual and the minority community over which they have no control. Any definition of health problems that is to serve as a point of departure for curative and preventive efforts *must* incorporate these relevant societal factors. Yet achieving the level of analytical sophistication that pinpoints the social origins of health problems is no guarantee of a successful assault on the pathologies themselves.

Although modern medicine treats their symptoms, counteracting the factors that contribute to high blood pressure and heart disease falls far outside the traditional physician-patient relationship. For example, biochemists, nutritionists, schoolteachers, home economists, sociologists, city planners, and psychologists can perform important roles in public education and in lessening the prevalence of many diseases. The actions of business persons, bankers, and other economic elites who make decisions about where to locate employment opportunities and what types of job skills will be used can have an important bearing on health issues because economic independence and a decent standard of living can go a long way toward promoting human dignity and thereby reducing stress. Legislators and administrators who control research budgets for the national institutes of health and other organizations that need funds to support both basic and applied research into the causes and treatment of circulatory diseases also play an important part in the process of reducing disability and death.

In the final analysis, however, circulatory pathologies will be little affected by education, research, or economic improvements because hypertension and related disorders stem from and are affected by the individual's attitudes, values, and behavior, and by social institutions. The tremendous costs of these diseases, in terms of human misery, economic goods and services consumed fighting them, and the unemployment they create, will not be reduced until reforms are made that change a good many of America's basic institutions. Cancer can be reduced dramatically by cleaning up the physical environment; smallpox and other infectious diseases can be eliminated by breakthroughs in science and technology. But most diseases of the circulatory system appear to be largely *social pathologies,* which can be affected or controlled only very marginally by scientific medicine and modern technology. They can be treated in the conventional manner, but their prevention, like the prevention of venereal disease, alcoholism, and most mental illness, awaits a reordering of society's institutions, priorities, and values.

Ethnic minorities may represent a special case in the array and severity of social factors that intervene to increase health risks. These social factors may be all the more destructive for being subtle and covert. However, when they are added to poor nutrition, ignorance of symptoms, inability or willingness to obtain treatment, and other disease-supporting conditions, levels of morbidity and mortality climb. The particular manner in which social stressors affect minorities creates for them a unique set of health risks—risks not open to correction by traditional curative procedures.

Conclusion

The preceding analysis suggests that social stressors play an important, if little understood, role in elevating the levels of heart disease and hypertension reported for minority communities. These psychosocial variables seem to combine with biological and cultural conditions to promote or exacerbate disease. This additive, interactive model of health risk does not prescribe the relative importance of its components, and in this regard, the model is clearly deficient as a guide to preventive and remedial action. The next step is to refine the model by determining the relative priorities or weights of institutional racism, health care subculture, financial barriers to care, absence of positive role models, and so forth. This will lead to information that can be the basis for living and collective corrective action.

References

Bennett, C., Tokuyama, G. H., & McBride, T. C. Cardiovascular renal mortality in Hawaii. *American Journal of Public Health,* 1962, *52,* 1418–1431.
Boyle, E., Jr. Biological patterns in hypertension by race, sex, body weight, and skin color. *Journal of the American Medical Association,* 1970, *213* (Sept. 7), 1637–1643.
Chang, S. Mental health in Chinatown. *Bridge,* 1974, *1,* 34–37.

Friedman, M., & Rosenman, R. *Type A behavior and your heart.* New York: Knopf, 1974.

Gordon, T. Mortality experience among the Japanese in the United States, Hawaii, and Japan. *Public Health Reports, 1957, 72,* 543–553.

Gordon, T. Further mortality experience among Japanese Americans. *Public Health Reports, 1967, 82,* 973–984.

Harburg, E., Erfurts, J. C., Hauenstein, L. S., Chape, C., Schull, W. J., & Schork, M. A. Socioecological stress, suppressed hostility, skin color and black-white male blood pressure. Detroit. *Psychosomatic Medicine, 1973, 35* (July-Aug.), 276–296.

Harburg, E. Erfurts, J. C., Hauenstein, L. S., Chape, C., Schull, W. J., & Schork, M. A. Socioecological stressor areas and black-white blood pressure: Detroit. *Journal of Chronic Diseases, 1973, 26* (Sept.), 595–611.

Henry, J. P., & Cassell, J. C. Psychosocial factors in essential hypertension: Recent epidemiologic and animal experimental evidence. *American Journal of Epidemiology, 1969, 90* (Sept.), 171–200.

Kato, H., Tillotson, J., Nichaman, M. Z., Rhoads, G. G., & Hamilton, H. B. Epidemiologic studies of coronary heart disease and stroke in Japanese men living in Japan, Hawaii, and California: Serum lipids and diets. *American Journal of Epidemiology, 1973, 97,* 372–385.

Keys, A. 10 heart attacks in the United States for 1 in Japan. *American Heart, 1966, 15,* 6.

Keys, A., Kimura, N., Kusukawa, A., Bronte-Stewart, B., Larsen, N., & Keys, M. H. Lessons from serum cholesterol studies in Japan, Hawaii, and Los Angeles. *Annals of Internal Medicine, 1958, 48,* 83–94.

Kiev, A. *Curanderismo: Mexican-American folk psychiatry.* New York: Free Press, 1968.

Kilcoyne, M. M. Hypertension and heart disease in the urban community. *Bulletin of the New York Academy of Medicine, 1973, 49* (June), 501–509.

Kleinman, A., Kunstadter, P., Alexander, E. R., & Gale, J. L. (Eds.). *Medicine in Chinese cultures: Comparative studies of health care in Chinese and other societies.* (Washington, D.C.: U.S. Government Printing Office, 1976.

Kramer, J. R. *The American minority community.* New York: Thomas Y. Crowell, 1970.

Lamont, J., & Tyler, C. Racial differences in rates of depression. *Journal of Clinical Psychology, 1973, 29,* 428–432.

Matsumoto, Y. S. Social stress and coronary heart disease in Japan: A hypothesis. *Milbank Memorial Fund Quarterly, 1970, 47,* 9–36.

McMahon, F. G., Cole, P. A., & Ryan, J. R. A study of hypertension in the inner city. A student hypertension survey. *American Heart Journal, 1973, 85* (Jan.), 69–70.

Moellering, R., & Bassett, D. R. Myocardial infarction in Hawaiian and Japanese males on Ohau—A review of 505 cases occuring between 1955 and 1964. *Journal of Chronic Diseases, 1967, 20,* 89–101.

Nutrition Newsletter, 1(1). Silver Spring, Md.: Food for Thought, 1977.

Oakes, T. W., Syme, S. L., Feldman, R., Friedman, G. D., Siegelaub, A. B. & Collen, M. F. Social factors in newly discovered elevated blood pressure. *Journal of Health and Social Behavior, 1973, 14* (Sept.), 198–204.

Okano, Y., & Spika, B. Ethnic identity, alienation, and achievement in Japanese-American families. *Journal of Cross-Cultural Psychology, 1971, 2,* 273–282.

Sanders, L., *Cultural differences and medical care: The case of the Spanish-speaking people of the Southwest.* New York: Russell Sage Foundation, 1954.

17 million Americans with hypertension. *Public Health Reports, 1966, 81* (March), 262.

Suchman, E. A. Socio-medical variations among ethnic groups. *American Journal of Sociology, 1964, 70* (Nov.), 319–331.

Suchman, E. A. Social patterns of illness and medical care. *Journal of Human Behavior, 1965, 6* (Spring), 2–16.

Sue, S., & Sue, P. Chinese-American personality and mental health. *Amerasia Journal, 1971, 1,* 36–49.

Syme, S. L., Oakes, T. W., Friedman, G. D., Feldman, R., Siegelaub, A. B., & Collen, M. Social class and racial differences in blood pressure. *American Journal of Public Health,* 1974, *64* (June), 619.

Tillotson, J. L., Kato, H., Nichaman, M. Z., Miller, D. C., Gay, M. L., Johnson, K. G., & Rhoads, G. G. Epidemiology of coronary heart disease and stroke in Japanese men living in Japan, Hawaii, and California: Methodology for comparison of diet. *American Journal of Clinical Nutrition,* 1973, *26,* 177–184.

Weaver, J. L. Mexican-American health care behavior: A critical review of the literature. *Social Seience Quarterly,* 1973, *53* (June), 85–102.

Weaver, J. L. *National health policy and the underserved: Ethnic minorities, women, and the elderly.* St. Louis: C. V. Mosby, 1976.

Wenkam, N. S., Wolff, R. J. A half century of changing food habits among Japanese in Hawaii. *American Dietetics Association Journal,* 1970, *57,* 29–32.

13

The Social and Psychological Aspects of Family Planning

Laurie Zivetz

It is widely recognized that the earth's population is growing at an unprecedented rate. In 1650 there were 500 million people in the world. By 1850 that number had doubled twice. In 1974 there were approximately 4 billion people. At present rates of population growth, it is estimated that 7 billion people will greet the 21st century.

While this surging population increase raises a number of important economic, social, and political issues, in this chapter we are going to focus on the psychological and cultural factors that impinge upon couples and shape their fertility behavior. Fertility behavior here means the decisions human beings make that affect the number of children they raise, the gender composition of their family, and their beliefs and practices concerning contraception. We shall see that there are widely differing attitudes, practices and beliefs from culture to culture, within a single group, and among different social classes.

It is important to begin our examination of family planning with the understanding that every society has a set of culturally derived behaviors related to fertility (Hines, 1963). For instance, the age at marriage that is acceptable in some African tribes, in which a young woman becomes part of her husband's household before she reaches puberty, gives the African a 5- to 15-year head start on her counterpart in the United States, where mar-

Laurie Zivetz • Research Triangle Institute, Office for International Programs, Research Triangle Park, Durham, North Carolina 27709.

riage is deferred until the late teens or 20s. Stigmas against the teen-age American who marries around puberty are as strong as those against the African adolescent who does not marry. Because of early marriage, the African woman may have borne two or three children by the time her American sister is bearing her first (United Nations, 1973).

Cultural practices relating to the role of women, division of labor, taboos against coitus and remarriage, as well as preference for male or female children, all impact upon fertility behavior (Hawthorn, 1970). These behaviors evolve in response to a particular set of circumstances. In a Darwinian sense, they do not arise randomly but are adaptations to the particular environmental "niche" in which the individuals live.

For instance, among nomadic tribes, child spacing is practiced to ensure that the mother will not be overly burdened with the physical weight and extra expenditure of labor that child-rearing entails. The survival of the group depends not only upon her role as child-bearer but also upon her contribution in gathering and preparing food, making clothes, erecting shelters, carrying common possessions, and so forth. The time and energy demands of children compete with the demands of these duties. In addition, young children represent added mouths at the communal pot that do not contribute additional economic resources. The survival of nomadic hunting peoples has made a 4-year birth interval necessary, as compared to 1–2 years among subsistence farmers. Subsistence farmers value the labor even 2- or 3-year-olds are able to contribute (Kolata, 1974).

Death rates in peasant societies have been very high historically. Therefore, great attention and emphasis continues to focus on reproduction as central to perpetuation of the community. Elaborate ritual, magic, and religious significances are attached to conception and birth. However, the balance between underpopulation and overpopulation has been tenuous in communities where famine and disease are constant threats to survival. Thus, the well-being of the group depends as much on procreation to produce labor as it does on fertility regulation to maintain the delicate balance between the food supply and the number of mouths to feed (Douglas, 1966).

Determinants of Contraceptive Use

Behaviors that involve the regulation of reproduction may be grouped into two categories: those practices dealing directly with conception (*fertility control*) and those culturally sanctioned behaviors that, directly or indirectly, affect group size (*population control*). Anthopological accounts of primitive societies reveal that abortion, infanticide, and postpartum abstinence are common, age-old forms of fertility control (Newman, 1972). In fact, recent studies from all over the world show that from one-tenth to one-quarter of all pregnancies end in spontaneous abortion (Newman, 1972). Chemical, mechanical, and magical means are the most common methods used to induce abortion, but throughout history, oils, earth, herb teas, animal parts, and other substances have been taken orally or rubbed on the outside of the body as abortifacients or to prevent conception. Activities such as running, jumping, beating the abdomen, or bleeding the pregnant women are common traditional modes of aborting. In general, however, mechanical rupturing of the amniotic membrane remains the most widespread method of abortion. Among traditional societies this is done in a number of ways, such as the use of leaves on the end of sticks. Intricate magical ceremonies involving the wearing of amulets are also prevalent (though questionable) methods used to interfere with conception or gestation of an unwanted fetus. (Himes, 1963).

Infanticide connected with ritual and magical beliefs is often encountered in primitive societies (Himes, 1963). Infanticide serves the dual purpose of limiting population while weeding out children who might prove to be unproductive or dependent members of the society because of some physical defect. Infanticide is also commonly gender-related in situations where either more mothers or, alternatively, more male warriors are needed. In some cultures, twins are received superstitiously and one or both may be killed. (Newman, 1972).

Infanticide may also be caused by indirect behavior. For instance, a common practice in some very poor nomadic and hunting groups is leaving an ailing child unattended or minimally cared for until it dies. Where food is in very short supply, some groups decide to support older children who have survived the rigors of infancy, to the detriment of the newest members. *Kwashiorkor*, literally "the child who has been replaced at the breast," is a severe form of protein malnutrition that accounts for a substantial percentage of infant and child mortality and morbidity in many developing countries. The older child, whose source of protein and calories has been abruptly cut off with the arrival of a new baby, becomes more vulnerable to disease from the environment and has to fend for itself at the common pot. (Huenemann, 1977).

Coitus interruptus is an ancient and still widely practiced coitus-related form of contraception (Firth, 1936). In communities where coitus interruptus is prescribed at appropriate times in the estrous cycle, this form of contraception may make a significant impact on fertility. Roman Catholic as well as Hindu and Moslem religious dictums urge members wishing to practice birth control to use withdrawal as a "natural," not physically intrusive form of contraception.

The use of bark, herbs, dung, seaweed, and later metal and plaster pessary devices or cervical blocks was once widely practiced and is still common in many societies. This technique of blocking the entrance to the uterus evolved into the cervical cap and eventually the modern diaphragm. (Himes, 1963).

More extreme irreversible modes of birth control such as male castration and female sterilization are not uncommon in the history of contraception. The ancient Egyptians removed the ovaries of some women and girls, ostensibly to prolong the bloom of youth (Himes, 1963). Castration of captured warriors was used in ancient China to humiliate prisoners while preventing the natural increase of the enemy. In many societies, slaves were castrated so they could not threaten their owner's women. Subincision of the penis, by which a small slit is cut in the urethral canal at the base of the penis, is practiced by some primitive tribes. This technique renders the male relatively infertile because little or no sperm is ejaculated into the vagina (Newman, 1972).

Contemporary Approaches to Family Planning

Methods of contraception vary from society to society as well as across time. We have witnessed a vast change in contraceptive technology during the post-1945 era, so that many of the forms mentioned above are now rarely encountered in industrialized societies. The rate at which old methods are displaced with new forms is largely determined by societal attitudes and norms as well as by availability of contraceptive alternatives.

Every culture has mores, norms, taboos, and laws that represent its "population policy." Forms of family planning that are not consonant with this code simply will not become widely accepted (Economic and Social Commission for Asia and the Pacific, 1974). For example, where strict taboos against gynecological examinations exist, the intrauterine device (IUD) is unpopular because it requires contact between the recipient and the person performing the insertion (Scrimshaw, 1976) If only male personnel have been trained to perform insertions, resistance to use of the IUD based on cultural modesty may effectively prohibit the widespread use of the IUD (Scrimshaw, 1976). In societies where placing any foreign substance in the womb is seen as an irreversible impairment to the women's ability to conceive, IUDs may be equally unacceptable. Advocacy of IUDs in such circumstances places a tremendous psychological burden on potential acceptors who cannot reconcile their belief system with the argument that fertility will be restored with the IUD's removal.

Sterilization is incompatible in several religious and cultural contexts. Islam prohibits "mutilation" of the body, while Catholicism forbids forms of contraception that are nonreversible. Despite this, sterilization is the growing choice of contraception for many couples in developing countries as well as in the Western world. It is popular primarily because it is relatively permanent, inexpensive, and noncoitus-related.

The introduction in the early 1960s of the birth control pill has revolutionized family planning around the world. Currently, over 50 million women worldwide regularly use the pill to control their fertility (Population Report, 1975). The near-universal acceptance of the pill reflects the fact that it is noncoitus-related, easily reversible, and 95% effective (Tietze, 1969). In addition, the pill is easily distributed even in the most primitive areas because it requires little or no specialized storage, handling, or reliance on medical personnel for its use.

Clinical research has pointed out that there are several health risks associated with the pill among certain classes of users. Among women over 40 years old or women who smoke tobacco, elevated blood pressure, kidney infection, heart attack, and blood clotting have been correlated with taking the pill.[1] However, both producers of the pill and international agencies that distribute billions of pill cycles worldwide believe that the risk of mortality or morbidity from too many pregnancies far exceeds risks from clinically demonstrated counterindications of the pill (see footnote 1).

Condoms are used throughout the world, particularly where IUDs and sterilization are frowned upon and where the pill is not widely available. The condom has the advantage of having traditional (penis sheath) counterparts in many societies. Where there are not enough medical personnel to insert IUDs or the supply system cannot deliver massive numbers of pill cycles regularly, the condom is often the method of choice because it requires no backup medication support or elaborate supply system. Hundreds of units may be dropped off at small shops or stores on an irregular basis. Where such small businesses are politically powerful, condoms that are sold for profit by merchants may make their way into more expanded private distribution networks than will IUDs or pills, which are usually distributed free of cost or at a very low price by public health or other government agencies.

Diaphragms are commonly used in the United States among middle- and upper- middle-class women who wish to control their fertility temporarily but who choose not to use the pill. In the developing world, however, where sanitary conditions make it difficult to protect the diaphragm and coitus-related contraception on the part of the woman is unacceptable, it is less popular. In cultures where females are prohibited from touching their own genitalia, the use of the diaphragm is effectively curtailed.

---

[1]Corea, G. *The hidden malpractice.* William Morrow, referencing 'Hearings before the Subcommittee on Small Businesses, United States Senate, Second Session on Present Status of Competition in the Pharmaceutical Industry, Parts 15, 16, 17, Oral Contraceptives, Vols. I, II, and II. January-March, 1970.

Abortion has been an acceptable form of birth control in most societies throughout history (Himes, 1963). As we saw above, traditional preindustrial societies practiced abortion through reliance on herbs, violent body movement, or mechanical rupturing of the amniotic membrane. In the 20th century, abortion is still widely practiced (Freedman, Coombs, & Friedman, 1966), although in some societies, notably those where the Roman Catholic church is politically powerful, laws make it virtually impossible to receive a legal medical abortion. Nevertheless, self-induced and illegally obtained abortions, often with great risk to the woman from unsanitary situations and unskilled personnel, are widely reported (Romero, 1966). It is estimated currently that between 30 and 55 million unwanted pregnancies are terminated worldwide each year (Draper World Population Fund Report, 1978). Approximately half of these abortions are illegal. In face of the legal barriers and health problems many women encounter in obtaining abortions, this figure, even if it is only indicative and not an accurate indicator of the extent of abortions, bespeaks a widespread acceptance of abortion throughout the world. This reliance on abortion also reflects the fact that historically there has been an absence of effective reliable means of birth control. Only through abortion has the woman been ensured against the birth of an unwanted child.

Today, abortion is most frequently the recourse of poorer or more isolated women who do not have access to other means of family planning. In Latin America, middle-class, urban women enter hospitals and doctors' offices to obtain contraceptives while their lower-class and rural sisters are brought in through the emergency room for treatment of vaginal hemorrhages and infections resulting from illegal abortions (Romero, 1966). Research that uncovered the tremendous mortality and morbidity rates from illegal abortions in the slums of Chilean cities was instrumental in the liberalization of Chile's laws governing the sale and distribution of contraceptives (Romero, 1966).

In the United States, abortion has become increasingly common. Improved technology of abortion techniques plus changing legislation makes abortion both a viable backup to contraceptive failure and an attractive alternative to an unwanted pregnancy. In the United States in 1974, 32% of all abortions were performed on women under 20 years of age (Center for Disease Control, 1974). Apparently, having an abortion is now an increasingly acceptable alternative to either early parenthood or early marriage.

Incentives to Control Fertility

Aside from taboos, customs, and laws that impinge upon the use of contraceptives, every society offers incentives to regulate fertility (Berelson, 1971). Sometimes these incentives are direct. In the United States, for instance, taxpayers receive an exemption for each child: an incentive for large families, all else being equal. However, there are also indirect incentives to have small or large families. In places where subsidized public housing is available but apartments have only two bedrooms, families with more than three or four children simply are not eligible. On the other hand, governments may offer incentives to settle in sparsely populated land where settlers are encouraged, by the economics of agriculture, to have large families in order to secure the needed labor (Nerlove, 1974).

Aside from government policies that act as incentives or disincentives to control fertility, societies reinforce collective mores, attitudes, and customs through informal but often highly effective sanctions. Each member of a society is exposed to models or behavioral traits that the group deems valuable (or unacceptable) (David & Lere, 1973). In the United States it is considered appropriate by most Americans for women to wear trousers but not for men to wear skirts; in Indonesia and Scotland it is perfectly acceptable for males to wear skirts. When members violate group mores, sanctions ranging from mild demonstrations of disapproval to physical violence are inflicted on the transgressor. Thus, the desire to be accepted, to be seen as a "good person," as well as fear of negative sanctions, bring most group members into conformity.

Perhaps the best example of how societal norms can effect fertility comes from the People's Republic of China (Tien, 1973). It is now widely accepted that marriage will be deferred until the individual's late 20s or early 30s. This practice, combined with severe taboos against illegitimacy plus the widespread use of contraceptives, allows Chinese women a far shorter effective fertility period than that of their counterparts in other developing countries where marriages are arranged for teen-aged women. The dramatic decline in China's population growth rate since 1960 is in large measure a reflection of the interaction of new legislation on abortion and contraception combined with the prevailing custom of late marriage (Tien, 1973).

China's preference for late marriage is part of the government's emphasis on the employment of women throughout the industrial and agricultural sectors. The entry of women into the Chinese labor force illustrates the fertility consequences of women taking on nontraditional economic roles. Rather than remaining in the home preparing food and tending children, woman are working for wages in jobs once restricted to men. These new activities tend to work against early and frequent maternity (Salaff, 1972).

In contrast to China's emphasis on new economic and social roles for women stand such countries as Pakistan, Afghanistan, and most of the Islamic world, where women are still rarely seen in business, commerce, or the professions. Here the barriers to nontraditional roles are especially strong for peasant and lower-class women. The popular perception of women as child-bearers and mothers leaves most Islamic women defining their worth to their husbands and the broader society in terms of their ability to bear and bring up children—especially male children (Boserup, 1970).

In the United States and Europe, the decline of traditional prohibitions against divorce, premarital sex, and illegitimacy, plus expanding education and employment opportunities, has produced a variety of economic roles for women. Today, women who wish to mix family and career are able to do so far more effectively than were previous generations. At the same time, it is increasingly acceptable by society for a woman not to have children. Taking on nontraditional roles varies considerably, however, among classes and regions in developed countries, with the level of education a powerful determinant of whether or not women place motherhood and having several children ahead of pursuing a career and having only one or two children. Religious preference is also a strong determinant of family size (Westoff, Potter, Sagi, & Mishler, 1961).

Changing attitudes about what is acceptable behavior for an American woman have come about in the context of a greater availability of safe and effective methods of birth control (Newman, 1972). From the ability to plan her family has come the potential for greater mobility—physical as well as social and economic. Moreover, greater access to education, plus recent antidiscriminatory legislation, have increased the range of alternatives to economic security both in and outside of marriage. As a result of this combination of circumstances, many more women are opting to space their children and to have smaller families.

An analogous situation can be observed in many developing countries where women from urban, middle-class backgrounds have greater access to education, jobs, and contraception than their rural and lower-class counterparts. The discrepancy in birth rates between these groups is common in less developed countries where birth rates among the rural poor are at the highest end of the spectrum, whereas those in the urban middle class are at the lowest.

Part of this discrepancy in fertility rates reflects the fact that children are often highly valued for the labor they provide the lower-class family. Such labor is especially valued in subsistence agriculture, as mentioned above, because it enables the household to secure workers without having to pay for them in cash or to become indebted to other families for reciprocal labor (Nerlove, 1974).

In cash economies, where the division of labor is extensive, there is less economic opportunity for children, especially if the family is outside the agricultural sector. In this case, the marginal utility of additional children declines because each child represents a consumer of cash-based goods and services who is unable to earn equivalent amounts of money.

Aside from the labor they represent, children are seen in many societies as a source of protection against the hardships of old age or incapacity.

Couples may wish to have many children, especially sons, so that several will survive into adulthood in order to be able to offer their parents food, shelter, personal services, and other basic human needs (McGreevy & Birdsall, 1974). The decline in birth rates in Japan, Korea, and Taiwan are thought to be in part a result of the growing recognition on the part of urban workers and peasants that formal institutions such as governmental social security systems, public hospitals and health posts, and retirement plans will remove the support burden once carried by family members (Population Council, 1975).

In the context of economic development and urbanization, it has become increasingly clear that economic and social advancement is tied to receiving formal education (Interdisciplinary Communications Program, 1974). In parts of West Africa, parents seek to secure postsecondary education for one or two sons because such training opens the doors to government employment and the learned professions. Parents recognize that a son or two safely within the educated urban middle class is a much richer source of support than a dozen children living as peasants. Since secondary and postsecondary education is expensive, smaller families mean that there will be proportionately more money available for education.

Of considerable significance to fertility behavior may be the fact that only in the past two or three decades has a rural or lower-class child had a reasonable chance of surviving to adulthood. The centuries-old stability of the earth's population growth is a result of high infant mortality and short life-span. Since World War II, however, there has been a revolution in public health and medical care. Traditional killers such as malaria and smallpox have been controlled or eliminated. Famines and severe malnutrition, which once killed hundreds or thousands of children annually, are less threatening because of better distribution and production systems. Public sanitation has been improved in most of the world, and nutrition and personal hygiene education have helped to reduce or control diseases. Although there is a tremendous gap between the health conditions of rural and urban indigents and between middle- and lower-class areas, as well as between the industrial nations and developing nations, recent improvements in individual health have been felt globally. Yet, while life expectancy has increased and deaths per age cohort have declined markedly, there has been little change in the traditionally high birth rates in the developing world over the past three or four decades.

Some observers of this phenomenon have argued that people wish to control their own fertility but lack the information and contraceptives to do so.[2] This line of reasoning has led international organizations such as the International Planned Parenthood Federation and the Population Office of

[2]This has been the contention of the Population Division of the United States Agency for International Development under R. Ravenhold to date (11/78).

the United States Agency for International Development to spend billions of dollars to send millions of cycles of pills, millions of condoms, and thousands of sterilization kits to Asia, Latin America, and Africa. But for all of this effort, there are few places where birth rates have fallen significantly after the introduction of large-scale family planning programs.

There are a number of factors related to this limited impact of commodity programs. Distribution has failed in some places. There has been corruption and mismanagement. In several cases (such as in India) some family planning programs have become so highly politicized that efforts have had to be discontinued. Nevertheless, the likelihood remains that decisions to use an IUD, the pill, or a condom are not much different from decisions to use traditional forms of birth control. They are made in the context of existing social and psychological institutions and attitudes, which, in turn, rest on cultural norms, economic and political processes, and prevailing levels of technology. It may take several decades or generations for the full impact of disease control, new economic opportunities, and improved technologies to be reflected in smaller families.

Conclusion

Family planning is often falsely construed as a by-product of development. Although it is true that safer, more reliable methods of birth control have been developed in first world countries in the last 40 years, family planning *per se* is not a new phenomenon. As we have seen, all cultures practice some form of fertility control (Himes 1963). However, the political, social, and psychological factors that condition fertility behaviors are as variable as the techniques employed to promote or control fertility.

Because reproduction is so central to the human experience, the social and psychological significance attached to conception, contraception, and childbearing are strong currents in all cultures. Positive or negative sanctions concerning fertility behavior are as much in evidence in the United States as they were among primitive nomadic peoples of Central Africa.

As we have seen, changes in fertility behavior most often occur in response to a change in ecological, political, social, or economic circumstances; historically, however, fertility behavior has lagged behind these other changes. For instance, during the Industrial Revolution, Europe experienced a surge in population based on a drop in mortality and increased life-span that persisted over a century before a slowdown in the birth rate was achieved (United Nations, 1965). Currently, conditions in developing countries are changing with unprecedented speed. Infant death rates have dropped and average life-span has increased in most areas. But birth rates have slowed only slightly. As we have seen, only when parents feel that in fact fewer children are more desirable will they begin to change their fertility behavior.

The impetus for changing a couple's desired family size is two-pronged: it hinges primarily upon the social sanctions and mores that condition a couple's desire to have children, and secondarily upon the availability, reliability, and acceptability of birth control. Because of the very personal nature of fertility behavior, modern contraception is not introduced as easily into traditional societies. Since sexuality is often a taboo topic of conversation in traditional cultures, particularly between men and women, information about new methods of family planning cannot rely on oral communication to facilitate acceptability and adoption.

Providing couples with safe, effective, and easily available family planning methods offers them a powerful means for controlling their individual and collective destinies. The availability of contraceptives gives the couple the freedom of choice in determining the size and spacing of their family while affording the woman control over her body. Yet this freedom and responsibility comes only when an understanding is achieved of what motivates people to practice contraception. Knowledge and means are important elements in this motivation, but the controlling elements are individual attitudes, values, and behavior, which stem from and reflect the social and cultural institutions within which they exist.

References

Berelson, B. Population policy: Personal notes. *Population Studies,* 1971, *25,* 173–182.

Boserup, E. *Women's role in economic development.* New York: St. Martin's Press, 1970.

Center for Disease Control, DHEW. *Abortion Surveillance, 1974.*

David, H., & Lere, S. J. (Eds.). *Social and psychological aspects of fertility in Asia. Proceedings of the Technical Seminar.* Choonchun, Korea, Nov. 1973.

Douglas, M. Population control in primitive groups. *British Journal of Sociology,* 1966, *17,* 263–273.

Draper World Population Report, The. Washington, D.C. Summer, 1978.

Economic and Social Commission for Asia and the Pacific, United Nations. *Report and Papers of the Expert Group Meeting on Social and Psychological Aspects of Fertility Behavior,* Bancock, June 10–19, 1974.

Firth, R. *We, the Tikopia: A sociological study of kinship in primitive Polynesia.* London: Allen and Unwin, 1936.

Freedman, R., Coombs, L., & Friedman, J. Social correlates of foetal mortality. *Milbank Memorial Fund Quarterly,* 1966, *44,* 327–344.

Hawthorn, G. *The sociology of fertility.* London: Collier–Macmillan, 1970.

Himes, N. E. *Medical history of contraception.* New York: Gamut, 1963.

Huenemann, R. L. Nutrition and family planning. In *Women in food production, food handling and nutrition.* Report of the United Nations Protein Advisory Group, June 1977.

Kolata, G. B.! Kung hunter gatherers: Feminism, diet and birth control. *Science,* 1974, *185* (Sept. 13).

McGreevy, W. P., & Birdsall, N. *The policy relevance of recent social research on fertility.* Occasional monograph series No. 2. Interdisciplinary Communications Program, Smithsonian Institution, 1974.

Nerlove, M. Household and economy: Toward a new theory of population and economic growth. In *Marriage, family, human capital and fertility,* Proceedings of a conference sponsored by the National Bureau of Economic Research and the Population Council, June 4–5, 1974.

Newman, L. F. Birth control: An anthropological view. *Addison-Wesley Module in Anthropology,* 1972, *27,* 1–21.

Population Council, The. *Studies in family planning,* 1975, *6*(8), August.

Population Report. Series A on oral contraceptives, 1975.

Remero, H. Chile. In B. Berelson (Ed.), *Family planning and population programs.* Chicago and London: University of Chicago Press, 1966.

Salaff, J. Institutionalized motivation for birth limitation in China. *Population Studies,* 1972, *26*(2), 233–262.

Scrimshaw, S. C. M. Women's modesty: One barrier to the use of family planning clinics in Ecuador. In J. F. Marshall & S. Polgar (Eds.), *Culture, natality, and family planning.* Chapel Hill, N.C.: Carolina Population Center, 1976.

Tien, H. Y. *China's population struggle, 1949–1969.* Columbus: Ohio University Press, 1973.

Tietze, C. Modern methods of birth control: An evaluation. In B. Berelson (Ed.), *Family planning programs.* New York: Basic, 1969.

United Nations. The determinants and consequences of population trends. *Population Studies,* No. 50, 1973.

United Nations. *Population Bulletin 7, 1963.* New York: United Nations, 1965.

Westoff, C. F., Potter, R. G., Jr., Sagi, P. C., & Mishler, E. G. *Family growth in metropolitan America.* Princeton: Princeton University Press, 1961.

14

Healthy Family Functioning: Cross-Cultural Perspectives

Henry P. David

Introduction

Writing about healthy family functioning is expected to provoke questions. What is it? How is it defined? What are its implications for public health services, training, and research in different lands? As will be seen, adaptation and coping with diverse forms of sociocultural, environmental, economic, and physical stress are not the province of any one discipline, research orientation, or ideology. The widely dispersed international, behavioral, and biomedical literature does not yield any shared or systematic conceptualization of healthy family functioning or its determinants. While environmental circumstances placing increasing stress on family functioning are generally recognized, and family dysfunction is of growing public health concern, there are few studies identifying elements likely to strengthen family capabilities for coping and prevention.

Within these constraints, the chapter will examine briefly diverse concepts of family health and likely parameters of healthy family functioning, including a suggested definition. This is followed by a discussion of prevention promotion and the social revolution in the distribution of health re-

Henry P. David • Transnational Family Research Institute, Bethesda, Maryland 20034. This chapter was adapted, with permission, from an overview prepared under contract with the Division of Mental Health, World Health Organization, Geneva, Switzerland.

sources and the delivery of services. Effective fertility regulation is suggested as one example of healthy family functioning. The family life cycle is reviewed, together with relevant findings from psychosocial studies and research on family coping with environmental stress, such as uprooting and migration and the interaction between the family and mentally ill family members. Communal coping is considered in terms of enhanced self-reliance and mutual help; examples are noted from the People's Republic of China. Cross-cultural perspectives are cited together with cooperative research prospects and the need for more efficient utilization of already available knowledge and the assessment of potential transferability of experience from one country to another. After the presentation of an evolving theory of healthy family functioning, studies of young families are suggested as particularly promising vehicles for cooperative and comparative cross-cultural research. The chapter concludes with 225 references to the international behavioral and biomedical literature.

Although the emerging perspective is influenced heavily by the traditions of North American researchers, it should not be assumed that the research style developed in North America is universally applicable or valid beyond the conditions studied. Although colleagues with different backgrounds might well prefer a different approach to the topic, they would, I hope, share in the growing recognition of the necessity to redirect health resources and priorities to meet the urgent needs of that 80% of the world's population living under conditions of deprivation and rapid socioeconomic and cultural change.

Healthy Family Functioning: An Elusive Concept

The Family

The concept of the family is universal and has existed throughout history, although its form varies and is changing within societies (Carballo, 1975; Elliott, 1970; Johnson, 1975). Although preoccupation with the family as a sociocultural institution is as ancient as humanity, its scientific study in the context of mental health and family functioning in coping with stress is far more recent in origin (Fleck, 1975a), evoking the attention of numerous learned disciplines, including behavioral and biomedical researchers.

The view is widely shared that the family has been and continues to be society's primary agency in satisfying common needs for survival, a sense of loving and belonging, status and self-esteem, and self-realization. The family provides for the child's biological needs and simultaneously directs its development toward becoming an integrated person capable of living in society and maintaining and transmitting culture (Lidz, 1963). There has been considerable discussion of positive mental health (Jahoda, 1958), but many clinicians would probably concur with Tolstoy's opening statement in *Anna Karenina* that all happy families are similar and that all unhappy families are unhappy in their own fashion (cited by Fleck, 1976). Mental health professionals continue to focus more frequently on family dysfunction and its eventual origins than on healthy family functioning and the likely determinants of successful coping with a variety of stressors in differing socioenvironmental circumstances.

Family Health

Although the concept of family health has been discussed widely in medicine, it is rarely applied in the delivery of health care (Manciaux, 1975; Miller, 1975). A cursory review of the massive tangential literature demonstrates the ambiguity of such terms as *family health, family mental health,* and *healthy family functioning.* For example, family health may refer to the health of individual family members, the health of the family as a unit, or the sum of the health statuses of the individual family members (WHO, 1976). The designation of "family physician" is usually based on performing in identical health services role with all members of the family; formal knowledge and understanding of family dynamics and their institutional characteristics is a fairly recent development. It was not until 25 years after Freud's initial accounts of family-related unconscious processes that Flugel (1921) published the first psychoanalytic effort to conceptualize family processes. Systematic clinical study and research on the family as a group did not begin until the 1940s (Fleck, 1975a). Even more recent is the growing recognition of health as a social value, the relationship of the family to community health, and the need for societal actions to enhance family health.

The past two decades have seen a rapidly increasing clinical, scientific interest and appreciation of the family as one of the most significant social forces in human development. Study of disturbed families stimulated consideration of the normal, e.g., Ackerman's (1958) findings that the families of disturbed children needed study and treatment as a group. In the meantime, sociologists (e.g., Parsons, Merton, and Rainwater) had elucidated some of the institutional characteristics of the family, and the health effects of socioeconomic status, while anthropologists wrote about family structure in diverse cultures and societies. Systematic attention began to be given to the role of the total family in individual illness, the impact of disorder on family life, and the way the family contributes to illness and health care (Litman, 1974; WHO, 1976). The traditional role of the family as a support system is being reexamined as more liberal definitions of male and female roles, and alternative life-styles are increasingly discussed (Carballo, 1976).

In his comprehensive social behavior overview of the family as a basic unit in health and medical care, Litman (1974) observed that considerable knowledge has been gleaned concerning familial interaction, power relations, kinship structure, and socialization patterns but that with few exceptions, such other major issues as familial responsibility, adjustment, and behavior in health and illness "have generally escaped the empirical involvement and theoretical interest of the family sociologist." The terms *family health, family mental health,* or *healthy family functioning* are not cited in the indices to the 12,850 references on marriage and the family, published between 1900 and 1964 and reviewed by Aldous and Hill (1967). They also do not appear in subsequent inventories compiled for the years 1965–1972 by Aldous and Dahl (1974) and for 1973–1974 by Olson and Dahl (1975). Aldous (1971) defined a family problem as "any situation or circumstance which threatens the family's values, or those of its members, requiring cognitive effort on the part of one or more of its members and interaction among family members to resolve the situation in a manner commensurate with their values." Lieberman (1975) suggests that any treatment is incomplete without attention to the family.

WHO and Social Health

Recent years have witnessed a gradual shift from concern with individual pathology (and its effects on family dysfunction). In the area of mental health, for example, there has been a shift from specific conditions of major public health importance (such as acute psychoses, alcoholism, and drug abuse) to the effects of social environmental changes, promotion of mental health, and the protection of the family from mental disturbance. The 1974 Technical Discussions of the 27th World Health Assembly reviewed "the role of health services in preserving or restoring the full effectiveness of the human environment in the promotion of health." The reports submitted by WHO member countries and the ensuing discussions reflect a growing recognition of the health effects of changes in family structure, sociocultural attitudes, and environmental stress (Mahler, 1975; Meyer and Sainsbury, 1975).

Psychosocial factors in health have continued to be given increasing consideration in the deliberations of the WHO Assembly (1975). In 1976, psychosocial factors were defined as those

> influencing health, health services, and community well-being stemming from the psychology of the individual and the structure and function of social groups. They include social characteristics such as patterns of interaction within kinship

or occupation groups; cultural characteristics such as traditional ways of solving conflict; and psychological characteristics such as attitudes, beliefs, and personality factors.

The director-general's report to the 29th World Health Assembly (1975) includes a selective review of psychosocial factors, health, and health services, with particular relevance to WHO activities. An initial WHO Centre on Research and Training on Psychosocial Factors in Health has been established in Stockholm. Thus far, most of its energies have been directed toward studies of pathological effects on individuals. Although the importance of the holistic approach is recognized, there has been less emphasis on the family as a unit (Levi & Andersson, 1975). The 29th World Health Assembly (1975) confirmed the importance of the relationship between psychosocial factors and health, and their implication for health services, particularly concerning the needs of uprooted persons and families in conditions of rapid social change.

A Proposed Definition

There is growing recognition that rapid cultural, social, economic, and technical changes are imposing increasing stress on family structures, traditional values, and ability to adapt to new environments in diverse societies (Coelho, Hamburg, & Adams, 1974). For the purposes of this chapter, it is proposed that healthy family functioning (HFF) be defined in terms of a family unit (however delineated in a given society), effectively coping with cultural-environmental, psychosocial, and socioeconomic stressors throughout the diverse phases of the family life cycle. Although the literature does not yield any indications of coordinated and cooperative cross-cultural studies of well-functioning families or HFF, the impression persists that cohesive family life can reduce tensions and improve family coping capabilities (Buckle, Hoffmeyer, Isambert, Knobloch, Knoblochova, Krapf, Lebovici, Pertejo de Alcami, Pincus, & Sandler, 1965; Lewis, Beavers, Gossett, & Phillips, 1976; May, 1974; Rabkin, 1976). As will be noted in subsequent sections, study of healthy family functioning has posed as many complications as the concept, in part because empirical inquiry has been theoretically eclectic. With different views on health and well-being in diverse societies, it is recognized that it is likely there will be more than one model of healthy family functioning.

Perceptions of families coping with stress have been sensitively portrayed in the arts and in clinical reports; however, there is as yet no widely accepted theory of HFF. Few testable hypotheses have emerged and only a beginning has been made toward developing cross-culturally adaptable assessment procedures (Lewis et al., 1976; WHO, 1976). Social researchers are groping toward a better understanding of the complex interrelationships among individuals, family, health, and society (Hansen & Hill, 1964), while public health administrators are exploring new ways of responding to service demands generated by rapid social and environmental changes (Lalonde, 1975; Meyer & Sainsbury, 1975; Newell, 1975). Of particular relevance are potentially transferable experiences from developing countries representing different sociopolitical structures and recognizing the influence on family well-being of changes in socioeconomic sectors of society, the priority given to preventive hygiene over curative medicine, and the enhancement of self-reliance while accepting lowered standards of comprehensiveness and professional skill (Djukanovic & Mach, 1975; Wilenski, 1976; Wolfson, 1976).

Prevention Promotion: An Evolving Concept

An Emerging Social Revolution

Recognition of the health sector impact of environmental change and stress is accompanied by a global concern with the eroding quality of life and an awareness that family well-being is linked to progress in social and economic development. The relevance of conventional health services is being reconsidered (Miller, 1971). Different concepts of health promotion and delivery of services are being tried, especially in the rural sectors of developing countries, where most of the world's population resides (Newell, 1975). As Mahler (1976a) wrote in the report of the WHO director-general to the 1976 World Health Assembly, "Because disease technology has been rather institutional and patient-oriented, it has been sorely lacking in preventive emphasis . . . perhaps we have to restate the case for public health in social terms that will be relevant to all societies throughout the world." This view was further expressed in talks to WHO regional committees (Mahler, 1976b). The WHO deputy director-general expressed similar concerns: "It has been made painfully clear in recent years that health services too frequently lack relevance to the total needs of people" (Lambo, 1975a); "a more balanced consideration of the biological, social, and cultural aspects of health is needed" (Lambo, 1975b); and "there is room for social revolution in health which should pave the way to a more equitable distribution of health resources" (Lambo, 1976).

Prevention Terminology

In public health terminology, distinctions are made among (a) primary prevention, referring to actions taken prior to the onset of disease; (b) secondary prevention, meaning early diagnosis and treatment; and (c) tertiary prevention or rehabilitation efforts (Leavell & Clark, 1965). In this conceptualization, primary prevention usually has two aspects: (a) health promotion, referring to efforts to improve the quality of life and general level of health, and (b) specific protection, denoting explicit procedures for disease prevention. To reduce semantic difficulties, Goldston (1977) advocates limiting mental health usage of the term *prevention* to actions that aim to anticipate potential mental and emotional disorder or foster optimal mental health, thus making prevention in mental health synonymous with prevention in public health. Goldston further suggests that

> primary prevention encompasses those activities directed to specifically identified vulnerable high-risk groups within the community who have not been labeled as psychiatrically ill and for whom measures can be undertaken to avoid the onset of emotional disturbance and/or enhance their level of positive mental health. Programs for the promotion of mental health are primarily educational rather than clinical in conception and operation with their ultimate goal being to increase people's capacities for dealing with crises and for taking steps to improve their own lives.

Goldston's concept of health promotion connotes a social-psychocultural-educational model with emphasis on social competence, coping capability, and self-strengthening measures.

The staff of the Hogg Foundation (1976), Huntington (1975), Vaughn (1975), and others advocate the concept of "proactive," meaning "moving forward or ahead of" or acting rather than waiting for something to happen and then treating the symptoms. A proactive system is designed to support individual and/or family strength and coping mechanisms. Cromwell and Thomas (1976) similarly recognized that the family provides an arena for education and growth seldom tapped by organized health programs. Although there has been much discussion and clinical experience with family action models, family life education, and family interaction, a 1971 review of United States research did not elicit any project assessing family strengths (Otto, 1971).

Effective Fertility Regulation: An Example of Healthy Family Functioning

With the evolving worldwide awareness of the interdependence of population growth and socioeconomic development, modifiability of fertility behavior, motivation for fertility regulation, and effective utilization of already available knowledge and service capabilities have become priority areas for social science and family research. In many countries, the present generation of families is perhaps the first to engage in the conscious process of deciding not just how many children to have, and when, but whether to have children at all. For many couples, such deliberate decisions are at times difficult to make, requiring a balance of personal values, anticipated costs and benefits, and perceived societal pressures (David & Johnson, 1977). Rational fertility behavior may well be one example of HFF.

The pleasures that parents experience in raising their children are highly valued, as demonstrated in the cross-national studies of the value of children (Arnold, Bulatao, Buripakdi, Chung, Fawcett, Iritani, Lee, & Wu, 1975). Although the economic utility of children was found to be a waning motivating factor for most parents, persisting primarily in more remote rural areas, the contributions that children made to parental well-being were most highly prized. How many children are needed to experience the emotional benefits of parenthood is open to further consideration in diverse societies. With rapid social change, it may well be that psychosocial perspectives on family resource allocations, emphasizing subjective assessments of costs and benefits, will determine fertility behavior. The escalating costs of child-rearing may help explain the sudden convergence on two children as the preferred family size (David & Johnson, 1977).

More than any other health-related activity, effective couple decision making in family planning can positively affect biological, psychological, sociocultural, and economic aspects of family health, family functioning, and family well-being. When wanted children are born at optimum times, the family environment is more likely to be conducive to normal growth and development (David, 1972; Dytrych, Matejcek, Schüller, David, & Friedman, 1975). In terms of HFF, the most important pregnancy may be the first one (Lieberman, 1975). The evidence from developed and developing countries is persuasive that effective family planning improves the quality of life and thus HFF (Katz, 1972; Mukherjee, 1975; Munandar, 1970; Omran, 1974; Park, Chung, & Han, 1975; Wishik & Bernard, 1969). Psychoeconomic determinants in fertility decision making, especially by younger couples, may be another important ingredient of HFF (Schultz, 1974).

The Family Life Cycle

Structure

Each family experiences its own dynamics of formation, growth, maturation, and dissolution. Crises confronted may be divided into those that are transitional in the family life cycle (e.g., birth of first child or loss of spouse) or nontransitional (e.g., acts of war, uprooting, mental disorder). Various classifications have been proposed and are reviewed by Hansen and Hill (1964) and in the 1975 WHO consultation on family health (WHO, 1975b). Family sociologists have studied effects of sudden shifts in economic status, migration, uprooting, disasters, physical change or incapacity of a family member, and the impact of crises at diverse stages of the family life cycle. It has been hypothesized that stress and health hazards are likely to increase when environmental changes cluster at critical developmental periods such as adolescence, first pregnancy, menopause, retirement, and other transitions in the life cycle. How effective coping patterns are in given situations depends, in part, on perception of threat, motivation and readiness to respond creatively, available emotional and social supports, and cultural provisions (Coelho et al., 1974). Reports in the literature stem largely from studies of individuals; the concept of HFF has been more a matter of speculation than research (Moos, 1976).

Compared with other social organizations, the average family has distinct disadvantages. Its age composition is heavily weighted with dependents and is of uncertain sex distribution. No other institution is so exposed to crises and life stressors, yet so potentially capable of resolving frustration and releasing tension. Parad and Caplan (1960) suggest the concept of "family life-style" as representative of a reasonably stable patterning of family organization, subdivided into three dependent elements: value system, communication network, and role system. However, as noted by Weiss (1975), subsequent research has not produced consensus regarding a conceptual or operational definition of "life-style" or how it develops in different societies.

Sociologists have long thought in terms of resources that might help a family to avoid the panic crisis in a stressful situation. Angell (1936) wrote about "family integration" and "family adaptability," forerunners of the "life-style" concept (Parad & Caplan, 1960). It was believed that a well-organized family would resist the formation of crises. Organization would include (a) agreement on role structure, (b) subordination of personal ambitions to family goals, (c) satisfaction with the family because it successfully meets the physical and emotional needs of its members, and (d) perceived and shared goals toward which the family is moving collectively. Lacking these, the family is inadequately organized and likely to succumb to stress (Hansen & Hill, 1964). Nye (1976) recently reviewed studies of the role structure and analysis of the American family.

Wesley and Epstein (1969) defined family organization as the durable modes of relationships between family members, involving power, psychodynamics, roles, status, and work. Other investigators demonstrated considerable consistency in their findings that families vary in the way power is distributed and that such differences are influenced by social class, ethnicity, individual competence, achievement, motivation, and psychopathology (Lewis et al., 1976). Miller (1975) described five areas of interdependent family functioning (biological/reproductive, psychological, sociocultural, economic, and educational) which interact to provide nutrition and family continuation, emotional security of family members, socialization of children and transfer of values, acquisition and distribution of resources, and preparation for adult life and responsibility. McEwan (1975) described the requirements for family health relating to the functions Miller cited. There is, however, no compilation of what is known in terms of the dynamics and determinants of healthy family functioning; problems of assessment are considerable, as reported by McEwan (1971 in a WHO document).

Another source of hypotheses about HFF stems from writings on systems theory (Buckley, 1968). In his challenge of the usefulness of the concept of homeostasis in the understanding of family systems, Speer (1970) reviews several interactional systems that support the postulated relationship between family system viability (health) and flexibility, autonomy, and absence of rigid constraint in system structure. Speer suggests that disturbances of homeostasis with the family may be positive and that homeostasis itself may be one form of dysfunction. He observes, "We know almost nothing about the satisfaction, closeness, meaning achieving, autonomy, problem-solving, communication, change, and basic relationship-organizing processes of exceptionally well-functioning, broadly and deeply satisfied families."

Childhood

As noted by Murphy (1974), Huntington (1975), and Rutter (1976), the literature on delinquency, psychiatric conditions, mental disorders, and other childhood disorders has produced considerable knowledge on *insecurity* and *incompetence*, and on the damage done by marital discord, parental rejection, and institutional rearing. Much less is known about conditions facilitating normal development or why some children experiencing stress and a variety of unfortunate disadvantages still manage to develop a healthy personality, emotional security, and social competence. Rutter's review suggests that "it is a question of age dependent susceptibilities." Children are better able to cope with some forms of stress at an older age. Also, coping with single, isolated, acute stresses is likely to be more successful and less damaging in terms of longer-term psychological development than facing recurrent, multiple acute stresses. Children from a disadvantaged family with chronic stresses are more likely than other children to experience recurrent and interacting multiple acute stresses and be damaged by them. "It is when several stresses occur in combination that the most damage results." Even in these difficult circumstances, however, children are more likely to experience normal development "if they have adaptive temperamental characteristics which make them easy to get along with, if they maintain a good relationship with one parent, if family circumstances change for the better, and if there are compensating good experiences outside the family, such as at school" (Rutter, 1976).

In November 1976, a WHO expert committee considered current trends in childhood mental health and psychosocial development (WHO, 1977). Persistent and socially handicapping mental disorders affect between 5 and 15% of all children aged 3 to 15 years—and there are 1.3 billion children under age 15 in the world. Concern with childhood mental disorders is especially appropriate in developing countries where children under age 15 account for about 40% of the population (compared to around 25% in developed countries). Poverty and low socioeconomic status appear to be associated with a greater incidence of mental disorder. The committee recommended that immediate steps be taken to forestall the rise in psychosocial problems that can be expected to occur in developing countries with increasing industrialization, urbanization, and affluence. "This can be done only if decision-makers are made aware of the psychosocial repercussions of socioeconomic policies." It was noted that the majority of effective interventions in childhood mental health are based on human interaction, which can occur in simple surroundings such as the home, the school, dispensary, or health center. The recommendation was made to involve families in treatment and to increase parental skills and confidence. "The aim is to enhance normal family functioning by helping parents to help their children" (WHO, 1977). Similar views have been expressed by other specialists, such as Hobbs (1976).

Parenting

In modern society, preparing for parenthood is a complex and changing task (Donner, 1972; Lambo, 1969; UNICEF, 1975). The family is "more than an evolutionary production line" (Fleck, 1976), but parenting skills do not necessarily come easily and naturally (Grams, 1970; Schaefer, 1972). In part, parents behave the way they do because of their own childhood experiences. Persons reared in unhappy, discordant, or disrupted homes are more likely to marry in their teens, to have out-of-wedlock children, and to experience unhappy marriages and difficulties in child-rearing (Rutter & Madge, 1976). It is equally apparent from the literature that such links between childhood experiences and subsequent parenting behavior are not inevitable. There appears to be considerable modifiability in parental behavior, as shown most frequently in the differential treatment of second children. Moreover, the Prague studies of children born to women twice denied abortion for the same pregnancy showed that many of the initially rejecting mothers subsequently experienced positive feelings and good relationships with their children, who then developed normally despite difficult beginnings (Dytrych et al., 1975).

Stereotypes of parenthood are losing validity amid cultural changes (Farber, 1973; Woody & Woody, 1975), as reflected in the increasing awareness of the father's role as women are encouraged to extend their activities beyond mothering (Benson, 1968; Lynn, 1974; Price-Bonham, 1976). Special stresses have received extensive review, e.g., parent–child communication when one parent dies (Furman, 1974), infant death in a family situation (Hardgrove & Warrick, 1974), early childhood intervention (Bronfenbrenner, 1975), single-parent families headed by women (Ross & Sawhill, 1975), and the relationship of family circumstances to the wider social environment (Rutter, 1976). Many of the studies are hampered by inadequate samples and research techniques. In sum, not nearly enough is known about factors modifying parental behavior or how to help parents improve healthy family functioning with their children, who compose nearly half of the world's population.

Adolescence

Although puberty and physical maturation are universal, adolescence as a stage of psychological growth is associated more closely with economic development, social and cultural values, and historical traditions. Ages defining this developmental phase may differ between countries within the same geographic region. Few nations have adequate information on drug abuse, sequelae of inappropriate sex behavior, alcoholism, and related difficulties. Innovative European youth advisory services have been described by Shore (1976a, b). The international situation on adolescent pregnancy and abortion in different cultural settings was considered at a 1974 WHO meeting (WHO, 1975). Coping problems of early adolescence (the junior high school period in the United States) have been summarized by Hamburg (1974). Ortutay (1970) has discussed the social and educational function of the family as reflected in the family laws promulgated in the socialist countries of Central and Eastern Europe. The changing family patterns in the Arab Middle East have been studied by Prothro and Diab (1974), while Oliensis (1967) has written about evolving East African patterns.

Aging

Psychosocial research on the second half of life is only beginning to elicit more interest, although demographic projections indicate that by the year 2000, 1 in every 20 Europeans will be aged 75 years or older, a 100% increase over the comparable 1950 situation. Similar increases in the population of older persons can be anticipated in other world regions (Carballo, 1975). While gerontologists have become increasingly concerned with patterns of social adaptation and the role of the family in the lives of older persons (Troll, 1971), the literature on mental health aspects of midlife crises is sparse. Neugarten (1968) has reviewed changing family roles during and after middle age in the American context. Mogey (1971) inventoried studies in the sociology of marriage and family behavior outside the United States. Glasser and Glasser (1970) and Neuhaus and Neuhaus (1974) review family crises in terms of disorganization and actualizing potentials. Family-focused mechanisms for coping with old age and death have been described by Fleck (1975b).

Psychosocial Studies of the Family

Classification

Existing studies of the family can be classified as (1) traditional psychosocial research and (2) reports of control families based on interactional studies concerned primarily with families of identified psychiatric patients. The different sources of information, hypotheses, and research often overlap, crossing disciplinary boundaries (Lewis et al., 1976). In their review of 12,850 research publications on marriage and the family printed during the period 1900 to 1964, Aldous and Hill (1967) noted an emphasis on microscopic studies of marriage and divorce, transactions with groups, and the family as a small unit. Most researchers assumed an individual-psychological perspective with limited consideration of HFF.

Psychological studies typically use interviews or tests of individuals in a family to construct a composite family picture. This approach relies on what family members are willing or able to share with researchers. There are few studies of couple communication, interaction, or marital power. The absence of simultaneous but separate interviews with spouses makes it difficult to predict behavior based on conjugal authority, influence, and decision making (Safilios–Rothschild, 1970). Retrospective interview data can be still further obscured by selective remembrance or misperceptions (Olson, 1969). However, in spite of methodological flaws in individual studies, a confirmation by consensus is being achieved through the gradual accumulation of comparable findings on key issues (David & Johnson, 1977).

In studies of patient families and control families (selected not on the basis of healthy family functioning but according to absence of an identified psychiatric patient), both sets of families are usually invited to respond to identical stimuli, solve an identical problem, or resolve intrafamilial disagreements. There is a search for provocative differences on such variables as intrusions, silences, communication sequences, and interruptions. The presumption that such differences are etiologic in regard to the identified patient's disturbance must be counterbalanced by the possibility that the differences either are responsive to the presence of the patient in the families of one group or reflect differences in "set" between the two groups (Lewis et al., 1976).

Cross-Cultural Aspects

Of particular concern in cross-cultural studies of the family are value perspectives (Lewis, 1959). What is the impact of contemporary societal trends, such as, for example, changing roles of women on traditional values and HFF? Mead (1970) writes of the passage of the American society and of societies generally from postfigurative through cofigurative to prefigurative cultures. In the postfigurative stage, models of behavior remain constant because life patterns remain constant; parents and grandparents can be effective models because they adapted successfully to similar life situations. When, however, there is a sudden break in cultural continuity, as for example in migration, uprooting, or rapid social change, parents no longer provide effective models for young couples. Peers negotiating the new cultures become sources of authority, forming a cofigurative culture. With the awareness and anticipation of continuing social change in the future, a prefigurative culture emerges and parents' capacity to function as models for children is severely undermined. In some cultures, parents of today's children are like immigrants to a new land who must learn from their children how to cope with the environment.

Current Studies

Following the WHO International Pilot Study of Schizophrenia and the Programme of Standardization of Psychiatric Diagnosis, Classification, and Statistics, the 1977–1979 WHO Collaborative Study extends the search for determinants of outcome of schizophrenia into the area of psychosocial factors, family life, and other potentially significant variables in different cultures. A social anthropological perspective has been added to the cross-cultural clinical approach. Of particular interest for study of healthy family functioning is a cooperative project to be conducted in Hawaii, Nagasaki, and Prague. The objective is to compare in each area the histories of families with schizophrenic patients with indices obtained from a comparison group of control families whose members coped successfully with similar stresses. A special focus of the study will be the comparison between groups of common ethnic extraction (Japanese) in the different culture settings of Hawaii and Nagasaki. Of related interest is an ongoing longitudinal study in Prague, Czechoslovakia, where married couples with children are required to inform their local social service agency if they are contemplating divorce. One objective of the research project, conducted by the Psychiatric Research Institute, is to compare those families repeatedly returning to the social service agency for assistance in coping with the social stress of divorce with those families who manage to cope without returning to the social agency after the initial mandatory visit.

A search for ongoing United States studies elicited seven relevant responses from the data bank of the National Clearinghouse for Mental
Health Information; others may be in progress. Reiss (1976) is studying
factors regulating the family's interaction with its social environment, comparing the family's performance in its home with that in the laboratory.
Family coping and effectiveness of social support relationships in reducing
the negative physical and psychological impact of job loss are examined in a
longitudinal study conducted by Ferman (1976). The interaction between
health and economic roles is analyzed in a variety of supportive contexts.
Rogler (1976) is examining the way in which Puerto Rican families in New
York City cope with life problems by turning to others for assistance;
specific interview schedules have been constructed. Mexican-American
family structure and coping behavior under stress are being analyzed in
California by Padilla (1976), including comparisons of families using and
not using public mental health facilities. Black families' survival style is one
of the segments of research conducted by King (1976). Eiduson (1976) is
observing children born and reared in "alternative" family settings, using
parent interviews and field and laboratory observations. Jacob (1976) is
exploring interaction patterns of families with disturbed and control children of preadolescent and adolescent age. Search of other data banks did
not yield any results, although it is quite likely that relevant studies are
under way in different countries.

Coping With Environmental Stress

Definitions

Stress has been defined as a nonspecific physical and/or emotional
response to a variety of psychosocial and environmental conditions of modern life (Levi & Andersson, 1975). The effects of stressful family life cycle
events are well documented in the clinical literature, particularly the impact
on high-risk groups such as, for example, the young and the uprooted.

Coping is defined as any action or intrapsychic attempt to alter a
troubled relationship with the environment (Lazarus, 1966, 1976). Coping
consists of problem-solving efforts of an individual or family faced with
demands highly relevant to their welfare but taxing adaptive resources
(Lazarus, Averill, & Opton, 1974). Efforts to identify and synthesize methodological and conceptual issues in coping and adaptation have been coordinated by Coelho et al. (1974). An overview of human competence and
coping by Moos and Tsu (1976) focuses on the individual rather than the
family. For White (1974), adaptation is the central concept and strategy of

adaptation is the superordinate category under which are subsumed such terms as *defense, mastery,* and *coping.*

Introduced by public health, the concept *at risk* has been adopted by the behavioral sciences. What makes for strength and mastery of risk? There is little available knowledge about multimodal coping strategies or common responses to varied stress categories. Coping behavior is influenced by the situation in which it occurs, but there is a paucity of information about how families develop coping competence. What kinds of life experiences are competency-promoting? How can coping skills be identified and taught? There are few suggestions in the biomedical, sociological, and anthropological literature.

The following sections on migration and uprooting and on family interaction effects in mental illness are cited as examples of family coping with environmental stress. Other high-risk groups, such as children, adolescents, and the aged have already been mentioned in previous sections.

Migration and Uprooting: Effects on Family Coping

The concepts of migration and uprooting have many meanings. Migration may be intercontinental, intracontinental, internal (e.g., within one country), or local (within the community). Movements may include brief visits, seasonal work, and/or seeking of a new habitat in city or country. Levi and Andersson (1975) reviewed recent research in terms of stress effects, primarily on the individual. Reasons for migration and uprooting range from environmental catastrophies, economic deprivation, and political and religious persecution to social and psychological upheavals and industrialization and urbanization often associated with temporary or longer term family separation (Pfister-Ammende, 1960; Zwingmann & Pfister-Ammende, 1973).

Men and women have been on the move since the dawn of human existence. Changing from one social environment to another is often provocative of social dislocation, with family adjustment becoming more difficult with the increasing complexity of urbanization and industrialization (Bernard, 1974). Studies of mental health/adaptation problems of involuntary migrants have usually been concerned with prevalence, incidence, etiology, and symptomatology, seldom with coping and family adjustment (Brody, 1970; David, 1970; Sanua, 1970). Particularly sparse is the literature on healthy family functioning among voluntary migrants moving from country to city and attempting to cope, whether, for example, in the United States (Schwarzweller & Brown, 1970) or abroad (Weisanen, 1970). Coping among families of European migrant workers was described by Underhill (1975); Bauernfeind (1975) contributed a case history of teaching a migrant family what to do to help themselves, an approach based on family systems theory.

By 1970, about 864 million (24% of the world's population) lived in 1,777 cities of more than 100,000 inhabitants. By the year 2000, 40% of the population is expected to live in urban areas, with 25% of the cities exceeding 1 million population (Segal, 1975). In developing countries, about one-third of the city dwellers live in slums and shantytowns; half of this population are children (UNICEF, 1975). With the accelerated process of urbanization and industrialization in these lands, traditional social systems are changing more rapidly than was the experience in developed nations. Patterns of family structure and control are being invalidated (WHO, 1975b). Many of the ensuing social problems and the related health care cost explosion have been inventoried by Levi and Andersson (1975) and by Ehrlich (1975). Rarely, however, is there any mention of family coping or HFF. Another neglected area is the growing struggle for family sustenance. Deteriorating rural areas mean less food production and often force people to abandon the land (Eckholm, 1976). Much more needs to be ascertained about family coping with limited food resources (WHO, 1972).

Considering the long history of migration and the magnitude of the problem, there is a surprising lack of systematically accumulated knowledge (Shaw, 1975). Discussions with representatives of international, national, and local service organizations suggest that field workers are often aware of likely adjustment problems and interested in supporting family coping efforts (Brody, 1970). There is, however, no source book of experience gained in diverse cultures with recommendations for assisting future waves of migrants (David, 1968).

Mental Disorder: Family Interaction Effects

Social science studies of families of mentally ill patients began in the 1950s, when theoretical interest in social deviance, control, and perception provided a conceptual framework. At about the same time, the then innovative programs of community care for mental patients in the United Kingdom and North America turned the attention of psychiatric researchers to families as agents of rehabilitation and bearers of burden. The family's affective responses have usually been assessed through direct questioning or by use of semistructured interviews. Kreisman and Joy (1975) noted that "it is difficult to draw any clear conclusions about the response of family members from these studies, but it would be unwarranted to underestimate the presence of negative affect even where data is reported to the contrary." Situations of any complexity are likely to distort single variable predictors. For example, a family may express much affection and warmth for a patient, indicating a desire for his return home. Yet, doubts about ability to care for the patient and fear of bizarre behavior may surface in stringent attempts to monitor behavior on release, thus effectively sabotaging the patient's efforts at rehabilitation.

Of particular interest is a series of studies conducted by Brown, Birkley, and Wing (1972) concerning the influence of family life on the course of schizophrenia. They rated the interaction of patient and a key relative in a joint interview. An emotional expression score was derived, using the number of comments denoting criticism, hostility, dissatisfaction, warmth, and emotional overinvolvement. Findings indicated that emotional expression, rather than previous work or behavioral impairment, was the best single predictor of symptomatic relapse. Results were replicated subsequently for two clinically different groups of psychiatric patients by Vaughn and Leff (1976).

Most available research confirms the need to examine complex interfamilial relationships. It is not enough, however, to relate family attitudes to outcome. Patient attitudes, their consequences for family attitudes, and patient behavior are equally important and need to be given more consideration (Kreisman & Joy, 1975).

In their review of British and North American studies on family attitudes toward returned patients and the outcome of release home, Kreisman and Joy (1975) also noted a paucity of systematic empirical investigations concerning such reality factors as, for example, economic and social pressures on the family, patient's role in the household, and life-cycle variables. While recent studies by Sainsbury (1975) and by Doll (1976) are more promising, there is a scarcity of significant results relating family attitudinal variables to successful outcome. Few studies have focused on complex interrelated variables, such as, for example, analysis of patient and family variables in conjunction with one another. Most investigations failed to establish comparative baselines of attitudes for families with a member exhibiting physical incapacity or for families without psychologically disordered members.

In a study marked by unusually precise methodology, Mishler and Waxler (1968) reported a long-range interactional project comparing three groups: (a) families with a schizophrenic child with a good premorbid social adjustment, (b) families with a schizophrenic child with a poor premorbid social adjustment, and (c) a control group with no child having a history of hospitalization for mental/psychiatric disorder. As summarized by Lewis et al. (1976), these families were observed in two sessions; one involved the parents with the schizophrenic child and the other involved the parents with a well sibling (never hospitalized for psychiatric illness). Strodtbeck's (1958) Revealed Differences Technique was used to generate discussion among the three family members. There were approximately 1,800 communication acts per session. The 20 different interaction codes applied to each act were designed to measure aspects of communication believed to be clinically relevant, including such variables as affective expressiveness, imperviousness, speech fragments, interruptions, and silences. It was found that the control families were more expressive and more positive in affect, unselective in the target toward whom feelings were expressed, and flexible in terms of roles. Generational boundaries were observed: father held the most power, mother somewhat less, and the child least. The parental coalition was strong, with a clear hierarchy, but power was not exercised authoritatively or rigidly, and communication was more disruptive than in the families with a schizophrenic child. Control families demonstrated greater responsiveness to each other's statements. The research involved was expensive and not easily applicable cross-culturally.

The key role of relatives participating in the treatment of family members in developing countries has been well described by Lambo (1966) and Carstairs (1973). A relative will stay near the patient day and night; if admitted to hospital, the relative sleeps on a mat beside the bed. The relative thus learns how to cope with someone in a state of distress and becomes better prepared for contributing to the patient's rehabilitation, thus strengthening the family's coping capabilities. Such studies need to be replicated in rural areas of other developing countries.

Although most of the published research views the patient as a reactor to the family's attitudes and behavior, there is growing evidence that family tolerance and expectations reflect patient functioning (Kreisman & Joy, 1975). Generally, research studies have concentrated on women's perceptions and expectations as related to male patients, but a wife's illness may have a more pervasive and destructive influence on family organization and coping if husbands are unwilling to assume traditionally female roles. There are few studies of effects of cultural changes on sex roles in adaptation to stressful family situations. Anthony (1970) observed no significant differences in impact on the families of mentally or physically ill family members. Family disruption, reintegration, or disintegration depended on family adjustment, socioeconomic and cultural level, and severity of illness.

The growing emphasis on community placement of persons handicapped by mental disorder and/or mental retardation has been accompanied by a gradual awareness of the increasing risk for unwanted fertility. Failure to provide family planning assistance has been ascribed to restrictive interpretations of existing policies, institutional inertia, or other people's presumed sensibilities. The literature has been summarized by Abernathy and Grunebaum (1972) for returning mental patients; David and Lindner (1975) extended the focus to mental retardation and family responsibilities. Cooperation between mental health and family planning services appears to be minimal in the United States and probably in other lands as well (David, 1971, 1972; Goldston, 1977).

In sum, research to date suggests a need for multivariate studies evaluating the family's responsibilities to its patient/relative along several dimensions, such as, for example, the personalities of family members, sociocultural position, prior and contemporaneous experience with the patient, attitudes and expectations, and stresses perceived at any particular time (Kreisman & Joy, 1975). Jackson's (1959) concept of familial homeostasis may be useful in considering the effects of stressful experience in strengthening or weakening familial interactions. Ideally, the ongoing WHO collaborative study will provide additional new knowledge.

Communal Coping

Paramedical Resources

Improving health care and health delivery systems, and strengthening the family, have long been a priority concern for WHO, especially in rural areas of developing countries (Newell, 1975). In 1973, only 30 of 137 WHO member countries were utilizing the services of medical assistants (Pitcairn & Flahault, 1974). It is well recognized that the definition of priority needs involves value judgments (Draper, 1973) and that improved health care is an important ingredient for improving family socioeconomic conditions (Smith, 1975). Since the great majority of mentally ill persons in developing countries "have no access to any kind of modern, effective mental health care" (Giel & Harding, 1976), there has been considerable review of needs, priorities, and suggestions for expanding the training and responsibilities of paraprofessional mental health workers (Baasher, Carstairs, Giel, & Hassler, 1975; David, 1966; Harding, 1975). These observations are further supported by regional reports, such as, for example, from Latin America (Gonzalez, 1976; Leon, 1972), Sub-Saharan Africa (German, 1972), Southeast Asia (Neki, 1973), and eastern Mediterranean countries (Baasher, 1976). A well-designed study of the prevalence of mental disorders in a South Indian village was reported by Carstairs and Kapur (1976). Descriptions of innovative mental health services have become available from, for example, Senegal (Collomb, 1965), Sarawak (Schmidt, 1969), Zambia and Uganda (Egdell, 1970), Colombia (Argandona & Kiev, 1972), Iran (Mehryar & Khajavi, 1974), Tanzania (Swift, 1972, 1975), Ethiopia (Lippman, 1976), and New Guinea (Watson, 1976). The important contributions of traditional healers to family well-being have been repeatedly stated (Dunlop, 1975; Kolman, 1976; Lambo, 1975a, 1966). Carstairs (1973) observes that "in developing countries there is no place for demarcation disputes of who should do what."

Giel and Harding (1976) note that "health care must be seen in the overall context of socioeconomic development and increased coverage can only be achieved through a considerable degree of community involvement and responsibility." It is, of course, realized that the structure and operation of health services, as well as its orientation to preventive hygiene or curative medicine, will be influenced by a country's political system and economic ideology in addition to realities related to health, manpower, and resources, especially in the rural areas of developing countries (Diop, 1974).

Self-Reliance and Mutual Help

Traditionally, health and community services have assumed a reactive posture, responding to requests for assistance. As shown in WHO deliberations and publications, there is increasing awareness of the inappropriateness for most developing countries of the western model of medicine with its emphasis on individual care by a highly trained physician or a small team functioning under his/her direction. It is seldom realized that issues of socioeconomic development were not a major consideration in the evolution of the Western model. The situation is quite different when policy makers are forced to make difficult choices in the allocation of scarce resources and must evaluate health sector priorities in terms of their impact on the rate of national economic development. This socioeconomic/political approach explains some of the emphasis on environmental hygiene for the many rather than curative medicine for a few, for encouraging citizen participation and community self-reliance, and for redefining the concept of service (Meyer & Sainsbury, 1975). Little research has been reported on the evolving perception of health policies and services as perceived by service providers and users (McKinlay, 1972; Peled & Friedman, 1976).

Mutual help is an alternate method of coping that involves the positive qualities of family and community. Most often mutual help groups develop around critical transition points in the family life cycle and are oriented to shared concerns (Katz, 1970, 1976; Levin, Katz, & Holst, 1976; Silverman, 1975). It may also be organized as a means of encouraging self-reliance and strengthening local resources for meeting health problems (Sidel & Sidel, 1975). In recent years considerable information has become available on the transformation of health services in the People's Republic of China with its emphasis on preventive and environmental hygiene rather than curative medicine, training of generalists, utilization of part-time paramedical auxiliaries, narrowing the gap between urban and rural health facilities, strengthening and integrating traditional medicine with Western medicine, and common identification and resolution of problems through fostering self-reliance within the family (Akhtar, 1975; Sidel & Sidel, 1974, 1975; Wilenski, 1976; Wolfson, 1976). The importance of motivational style and total organizational effort is noted repeatedly in such areas as changing roles of women and children (Sidel, 1973), the family (Chomel, Perez, & Samuel, 1973), population planning (Orleans, 1975), training of barefoot doctors (Wang, 1975), revision of medical education and service delivery (Cheng, Axelrod, & Leaf, 1975), community action (Horn, 1975), and health education (Wang, 1976). Many efforts succeeded because personal and social activities became synonymous in the dedication of "service to the people," and because of a remarkable emphasis on "self-reliance." The organizational system ensures that every individual family is reached (Wolfson & Kane, 1976). Identification of transferable ingredients is of major import in viewing innovations from the PRC and their possible applicability in other lands (Chen, 1975; Wilenski, 1976).

Cross-Cultural Perspectives

There is little information on whether features of family interaction that appear to characterize dysfunctional families occur as often, to a lesser degree, or not at all in healthy family functioning in different cultures. In the absence of research findings, clinicians speculate on whether healthy families invariably demonstrate a single feature, a limited group of features, or a wide variety of interactional features that distinguish them from dysfunctional families. Families in developing countries are experiencing currents of social change that present them constantly with new problems to solve and with new options for problem solving (Allman & Mathson, 1975).

Because healthy family functioning is an interacting dynamic, it is rarely possible to study selected determinants in isolation. A holistic approach to social change offers social scientists a unique way for elucidating determinants and effects of HFF. This means going beyond traditional variables such as, for example, socioeconomic status, urbanization, and education, and using in-depth microanalytical approaches to understand the components of HFF under diverse circumstances reflecting the social, economic, and cultural aspects of a given society. There is much to be learned, for example, from the in-depth case studies of Mexican families by Lewis (1959). HFF will then be viewed as representing one of the ways in which families respond to their social and economic situation or, rather, their perception or view of that situation. Within such a research context, case studies might well be conducted in rural villages experiencing agrarian reform, mushrooming urban slum communities, middle-class areas integrating into modern life, etc. Although quantitative data are necessary for comparisons over time, research combining qualitative elements can be particularly important in clarifying the concept of HFF in diverse segments of changing societies and assessing the eventual transferability of concepts.

Research Utilization and Dissemination

WHO member countries represent varied sizes and environments, stages of economic and technical development, political systems and values, social systems and traditions, and varied environmental pressures from industrialization, urbanization, and changing life-styles. They also share the similarity of human problems and their influence on HFF. Although solutions must be country-specific, the commonality of stressors is conducive to coordinated and cooperative transnational research. For example, the patterns of communal psychiatric care in Nigeria (Lambo, 1966) are slowly being replicated in other developing countries. Similarly, the Israeli systems of communal coping (David, 1968; Gratch, 1973) and the European experiences with youth advisory services (Shore, Robert, & Jeanneret, 1977) might well be appropriate in other settings. Assessment of the transnational transferability of experience remains an area for priority research.

Another major need is more efficient utilization of already available knowledge. The capability of information clearinghouses has been well demonstrated in several areas of health education and research; a relatively modest investment is likely to produce a high yield. A related route for wider dissemination of health information to the public is the enlightened enlistment of media resources. Inexpensive transistor radios have already proven their value in several countries of Asia and Latin America where low literacy limits dissemination of the written word. Counseling can be offered in imaginative "down-to-earth" ways, thus strengthening self-reliance and family and communal coping.

Assessment Approaches

Reviews

Assessment techniques relevant to the conceptualization and measurement of adaptive behavior have been reviewed extensively by Moos (1974). Analysis of more than 300 references suggests "a rapidly expanding area of inquiry still in its developmental infancy." Investigators concerned with understanding the coping process have tended to rely on more complex, intuitive, clinical, and global assessment methods that permit intensive and detailed observations. Researchers interested primarily in accurate prediction have emphasized simple, objective, specific, and actuarial methods. Major goals of research have been to identify adaptation, prevent maladaptation, and effect changes in adaptive behavior and coping processes.

Moos (1974) offers descriptive comparisons of a variety of techniques, including interviews, tape recordings, films, essays, short-story and problem situations, and objective assessment methods. In his view "the field of inquiry is very new and there are few established methods; it is thus too early to attempt a highly critical review." A similar opinion was expressed previously by Straus (1969); he compiled a comprehensive inventory of 319 assessment techniques published between 1935 and 1965 for quantitatively measuring the properties of the family or the behavior of people in family roles. Only 56% of the methods reviewed had acceptable standards of reliability or validity. Nearly all the schedules, inventories, scales, and other assessment techniques mentioned by Straus and/or Moos are derived from North American experience.

Family Interaction

"The systematic use of family interactions in the study of coping patterns is still relatively rare" (Moos, 1974). One example is the Goldstein, Judd, Rodnick, Alkire, and Gould (1968) methodology for combining the advantages of relatively free responses to natural situations with standardization of the interview conditions and presenting problems. The aim is to determine whether there are consistent coping styles among family members confronting adolescent psychopathic behavior. One of the earlier approaches to this area was the "Revealed Differences Technique" of Strodtbeck (1958).

A review of assessment devices discussed by Moos (1974) and by Straus (1969) confirms the paucity of techniques oriented to family coping with stress imposed by environmental conditions and societal circumstances. Primary emphasis is on intrafamilial communication, conflicts, and interactions, most often between parents and children or between spouses. Straus (1975) concurs with the view that methodologies for assessing family functioning are still largely in the developmental stage. Brown and Rutter (1976) reviewed the methodological problems of measuring family activities and relationships, and then demonstrated the utility of the family interview as a research tool. Fleck (1976) considers a general systems approach to understanding severe family pathology. One of the more promising approaches in recent literature is the Beavers-Timberlawn Family Evaluation Scale (Lewis et al., 1976), based on a systems theory of healthy family functioning and encompassing longitudinal and empirical aspects with consideration of statistical control problems.

Social Indicators

Inferences drawn from descriptive statistics found in public records and reports have sparked research on social indicators of the quality of life and societal well-being and concerns in diverse lands (de Neufville, 1975; Ornauer, Wiberg, Sicinski, & Galtung, 1976; Van Dusen, 1974). Other forms of needs assessments have been reviewed by Warheit, Bell, and Schwab (1975). Thus far, however, there is little substantial knowledge on the life experiences of families in different cultures. Major dimensions of well-being remain to be identified, as do instruments for measuring them, analyzing their relationship to each other, and building time series for the study of the nature of change (Campbell, 1976; Campbell, Converse & Rodgers, 1976; WHO, 1976). It remains to be determined whether a conceptualization of the quality of life, without grounding in a theory of social change, provides a basis for effectively monitoring and accounting for change (Glock, 1976).

WHO Endeavors

Several WHO divisions have from time to time convened study groups and technical seminars on the family as a unit in health studies. For example, the Division of Health Statistics organized consultations on statistical aspects (WHO, 1972) and on statistical indices of family health (WHO, 1976), while the Division of Family Health considered implications for the training of health workers and the provision of services (WHO, 1975b). Extensive consideration was given to epidemiological, social, economic, and demographic approaches to the study of the family. Problems of measurement and of information collection and treatment were reviewed, with particular emphasis on demographic structures of the families and indices of family health (Herberger, 1974a, b). McEwan (1975) eventually described family health and its social indices as "a multifactorial jungle." This is in part because each of the concepts is ambiguous and "because for any specific connotation there is a multitude of dynamically interacting factors."

The 1973 WHO Report on Consultation on Family Health (WHO, 1975b), summarized by McEwan (1975) and by Miller (1975), noted the ambiguity of concepts and terms as cited by McEwan (1973). It was suggested that each family has its own dynamics of formation, growth, maturation, and dissolution, affected by numerous biological, psychological, sociocultural, economic, and educational variables. It was recognized that not all families have functions in every area and that not all areas appertain to each family for the whole of its natural history. "All areas are interdependent and dynamic; the family is not a stable system" (McEwan, 1975).

The 1975 WHO Study Group on Statistical Indices of Family Health noted that over the past two decades the family has been treated variously as an independent, dependent, and intervening variable, as well as a precipitating, predisposing, and contributing factor in the etiology, care, and treatment of both physical and mental illness, and as a basic unit of interaction and transaction in health care (WHO, 1976). It was concluded that "no satisfactory measure of family effectiveness has yet been developed" and that the concept of family functioning "remains ill-defined." Further, "most attempts have focused on fragmented aspects of family life which, although dynamic and interactive, has to be assessed holistically if it is to be evaluated in a manner accurate and sensitive enough for use in health studies." As McEwan (1975) noted, "considerable research is needed in the development of instruments more appropriate, more sensitive, and more useful than so far produced."

Methodological Considerations

There are major pitfalls in devising methodologically sound, administratively feasible, and cross-culturally relevent assessment techniques. For example, Whiteley and Watts (1969) noted that decision-making styles correlated significantly with actual behavior only when the decision had no personal consequence. The complexity of the relationship between attitudes and behavior, and the influence of intervening variables, has also been discussed by Warner and DeFleur (1969). Other methodological weaknesses, systematically reviewed by Lake, Miles, and Earle (1973) in their report on 84 instruments for assessing diverse aspects of social functioning, are cited by Cromwell, Olson, and Fournier (1976) in their discussion of tools and techniques for diagnosis and evaluation in marital and family therapy.

Reviewers mention repeatedly that methodological research is needed at all levels of the assessment process (Moos, 1974; Straus, 1964; WHO, 1976). Studies should be designed not merely to predict a criterion but to compare the efficacy of alternative methods of assessment and prediction. Coping and adaptive behavior cannot be studied apart from the environmental context and situational determinants (Lazarus et al., 1974; Lazarus, 1976; Moos, 1974). Particularly relevant is Mechanic's (1974) call for behavioral tests closely approximating real-life tasks, and Goldfried's and D'Zurilla's (1969) emphasis on studies assessing the task requirements of different types of naturally occuring situations.

Ethical Issues

Questions of ethics and protection of the rights of human subjects have risen to renewed prominence. For example, descriptively labeling family behavior as "healthy" or "dysfunctional" has great potential for misuse. There is the danger of projecting subjective values, rediscovering them as "objective" criteria of health, and then using them in conflict with others holding different value orientations. The role of the family as a social unit within society is interwoven with ideological concepts; normalcy may be defined as what is expected rather than what exists (Offer & Sabshin, 1966). The impact of culture, history, and social class is particularly relevant for defining family health. What is adaptive or creative in one era, culture, or socioeconomic class may be maladaptive in another. In this period of rapid social change, the societal relevance of the research approach must be scrutinized carefully in each country.

Cross-Cultural Aspects

There is little evidence of cooperative cross-cultural or transnational research involving assessment of healthy family functioning or coping with environmental threats. This is of particular importance when comparing "social stress" among inhabitants of various countries and regions. It would be a major advance in cross-cultural research if generalizations could be safely made regarding the relative significance of various life cycle stages, rapid social change, and environmental stresses. Cross-cultural relevance should be considered early in the development process of each new assessment area (Moos, 1974). Although it has not been used widely in the area of family functioning, Cantril's (1965) Self-Anchoring Scale offers an approach for obtaining a quantitative assessment of respondents' perceptions of their reality world, concerns, and future expectations, with the added advantage of empirical findings from different countries (Ornauer et al., 1976). The validity of measures of self-reported well-being has been reviewed by Andrews and Crandall (1976). International cooperation will be essential in reaching consensus on standards (WHO, 1976), maintaining sensitivity to mental health policy (Davis & Salasin, 1975), and effectively utilizing technical assistance (Thorne, 1975).

Toward a Theory of Healthy Family Functioning

Choice Behavior

Individuals constituting a family unit are constantly faced with choices and alternative courses of action that will determine, at least in part, healthy family functioning and coping with stress. The awareness of these choice points, the extent to which alternative courses are recognized, and the degree to which choices are based on realistic appraisals of varied costs and consequences are believed to be the keystones of healthy family functioning. Public policies and their implementation, the provision of information, education, and services, and the social-motivational factors that encourage or discourage various alternatives are subjective aspects of the environment that must be appraised by family members along with their own needs and desires. Family functioning involves more than one person and is subject to change over time. Understanding the communication process and the perceptions of family members is essential to an understanding of healthy family functioning.

Decision-Making Process

A study of healthy family functioning requires a closer look at the family constellation and decision-making process. In nearly all sociocultural contexts, an individual's idea of his or her partner's perceptions are of critical importance. However clever social scientists may be in unearthing valid information about knowledge, attitudes, and even individual practices of one person, false conclusions may be drawn about the behavior of this individual in conjunction with his/her partner and, consequently, on how healthy family functioning behavior is determined or modified. Valuable lessons can be drawn from the psychosocial model of fertility choice behavior that emphasizes the subjective assessment of the environment by the individual and the importance of the two partners in a couple in determining each other's choice behavior (Friedman, Johnson, & David, 1976). Where possible, both parental members of a nuclear family should be included in a research study of family decision making. Studies of conjugal authority, influence, and decision making have rarely obtained data from both husband and wife (Safilios-Rothschild, 1970). Examples of studies involving separate but simultaneous interviews with both marital partners have been reported from Israel (Peled, 1970) and from Sweden (Trost, personal communication, 1977).

Research Planning

In studies of healthy family functioning, it is critical to know not only what is available in the environment of the community but, even more critically, what family members believe to be available. Openness to health information can be constricted by conceptually elusive yet nonetheless powerful psychological forces, such as, for example, alienation. Similarly, decisions will have to be reached on how populations for study might be defined, the stage in the family life cycle of the population groups studied, the nature of the data that need to be collected, and methodological design factors.

The possibility of defining populations for study on the basis of self-selecting biopsychosocial dimensions makes cross-cultural comparisons more meaningful. While cultural and environmental factors differ, principles of the dynamics of healthy family functioning are held in common. It is these principles that form part of the theory of healthy family functioning and, in a classical pattern, the development of new hypotheses for behavioral testing (Friedman *et al.*, 1976).

The Young Family: A Proposal for Cooperative Cross-Cultural Research

The Basic Unit of Healthy Family Functioning

Whereas much attention has been devoted to the relationship between sociodemographic variables and indicators of dysfunction, relatively little consideration has been given to mutable psychosocial variables such as healthy family functioning, health maintenance, and coping behavior. Already available knowledge is used primarily by a minority of families who appear to engage in planning behavior encompassing all parts of family life, including health. To gain a comparative cross-cultural perspective, it is proposed that a coordinated research approach focus on the behavioral attributes of healthy family functioning in the early years of marriage (or consensual unions or alternate marriagelike, longer-term relationships). What distinguishes effectively planning young families from others at similar stages of the life cycle in diverse cultures experiencing rapid social change? What information and practical recommendations can be provided to policy makers to enlarge this group of effective early planners and copers? How can successful coping be defined, taught, and communicated?

The basic unit of successful coping and healthy family functioning is likely to be the young family. Categories of variables of seemingly universal relevance will have to be delineated and a set of structured data needs prepared to test hypotheses concerned with coping behavior in developed and developing countries. The focus can be on coping with specific concerns ranging from migration and uprooting to fertility regulation. Even though cultural differences exist, differentially influencing behavior, comparisons within and between cultures offer tests for hypotheses, especially if selected families can be followed through the family life cycle.

Methodological Advantages

There are major methodological advantages to studying recently formed family units. This population is relatively small in any given society, is usually definable, and (with proper precautions) can be approached. It is likely that a proportionately large, representative, and relatively good sample can be obtained in most countries willing to cooperate. Since in most societies nearly all individuals "marry," the proposed group usually represents a thorough cross section of the population (albeit at one point in their life cycles) so that information about them is likely to cut across all socioeconomic classes and provide useful information for the nation as a whole. At this stage in the life cycle, the couple is also a self-determining social unit, comparable across cultures, because the basis for the group is a universal stage in man's (and woman's) existence. By letting the group "self-select" rather than selecting them on the basis of age or other variables, which have different social significance in different cultures, more cross-culturally comparable populations are obtained.

Now in progress in Geneva, Switzerland, is a research study of 600 couples married for the first time (Kellerhals, personal communication, 1977). Initial contact was made 2 months after the marriage, including separate but simultaneous interviews with both marital partners. Initiated in 1974 with support from the Swiss National Fund, two rounds of interviews have been completed, with a third scheduled for 1978. Related studies comparing newly married couples with couples living in stable, marriage-like unions of unmarried cohabitation are being conducted in Sweden by Trost (personal communication, 1977) and his associates. They are also using separate but simultaneous interviews.

Summary

It is increasingly recognized that rapid cultural, social, economic, and technological changes are imposing increasing stress on family structures, traditional values, and ability to adapt to new environments in diverse societies. For the purposes of this chapter, "healthy family functioning" is defined in terms of a family unit (however delineated in a given culture), effectively coping with cultural-environmental, psychosocial, and socio-economic stressors throughout the family life cycle. While a review of international literature in the behavioral and biomedical sciences yields limited evidence of comparative studies, there is growing awareness of the need for cooperative transnational research on family coping mechanisms and determinants of self-reliant communal coping behavior, as well as more efficient utilization of already available knowledge. After consideration of methodological pitfalls of assessment procedures, there is a presentation of an evolving theory of healthy family functioning with the suggestion that studies of young married couples constitute a particularly promising vehicle for developing needed cooperative cross-cultural research.

ACKNOWLEDGMENTS

I am pleased to acknowledge the constructive suggestions of George Coelho, Stephen Goldston, Assen Jablensky, Norman Sartorius, and Milton Shore. I am solely responsible for the content of this chapter and no endorsement from the World Health Organization is assumed or implied.

References

Abernathy, V. D., & Grunebaum, H. Toward a family planning program in psychiatric hospitals. *American Journal of Public Health*, 1972, *62*, 1638–1646.

Ackerman, N. W. *The psychodynamics of family life*. New York: Basic, 1958.

Akhtar, S. *Health care in the People's Republic of China*. Ottawa: International Development Research Centre, 1975.

Aldous, J. A framework for the analysis of family problem solving. In J. Aldous, T. Condon, R. Hill, M. Strauss, & I. Tallman (Eds.), *Family problem solving: A symposium on theoretical, methodological and substantive concerns*. Hinsdale, Ill.: Dryden, 1971, pp. 265–281.

Aldous, J., & Dahl, N. *International bibliography of research in marriage and the family: 1965–1972* (Vol. 2). Minneapolis: University of Minnesota Press, 1974.

Aldous, J., & Hill, R. *International bibliography of research in marriage and the family: 1900–1964*. Minneapolis: University of Minnesota Press, 1967.

Allman, J., & Mathson, B. Social science research on family planning in developing countries. *International Social Science Journal*, 1975, *27*, 174–182.

Andrews, F. M., & Crandall, R. The validity of measures of self-reported well-being. *Social Indicators Research*, 1976, *3*, 1–19.

Angell, R. C. *The family encounters the depression*. New York: Scribner, 1936.

Anthony, E. J. The impact of mental and physical illness on family life. *American Journal of Psychiatry*, 1970, *127*, 138–146.

Argandona, M., & Kiev, A. *Mental health in the developing world: A case study in Latin America*. New York: Free Press, 1972.

Arnold, F., Bulatao, R. A., Buripakdi, C., Chung, B. J., Fawcett, J. T., Iritani, T., Lee, S. J., & Wu, T. S. *The value of children: A cross-national study* (Vol. 1). Honolulu: East-West Population Institute, 1975.

Baasher, T. A. Mental health services in eastern Mediterranean countries. *WHO Chronicle*, 1976, *30*, 234–239.

Baasher, T. A., Carstairs, G. M., Giel, R., & Hassler, F. R. (Eds.). *Mental health services in developing countries*. Geneva: World Health Organization, 1975. (Offset Publication No. 22)

Bauernfeind, L. Strengthening a disorganized family. *American Journal of Nursing*, 1975, *75*, 2198–2201.

Benson, L. *Fatherhood: A sociological perspective*. New York: Random House, 1968.

Bernard, W. S. Orientation and counseling; their nature and role in the adaptation and integration of permanent immigrants. *International Migration*, 1974, *12*, 182–200.

Brody, E. B. (Ed.). *Behavior in new environments: Adaptation of migrant populations*. Beverly Hills: Sage Publications, 1970.

Bronfenbrenner, U. Is early intervention effective? In M. Guttentag & E. L. Struening (Eds.), *Handbook of evaluation research* (Vol. 2). Beverly Hills: Sage Publications, 1975, pp. 519–603.

Brown, G. W., Birkley, J. L. T., & Wing, J. K. Influence of family life on the course of schizophrenic disorders: A replication. *British Journal of Psychiatry*, 1972, *121*, 241–258.

Brown, G. M., & Rutter, M. The measurement of family activities and relationships: A methodological study. *Human Relations*, 1976, *19*, 241–243.

Buckle, D., Hoffmeyer, H., Isambert, A., Knobloch, F., Knoblochova, J., Krapf, E. E., Lebovici, S., Pertejo de Alcami, J., Pincus, L., & Sandler, J. *Aspects of family mental health in Europe*, Public Health Papers, No. 28. Geneva: World Health Organization, 1965.

Buckley, W. (Ed.). *Modern systems theory for the behavioral scientist*. Chicago: Aldine, 1968.

Campbell, A. Subjective measures of well-being. *American Psychologist*, 1976, *31*, 117–124.

Campbell, A., Converse, P. E., & Rodgers, W. E. *The quality of American life: Perceptions, evaluations, and satisfactions*. New York: Russell Sage Foundation, 1976.

Cantril, H. *The patterns of human concerns*. New Brunswick: Rutgers University Press, 1965.

Carballo, M. Need for adaptation. *World Health*, September 1975, pp. 34–37.

Carballo, M. A promise unfulfilled. *World Health*, August/September 1976, pp. 16–21.

Carstairs, G. M. Psychiatric problems of developing countries. *British Journal of Psychiatry*, 1973, *123*, 271–277.

Carstairs, G. M., & Kapur, K. L. *The great universe of Kota: Stress, change and mental disorder in an Indian village*. Berkeley: University of California Press, 1976.

Chen, P. C. Lessons from the Chinese experience: China's planned birth program and its transferability. *Studies in Family Planning*, 1975, *6*, 354–366.

Cheng, T. O., Axelrod, L., & Leaf, A. Medical education and practice in the People's Republic of China. *Annals of Internal Medicine*, 1975, *83*, 716–724.

Chomel, M. C., Perez, C., & Samuel, A. The new Chinese family. *International Child Welfare Review*, 1973, *19/20*, 47–52.

Coelho, G. V., Hamburg, D. A., & Adams, J. H. (Eds.). *Coping and adaptation*. New York: Basic, 1974.

Collomb, H. Assistance psychiatrique en Afrique: Expérience sénégalaise. *Revue de la Psychopathologie Africaine*, 1965, *1*, 11–84.

Cromwell, R. E., & Thomas, W. L. Developing resources for family potential: A family action model. *Family Coordinator*, 1976, *25*, 13–20.

Cromwell, R. E., Olson, D. H., & Fournier, D. Tools and techniques for diagnosis in marital and family therapy. *Family Process*, 1976, *15*, 1–49.

David, H. P. (Ed.). *International trends in mental health*. New York: McGraw-Hill, 1966.

David, H. P. (Ed.). *Migration, mental health and community services*. Geneva: American Joint Distribution Committee, 1968.

David, H. P. Involuntary international migration. In E. B. Brody (Ed.), *Behavior in new environments*. Beverly Hills: Sage Publications, 1970, pp. 73–95.

David, H. P. Mental health and family planning. *Family Planning Perspectives*, 1971, *3*(2), 20–23.

David, H. P. Unwanted pregnancies: Costs and alternatives. In C. F. Westoff & R. Parke, Jr. (Eds.), *Demographic and social aspects of population growth*. Washington: U.S. Government Printing Office, 1972, pp. 439–466.

David, H. P., & Johnson, R. L. Fertility regulation in early childbearing years: Psychosocial and psychoeconomic aspects. *Preventive Medicine*, 1977, *6*, 52–64.

David, H. P., & Lindner, M. A. Family planning for the mentally handicapped. *Bulletin of the World Health Organization*, 1975, *52*, 155–161.

Davis, H. R., & Salasin, S. E. The utilization of evaluation. In M. Guttentag & E. L. Struening (Eds.), *Handbook of evaluation research* (Vol. 2). Beverly Hills: Sage Publications, 1975, pp. 621–676.

de Neufville, J. I. *Social indicators and public policy: Interactive processes of design and application.* New York: Elsevier, 1976.

Diop, S. M. B. *The place of mental health in the development of public health services.* Brazzaville: World Health Organization, AFRO Technical Papers, No. 8, 1974.

Djukanovic, V., & Mach, E. P. *Alternative approaches to meeting basic health needs in developing countries.* Geneva: World Health Organization, 1975.

Doll, W. Family coping with the mentally ill: An unanticipated problem of deinstitutionalization. *Hospital and Community Psychiatry,* 1976, *27,* 183–185.

Donner, G. J. Parenthood as crisis: A role for the psychiatric nurse. *Perspectives in Psychiatric Care,* 1972, *10*(2), 84–87.

Draper, P. Value judgments in health planning. *Community Medicine,* 1973, *129,* 372–374.

Dunlop, D. W. Alternatives to "modern" health delivery systems in Africa: Public policy issues of traditional health systems. *Social Science and Medicine,* 1975, *9,* 581–586.

Dytrych, Z., Matejcek, Z., Schüller, V., David, H. P., & Friedman, H. L. Children born to women denied abortion. *Family Planning Perspectives,* 1975, *7,* 165–171.

Eckholm, E. P. *Losing ground: Environmental stress and world food prospects.* New York: Norton, 1976.

Egdell, H. G. A rural psychiatric service in Uganda. *Psychopathologie Africaine,* 1970, *6,* 87–94.

Ehrlich, D. A. (Eds.). *The health care cost explosion: Which way now?* Bern: Hans Huber Verlag, 1975.

Eiduson, B. P. *Child mental health in alternative family styles.* Rockville, Md.: National Clearinghouse for Mental Health Information, 1976. (Project No. MH 24947)

Elliott, K. *The family and its future.* London: Churchill, 1970.

Farber, B. *Family and kinship in modern society.* Glenview, Ill.: Scott, Foresman, 1973.

Ferman, L. A. *Family adjustment and unemployment.* Rockville, Md.: National Clearinghouse for Mental Health Information, 1976. (Project No. MH 26546)

Fleck, S. The family and psychiatry. In A. Freedman, H. Kaplan, & B. Sadock (Eds.), *Comprehensive textbook of psychiatry* (2nd ed). Baltimore: Williams and Wilkins, 1975. (a)

Fleck, S. Unified health services and family-focused primary care. *International Journal of Psychiatry in Medicine,* 1975, *6,* 501–515. (b)

Fleck, S. A general systems approach to severe family pathology. *American Journal of Psychiatry,* 1976, *133,* 669–673.

Flugel, J. *The psychoanalytic study of the family.* London: Hogarth, 1921.

Friedman, H. L., Johnson, R. L., & David, H. P. The dynamics of fertility choice behavior. A pattern for research. In S. Newman & V. Thompson (Eds.), *Population psychology: Research and educational issues.* Bethesda, Md.: Center for Population Research, 1976, pp. 171–198.

Furman, E. *A child's parent dies: Studies in childhood bereavement.* New Haven: Yale University Press. 1974.

German, A. Aspects of clinical psychiatry in Sub-Saharan Africa. *British Journal of Psychiatry,* 1972, *121,* 461–479.

Giel, R., & Harding, T. W. Psychiatric priorities in developing countries. *British Journal of Psychiatry,* 1976, *128,* 513–522.

Glasser, P. H., & Glasser, L. N. (Eds.). *Families in crisis.* New York: Harper & Row, 1970.

Glock, C. Y. The sense of well-being: Developing measures. *Science,* 1976, *194,* 52–54.

Goldfried, M. R., & D'Zurilla, T. J. A behavioral, analytic model for assessing competence. In C. T. Spielburger (Ed.), *Current topics in clinical and community psychology* (Vol. 1). New York: Academic, 1969.

Goldstein, J. J., Judd, L., Rodnick, E., Alkire, A., & Gould, E. A method for studying social influence and coping patterns within families of disturbed adolescents. *Journal of Nervous and Mental Disease*, 1968, *147*, 233–251.

Goldston, S. E. Primary prevention: A view from the federal scene. In G. W. Albee & J. M. Joffe (Eds.), *Primary prevention in psychopathology*. Hanover: University Press of New England, 1977.

Gonzalez, R. Tendencias de la salud mental in America Latina (Mental health trends in Latin America). *Acta Psiquiatrica y Psicologica de America Latina*, 1976, *22*, 232–237.

Grams, A. Fatherhood and motherhood in a changing world. *International Child Welfare Review*, 1970, *8*, 18–23.

Gratch, H. (Ed.). *Twenty-five years of social research in Israel*. Jerusalem: Jerusalem Academic Press, 1973.

Hamburg, B. Early adolescence: A specific and stressful stage of the life cycle. In G. V. Coelho, D. A. Hamburg, & J. E. Adams (Eds.), *Coping and adaptation*. New York: Basic, 1974, pp. 101–124.

Hansen, D. A., & Hill, R. Families under stress. In H. T. Christensen (Ed.), *Handbook of marriage and the family*. Chicago: Rand McNally, 1964, pp. 782–819.

Hardgrove, C., & Warrick, L. H. Coping with infant death in a family situation. *American Journal of Nursing*, 1974, *74*, 448–450.

Harding, T. W. Mental health services in the developing countries: The issues involved. In T. A. Baasher, G. M. Carstairs, R. Giel; & F. R. Hassler (Eds.), *Mental health services in developing countries*. Geneva: World Health Organization, 1975, pp. 1–5.

Herberger, L. *Methodological implication*. Geneva: World Health Organization, 1974, Document DSI/SAF/71.2. (a)

Herberger, L. *Demographic structures of family and indices of family health*. Geneva: World Health Organization, 1974, Document DSI/WP/74.4. (b)

Hobbs, N. *Mental health, families and children*. Austin: Hogg Foundation for Mental Health, 1976.

Hogg Foundation for Mental Health. *Publications List and Cassette Series*. Austin, Tex.: Hogg Foundation, P.O. Box 7998, 1976.

Horn, J. S. Community action pays off. *World Health*, December 1975, pp. 22–25.

Huntington, D. S. Learning from infants and families. *Journal of the Association for Care of Children in Hospital*, 1975, *4*(1), 5–38.

Jackson, D. D. Family interaction, family homeostasis, and some implications for conjoint family psychotherapy. In J. Masserman (Ed.), *Individual and familial dynamics*. New York: Grune and Stratton, 1959.

Jacob, T. *Family interaction, child age, and diagnostic status*. Rockville, Md.: National Clearinghouse for Mental Health Information, 1976. (Project No. MH 25802)

Jahoda, M. *Current concepts of positive mental health*. New York: Basic, 1958.

Johnson, B. C. A. Changing patterns. *World Health*, September 1975, p. 16.

Katz, A. H. Self-help organizations and volunteer participation in social welfare. *Social Work*, 1970, *15*, 51–60.

Katz, A. H., with Bender, E. *The strength in us: Self help in the modern world*. New York: Franklin-Watts, 1976.

Katz, J. Family planning, mental health, and preventive psychiatry. *Mental Health in Australia*, 1972, *4*, 138–143.

Kellerhals, J. Personal communication, 1977.

King, L. M. *Fanon Mental Health Research and Development Center*. Rockville, Md.: National Clearinghouse for Mental Health Information, 1976. (Project No. MH 25580)

Kolman, B. R. A study of psychiatric patients at the University of Malaya Medical Centre who also consult indigenous healers. *Social Psychiatry*, 1976, *11*, 127–134.

Kreisman, D. E., & Joy, V. D. The family as reactor to the mental illness of a relative. In M. Guttentag & E. L. Struening (Eds.), *Handbook of evaluation research* (Vol. 2) Beverly Hills: Sage Publications, 1975, pp. 483–516.

Lalonde, M. *A new perspective on the health of Canadians.*Ottawa: Information Canada, 1975.

Lake, D. G., Miles, M. B., & Earle, R. B. (Eds.). *Measuring human behavior.* New York: Teachers College Press, 1973.

Lambo, T. A. Patterns of psychiatric care in developing African countries: The Nigerian village program. In H. P. David (Ed.), *International trends in mental health.* New York: McGraw-Hill, 1966, pp. 147–153.

Lambo, T. A. The child and the mother–child relationship in major cultures of Africa. *Les carnets de l'enfance/Assignment children.* France: Neuilly-sur-Seine, 1969, No. 10, pp. 61–75.

Lambo, T. A. Foreword. In *Promoting health in the human environment.* Geneva: World Health Organization, 1975. (a)

Lambo, T. A. Total health. *World Health,* December 1975, No. 3. (b)

Lambo, T. A. The world situation. *Royal Society of Health Journal,* 1976, *96,* 243–245.

Lazarus, R. S. *Psychological stress and the coping process.* New York: McGraw-Hill, 1966.

Lazarus, R. S. Psychological stress and coping in adaptation and illness. In S. M. Weiss (Ed.), *Proceedings of the National Heart and Lung Institute Working Conference on Health Behavior,* May 1975, Washington: DHEW Publication (NIH) 76–868, 1976, pp. 199–214.

Lazarus, R. S., Averill, J. R., & Opton, E. M., Jr. The psychology of coping: Issues of research and assessment. In G. V. Coelho, D. A. Hamburg, & J. E. Adams (Eds.), *Coping and adaptation.* New York: Basic, 1974, pp. 249–315.

Leavell, H. R., & Clark, E. G. *Preventive medicine for the doctor in his community* (3rd ed.). New York: McGraw-Hill, 1965.

Leon, C. Psychiatry in Latin America. *British Journal of Psychiatry,* 1972, *121,* 121–136.

Levi, L., & Andersson, L. *Psychosocial stress: Population, environment, and quality of life.* New York: Spectrum Publications, 1975.

Levin, L. S., Katz, A. H., & Holst, E. *Self care: Lay initiatives in health.* New York: Prodist, 1976.

Lewis, J. M., Beavers, W. R., Gossett, J. T., & Phillips, V. A. *No single thread: Psychological health in family systems.* New York: Brunner/Mazel, 1976.

Lewis, O. *Five families: Mexican case studies in the culture of poverty.* New York: Basic, 1959.

Lidz, T. *The family and human adaptation.* New York: International Universities Press, 1963.

Lieberman, E. J. Family formation and development: The primary institution. In E. J. Lieberman (Ed.), *Mental health: The public health challenge.* Washington: American Public Health Association, 1975, pp. 59–62.

Lippman, D. Psychiatry in Ethiopia. *Canadian Psychiatric Association Journal,* 1976, *21,* 383–388.

Litman, T. J. The family as a basic unit in health and medical care: A social behavioral overview. *Social Science and Medicine,* 1974, *8,* 495–519.

Lynn, D. B. *The father: His role in child development.* Monterey, Cal.: Brooks/Cole, 1974.

Mahler, H. A moral revolution. *World Health,* September 1975, No. 3.

Mahler, H. *The work of WHO, 1975.* Annual report of the Director-General to the World Health Assembly. Geneva: World Health Organization Official Records, No. 229, 1976. (a)

Mahler, H. A social revolution in public health. *WHO Chronicle,* 1976, *30,* 475–480. (b)

Manciaux, M. The health of the family. *World Health,* September 1975, Nos. 4–9.

May, J. T. (Ed.). *Family mental health: Annotated bibliography.* Rockville, Md.: National Institute of Mental Health, 1974.

McEwan, P. J. M. *The social approach.* Geneva: World Health Organization, 1971, Document DS/SAF/71.4.

McEwan, P. J. M. *Psycho-social aspects of the family and health care.* Geneva: World Health Organization, 1973, Document MCH/WP/73.11.

McEwan, P. J. M. *The search for social indices of family health.* Geneva: World Health Organization, 1975, Document DSI/WP/75.6.

McKinlay, J. B. Some approaches and problems in the study of the use of services: An overview. *Journal of Health and Social Behavior,* 1972, *18,* 115–145.

Mead, M. *Culture and commitment.* New York: Natural History Press, 1970.

Mechanic, D. Social structure and personal adaptation: Some neglected dimensions. In G. V. Coelho, D. A. Hamburg, & J. E. Adams (Eds.), *Coping and adaptation.* New York: Basic, 1974, pp. 32–44.

Mehryar, A., & Khajavi, F. Some implications of the community mental health model for developing countries. *International Journal of Social Psychiatry,* 1974, *21,* 45–52.

Meyer, E. E., & Sainsbury, P. (Eds.). *Promoting health in the human environment.* Geneva: World Health Organization, 1975.

Miller, F. J. W. The target. *World Health,* September 1975, pp. 10–15.

Miller, L. (Ed.). *Mental health in rapid changing society.* Jerusalem: Academic, 1971.

Mishler, E., & Waxler, N. *Interaction in families.* New York: Wiley, 1968.

Mogey, J. *Sociology of marriage and family behavior.* The Hague: Mouton, 1971.

Moos, R. H. Psychological techniques in the assessment of adaptive behavior. In G. V. Coelho, D. A. Hamburg, & J. E. Adams (Eds.), *Coping and adaptation.* New York: Basic, 1974, pp. 334–399.

Moos, R. H. (Ed.) *Human adaptation: Coping with life crises.* Lexington, Mass.: Heath, 1976.

Moos, R. H., & Tsu, V. D. Human competence and coping: An overview. In R. H. Moos (Ed.), *Human adaptation: Coping with life crises.* Lexingtion, Mass.: Heath, 1976, pp. 3–16.

Mukherjee, B. N. Marital decision-making and family planning. *Journal of Family Welfare,* 1975, *21,* 77–101.

Munandar, S. C. U. Family planning, *Psychologi (Jakarta),* 1970, *2,* 38–47.

Murphy, L. B. Coping, vulnerability, and resilience in childhood. In G. V. Coelho, D. A. Hamburg, & J. E. Adams (Eds.), *Coping and adaptation.* New York: Basic, 1974, pp. 69–100.

Neki, J. S. Psychiatry in South-East Asia. *British Journal of Psychiatry,* 1973, *123,* 257–269.

Neugarten, B. L. *Middle age and aging.* Chicago: University of Chicago Press, 1968.

Neuhaus, R., & Neuhaus, R. *Family crises.* Columbus, Ohio: Merrill, 1974.

Newell, K. W. (Ed.). *Health by the people.* Geneva: World Health Organization, 1975.

Nye, F. I. *Role structure and analysis of the family.* Beverly Hills: Sage Publications, 1976.

Offer, D., & Sabshin, M. *Normality,* New York: Basic, 1966.

Oliensis, D. East African psychological patterns. *Journal of the American Academy of Child Psychiatry,* 1967, *6,* 551–572.

Olson, D. H. The measurement of family power by self-report and behavioral methods. *Journal of Marriage and the Family,* 1969, *31,* 545–550.

Olson, D. H., & Dahl, N. S. (Eds.). *Inventory of marriage and family literature.* St. Paul: University of Minnesota, 1975.

Omran, A. R. Health benefits for mother and child. *World Health,* January 1974, pp. 6–13.

Orleans, L. A. China's experience in population control: The elusive model. *World Development,* 1975, *3,* 497–525.

Ornauer, H., Wiberg, H., Sicinski, A., & Galtung, J. (Eds.). *Images of the world in the year 2000: A comparative ten nation study.* Atlantic Highlands, N.J.: Humanities, 1976.

Ortutay, Z. The educational function of the family. *International Child Welfare Review,* 1970, *8,* 11–23.

Otto, H. A. A new light on human potential. In Iowa State University (Ed.), *Families of the future*. Ames: Iowa State University Press, 1971, pp. 14–25.

Padilla, A. M. *Mental health service utilization by Mexican-Americans*. Rockville, Md.: National Clearinghouse for Mental Health Information, 1976. (Project No. MH 26099)

Parad, H. J., & Caplan, G. A framework for studying families in crisis. *Social Work*, 1960, *5*, 3–15.

Park, H. J., Chung, K. K., & Han, D. S. A study of some behavioral problems in sequential processes of adoption in family planning. *International Journal of Health Education*, 1975, *18*, 229–240.

Peled, T. *Family planning behavior and preferences: Patterns of the well-to-do social strata in Israel*. Jerusalem: Israel Institute of Applied Social Research, 1970.

Peled, T., & Friedman, H. L. *Public and professional perception and response to population policy in Israel*. Research report from the Israel Institute of Applied Social Research, Jerusalem, 1976.

Pfister-Ammende, M. *Uprooting and resettlement as a sociological problem*. Geneva: World Federation for Mental Health, 1960.

Pitcairn, D. M., & Flahault, D. *The medical assistant: An intermediate level of health care personnel*. Geneva: World Health Organization, 1974.

Price-Bonham, S. Bibliography of literature related to roles of fathers. *Family Coordinator*, 1976, *25*, 489–518.

Prothro, E. T., & Diab, L. N. *Changing family patterns in the Arab East*. Beirut: American University, 1974.

Rabkin, L. Y. The institution of the family is alive and well. *Psychology Today*, February, 1976, pp. 66–73.

Reiss, D. *Factors regulating family–environment interaction*. Rockville, Md.: National Clearinghouse for Mental Health Information, 1976. (Project No. MH 26711)

Rogler, L. H. *Help patterns in intergenerational Puerto Rican families*. Rockville, Md.: National Clearinghouse for Mental Health Information, 1976. (Project No. MH 26314)

Ross, H. L., & Sawhill, I. V. *Time of transition: The growth of families headed by women*. Washington: Urban Institute, 1975.

Rutter, M. *Early resources of security and competence*. Unpublished lecture, February 1976.

Rutter, M., & Madge, N. *Cycles of disadvantage*. London: Heinemann, 1976.

Safilios-Rothschild, C. The study of family power structure: A review, 1960–1969. *Journal of Marriage and the Family*, 1970, *32*, 539–552.

Sainsbury, P. Evaluation of community mental health programs. In M. Guttentag & E. L. Struening (Eds.), *Handbook of evaluation research* (Vol. 2). Beverly Hills: Sage Publications, 1975, pp. 125–159.

Sanua, V. Immigration, migration, and mental illness. In E. B. Brody (Ed.), *Behavior in new environments*. Beverly Hills: Sage Publications, 1970, pp. 291–352.

Schaefer, E. S. Parents as educators: Evidence from cross-sectional, longitudinal, and intervention research. *Young Children*, 1972, *23*, 227–239.

Schmidt, K. E. Mental health services in a developing country in South-East Asia (Sarawak). In H. L. Freeman & J. Farndale (Eds.), *New aspects of the mental health services*. Oxford: Pergamon, 1969, pp. 213–236.

Schultz, T. W. (Ed.). *Economics of the family: Marriage, children, and the human capital*. Chicago: University of Chicago Press, 1974.

Schwarzweller, H. K., & Brown, J. S. Social class origins and economic, social, and psychological adjustment of Kentucky mountain migrants: A case study. In E. B. Brody (Ed.), *Behavior in new environments*. Beverly Hills: Sage Publications, 1970, pp. 117–144.

Segal, J. (Ed.). *Research in the service of mental health*. Rockville, Md.: National Institute of Mental Health, 1975.

Shaw, R. P. *Migration theory and fact: A review and bibliography of current literature.* Philadelphia: Regional Science Research Institute, 1975.

Shore, M. F. Mental health services for youth: What we can learn from the Europeans. *Journal of Clinical Child Psychology, 1976,* Spring, 10–13. (a)

Shore, M. F. Youth advisory services in six European countries. *Children, 1976, 5*(1), 23–27; 35. (b)

Shore, M. F., Robert, C-N., & Jeanneret, O. *Patterns of youth advisory services.* Copenhagen: World Health Organization Regional Office for Europe, 1977, ICP/MNH 016 III.

Sidel, R. *Women and child care in China.* Baltimore: Penguin, 1973.

Sidel, V. W., & Sidel, R. The delivery of medical care in China. *Scientific American, 1974, 230*(4), 1–8.

Sidel, V. W., & Sidel, R. The health care delivery system of the People's Republic of China. In K. W. Newell (Ed.), *Health by the people.* Geneva: World Health Organization, 1975, pp. 1–12.

Silverman, P. R., et al. *Helping each other in widowhood.* New York: Health Sciences, 1975.

Smith, K. A. Health priorities in the poorer countries. *Social Science and Medicine, 1975, 9,* 121–132.

Speer, D. C. Family systems: Morphostasis and morphogenesis, or is homeostasis enough? *Family Process, 1970, 9,* 259–278.

Straus, M. A. Measuring families. In H. T. Christensen (Ed.), *Handbook of marriage and the family.* Chicago: Rand McNally, 1964, pp. 335–400.

Straus, M. A. *Family measurement techniques.* Minneapolis: University of Minnesota Press, 1969.

Straus, M. A. Husband–wife interaction in nuclear and joint households. In D. Narain (Ed.), *Explorations in the family and other essays: Prof. K. M. Kapidia Memorial Volume.* Bombay: Thalker, 1975, pp. 134–150.

Strodtbeck, F. Family interaction, values, and achievement. In D. McClelland, A. Baldwin, H. Bronfenbrenner, & F. Strodtbeck (Eds.), *Talent and society.* Princeton: Van Nostrand, 1958.

Swift, C. R. Mental health programs in a developing country: Any relevance anywhere? *American Journal of Orthopsychiatry, 1972, 42,* 517–526.

Swift, C. R. The training of mental health workers: Types and roles of auxiliaries. In T. A. Baasher, G. M. Carstairs, R. Giel, & F. R. Hassler (Eds.), *Mental health services in developing countries.* Geneva: World Health Organization, 1975, pp. 89–100.

Thorne, M. C. Decision-making theory: A consultant's guide to getting technical information used. *Health Education Monographs, 1975, 3,* 372–384.

Troll, L. E. The family of later life: A decade review. *Journal of Marriage and the Family, 1971, 33,* 263–290.

Trost, J. Personal communication, 1977.

Underhill, E. The living conditions and family life of migrants and their children in the main countries of Europe. *International Child Welfare Review, 1975,* No. 26, pp. 28–33.

UNICEF. Twelve facts about the state of children in developing countries. *International Child Welfare Review, 1975,* No. 25, p. 24.

Van Dusen, R. A. *Social indicators, 1973: A review symposium.* Washington: Social Science Research Council, 1974.

Vaughn, C. E. & Leff, J. P. The influence of family and social factors on the course of psychiatric illness: A comparison of schizophrenic and depressed neurotic patients. *British Journal of Psychiatry, 1976, 129,* 125–137.

Vaughn, W. T., Jr., Huntington, D. S., Samuels, T. E., Bilmes, M., & Shapiro, M. I. Family mental health maintenance: A new approach to primary prevention. *Hospital and Community Psychiatry, 1975, 26,* 503–508.

Wang, V. L. Training of the barefoot doctor in the People's Republic of China: From prevention to curative service. *International Journal of Health Services*, 1975, *5*, 475–488.

Wang, V. L. Application of social science theories to family planning health education in the People's Republic of China. *American Journal of Public Health*, 1976, *66*, 440–445.

Warheit, G. J., Bell, R. A., & Schwab, J.J. *Planning for change: Needs assessment approaches*. Rockville, Md.: National Institute of Mental Health, 1975.

Warner, L., & DeFleur, M. Attitude as an interactional concept: Social constraint and social distance as intervening variables between attitudes and action. *American Sociological Review*, 1969, *34*, 153–169.

Watson, E. J. Meeting community health needs: The role of the medical assistant. *WHO Chronicle*, 1976, *30*, 91–96.

Weisanen, F. B. Coping with urbanity: The case of the recent migrant to Santiago de Chile. In E. B. Brody (Ed.), *Behavior in new environments*. Beverly Hills: Sage Publications, 1970, pp. 189–202.

Weiss, S. M. (Ed.). *Proceedings of the National Heart and Lung Institute Working Conference on Health Behavior*, Basye, Virginia, May 1975. Washington: DHEW Publication No. (NIH) 76–868, 1975.

Wesley, W. A., & Epstein, N. B. *The silent majority*. San Francisco: Jossey-Bass, 1969.

White, R. W. Strategies of adaptation: An attempt at systematic description. In G. V. Coelho, D. A. Hamburg, & J. E. Adams (Eds.), *Coping and adaptation*. New York: Basic, 1974, pp. 47–68.

Whiteley, R., & Watts, W. Information cost, decision consequence, and selected personality variables as factors in pre-decision information seeking. *Journal of Personality*, 1969, *37*, 325–341.

Wilenski, P. *The delivery of health services in the People's Republic of China*. Ottawa: International Development Research Centre, 1976.

Wishik, S., & Bernard, V. W. Family planning, population policies, and mental health. In S. E. Goldston (Ed.), *Mental health considerations in public health*. U.S.P.H.S. Publication No. 1898, May 1969, pp. 161–180.

Wolfson, M. Environment: A key to health. *People*, 1976, *3*(3), 12–14.

Wolfson, M., & Kane, P. Learning from the Chinese lesson. *People*, 1976, *3*(3), 22.

Woody, R. H., & Woody, J. D. Parenthood. In E. J. Lieberman (Ed.), *Mental health: The public health challenge*. Washington: American Public Health Association, 1975, pp. 130–135.

World Health Organization. *Report on consultation on the statistical aspects of the family as a unit in health studies*. Geneva, December 14–20, 1971. Geneva: World Health Organization, 1972. Document DSI/72.6.

World Health Organization. *Pregnancy and abortion in adolescence*. Geneva: WHO Technical Report Series, No. 583, 1975. (a)

World Health Organization. *Report on consultation on family health*. Geneva, November 5–12, 1973. Geneva: World Health Organization, 1975. Document FHE/75.4. (b)

World Health Organization. *Statistical indices of family health; report of a WHO Study Group*. Geneva: WHO Technical Report Series, No. 587, 1976.

World Health Organization. Child development: Separating fact from fiction. *WHO Chronicle*, 1977, *31*, 18–22.

World Health Organization Assembly. *Psychosocial factors and health*. WHO Executive Board Document EB 57/22, November 20, 1975.

World Health Organization Scientific Group. *Human development and public health*. Geneva: WHO Technical Report Series, No. 485, 1972.

Zwingmann, C., & Pfister-Ammende, M. *Uprooting and after*. New York: Springer Verlag, 1973.

15

Urban Health Services in Developing Countries: Culture, Technology, and Politics

Paul I. Ahmed and Robert Davis

This discussion begins from the premise that there is a web of interconnected health problems associated with urbanization. The purpose of this chapter is to set forth a partial explanation of those problems, especially as regards the less developed countries, and to suggest some strategies for their solution.

Dimensions of the Problem

Cities are home to a major part of the world population and host to its health problems. The developed world is already heavily urbanized, and the population of the less developed world will increase by some 1.3 billion in the next 25 years to become 42% of the total. Almost 300 third world cities

Paul I. Ahmed and Robert Davis • Office of International Health, U.S. Department of Health, Education and Welfare, Rockville, Maryland 20857. An earlier version of this chapter was presented by Paul I. Ahmed at the International Colloquium on Comparative Urbanization and Regionalization sponsored by the National Institutes of Public Management of Mexico, and the United States of America at the U.S. Department of Commerce, Washington, D. C., October 13, 1978. This paper represents the professional views of the authors and does not imply endorsement by the Office of International Health.

will have populations greater than 1 million by that time, with urbanization being greatest in Latin America (England, 1978). The already considerable health problems of city people will command even greater attention with growing urbanization, especially among poor rural migrants. Special attention will focus on the higher urban death rate deriving from such causes as cancers and suicides, which has been documented many times for the less developed countries (Federici, de Sarno Prignano, Pasquali, Cariani, & Natale, 1976).

The third world city is, if anything, more heterogeneous than its Western counterpart, containing as it does elements of the village and the preindustrial, industrial, and postindustrial worlds.

The problems of urban health are correspondingly complex and interconnected. To categorize them is to assure oversimplification. With that *caveat* in mind, the following ideas are offered as a framework for understanding the health problems of the city, particularly the third world city.

Demographic, Socioeconomic, and Political Influences on Health

Population, socioeconomic, and political forces all play a leading role in shaping the health status of city people and the health system that is meant to serve them. These influences may bear more heavily on the health of city dwellers than the medical and public health activities that are aimed specifically at promoting health.

The most notable impact of cities on population is the pressure of population. The impact of excessive population growth on health has been reviewed elsewhere by Wray (1971); our purpose here is to touch on its causes and treatment. Urban growth stems partly from migration and partly from natural increase among urban residents. No non-Communist country has succeeded in stemming immigration, although the degree of immigration may vary with the extent to which rural life is made more attractive through such things as land reform and economic regionalization.

The socioeconomic forces that impact on health fall in some cases on both the poor and the well-to-do. Where industrial and automobile emissions are uncontrolled, rich and poor breathe the same dirty air. Where the environment of the street is hectic, both suffer the same stresses. Some health problems, however, fall more heavily on the disadvantaged, so the following discussion will focus on the situation of rural migrants to the city and other members of the urban poor.

New migrants are susceptible to higher levels of stress and to increased infection. Higher rates of lung cancer and coronary diseases have been found among the new migrants (Tyroler & Cassel, 1964). The cumulative psychosocial stresses and impact of overcrowding and uprooting on populations in a rapidly urbanizing world have been affirmed by Coelho and Stein (1978).

Poorer ethnic minorities tend to have higher disease rates than the better-off nonminorities; they tend to have higher rates of tuberculosis (Holmes, 1956) than others in the urban population. Malnutrition rates in urban shantytowns can be higher than in rural populations. An estimated 30 to 40% of the clinic patients studied in Bogota could not be "cured" because of the treatment, or because of the poor home hygienic milieu that counteracted the effects of the drugs (Press, 1969).

Urban health hazards include water, which is affected by sewage, industrial waste, urban runoff, and chemicals. Waterborne organisms carry such diseases as cholera, typhoid, dysentery, infectious hepatitis, and guinea worm. These infectious diseases, usually associated with rural poverty, are found wherever people cannot afford clean water. Poverty is a health problem regardless of residence; to an extent, the health problems of the urban and the rural poor are all of a piece.

The economic causes of poor health are part of the economic structure of the city. For example, high unemployment keeps wages down, both parents must work, and the preschool child is left unattended and prematurely weaned. Low income limits access to medical services among the poor, and rapid urbanization of these groups leads to inadequate provision of water, electricity, education, and preventive health services in new settlements.

Just as socioeconomic conditions promote poor health among the poor, they also affect the medical system whose function is to make them well. While the urban hospital system is often a clone of a Western model, the rural medical system familiar to the migrant tends to be a smaller and simpler system where healer, patient, and patient's relatives all know each other. Modern medicine, which is "based on precisely defined knowledge, technique and procedures all of which are discontinuous from ordinary social process" (Manning & Fabrega, 1973) tends to isolate migrants from their social and cultural environment. The migrant, who is often accustomed to a folk healer, and who is having a traumatic adaptation to city culture, may find modern medicine to be more threatening than his disease. He may refuse modern medical care because of its procedures and style, or because of its inflexibility, "not altered by time and place of treatment or by personality of physician" (Manning & Fabrega, 1972). To an economically and perhaps culturally marginal migrant experiencing discomfort of illness or disability, the threat of disruption of income and expected role performance, along with fees for modern medicine, is much more important than the illness itself. The migrant may reject modern medicine for other reasons, such as what he perceives as its denial of God, denial of a role for the family in diagnosis and treatment, or desire for more ego-focused attention.

The patient may want a curer who is not "god" himself, who takes care of him, accepts his symptoms at face value, thus accepting his anxieties about acculturation, and validates his sick role performance (Press, 1978).

Traditional Medicine

The documented persistence of traditional medicine in urban societies (Boesch, 1972) illustrates an attraction that would not persist but for the failure of modern medical services to provide the patient with the psychic satisfactions of traditional care. Those satisfactions should be seen from the perspective of the patient's view of illness.

The peoples of some developing countries have a strong traditional culture. They tend to view disease as the result of a falling out of harmony with the world, for example, by the irritation of a living individual who then casts the evil eye or by the annoyance of an ancestor or dead soul who then seeks retribution. This commitment to their world view is supported by history, tradition, custom, and the need for psychological well-being. It is a view with two important behavioral consequences. One is a fatalistic attitude, an acceptance of disease and death as the will of God. The other is the importance that is perceived and attached by them to the preconditions and consequences of the illness, which bode larger in the patient's mind than its distinctive features or how it operates in the body.

These conceptions of disease are very different from those of modern medicine, but the approach represents a functional adjustment to the immediate situation. In most developing areas a very low degree of mastery over nature and social conditions has been achieved. Hence, devastating natural occurrences are seen as visitations from gods or evil spirits that can be propitiated but not controlled. People who live on bare subsistence view death and disease as common events, not subject to control. This attitude affects the use of modern medical services. People reared in a culture of fatalism tend to favor the traditional practitioner of like beliefs, who can share their love of God and sense of destiny, serving as advisor and healer as well as doctor. Medical care that overlooks these facts of cultural life runs the risk of treating disease without treating the patient. This leaves the patient an alien in a strange new system and drives him away from the modern medical care that could offer much to help him if it were presented in a sympathetic cultural context. Reform of medical curricula and of medical institutions is essential to correcting this situation.

Political Reform

Just as health and health care are parts of the socioeconomic system, so, too, they are parts of the political system. This sometimes shows itself in dramatic ways, like the curtailing of health services following the fall of the Allende government in Chile. Where political inequities persist, unrepresented groups get fewer health services through such practices as pricing, facilities location, the erection of social barriers between provider and patient, and the failure to provide such essential services as industrial hygiene. Inequities persist where politics are dominated by urban elites. The solution to such problems cannot move forward outside the context of larger political change.

Prevention in Context

Certain types of health problems can be eliminated only through demographic, economic, and political reforms. The influence of those forces in macroinstitutional reforms cannot be underestimated. In this connection it is instructive to remember that in developed countries, death rates began their decline before, not after, the scientific advances in understanding of disease causation that led to specific preventive and curative intervention. Tuberculosis in New York had declined to scarcely half its former incidence by the isolation of the tubercle bacillus in 1880. It had declined even further before the introduction of sanitoria, the widespread use of BCG immunization, and the introduction of effective drug therapy (Illich, 1977). Higher income, better sanitation, and improved nutrition tend in all urban societies to bring about a decline in death rates from infectious disease. Rises occur in life expectancy and the chronic degenerative diseases of aging replace the acute infectious diseases as major causes of death, as Bryant (1969) has shown from Hong Kong data.

Although the influence of external forces on general health status cannot be denied, there are many urban health problems that are amenable to specific public health interventions. The Pan American Health Organization has studied patterns of mortality in 12 cities, mostly in Latin America, and has concluded that, among adults, 39% and 29% of all deaths in males and females, respectively, are due to causes amenable to preventive action and treatment (Puffer & Griffith, 1967). Table I shows the major causes of preventable death discovered in the PAHO study. Since its publication, advances in such areas as the epidemiology of industrial cancers have probably raised the proportion of deaths amenable to preventive action. The range of preventive measures available is very wide and lies partly outside the scope of conventional public health programs. Industrial accidents and some forms of cancer fall within the province of industrial hygiene. The incidence of cirrhosis can be reduced through higher liquor taxes, as has been done successfully in England, and through specific treatment programs. Respiratory diseases can be reduced through clean air legislation and through no-smoking campaigns. Certain forms of cancer can be de-

Table I. Number of Deaths from Causes Amenable to Preventive Action and Treatment in Three Age Groups from 15 to 74 Years with Percentages, by Sex, in 12 Cities, 1962–1964[a]

Cause	Total		15–34 years		35–54 years		55–74 years	
	N	%	N	%	N	%	N	%
Male								
All causes	24,366	100.0	3,496	100.0	7,095	100.0	13,775	100.0
Causes amenable to preventive action and treatment	9,502	39.0	2,433	69.6	3,319	46.8	3,750	27.2
Infective and parasitic diseases	1,921	7.9	454	13.0	814	11.5	653	4.7
Alcoholism, cirrhosis of liver, and external causes	5,536	22.7	1,934	55.3	2,086	29.4	1,516	11.0
Bronchitis and cancer of lung	1,559	6.4	20	.6	294	4.1	1,245	9.0
Diabetes mellitus	486	2.0	25	.7	125	1.8	336	2.4
Other causes								
Other malignant neoplasms	3,309	13.6	216	6.2	848	12.0	2,245	16.3
Cardiovascular diseases	7,715	31.7	290	8.3	1,757	24.8	5,668	41.1
Other	3,840	15.8	557	15.9	1,171	16.5	2,112	15.3
Female								
All causes	18,932	100.0	2,680	100.0	5,100	100.0	11,152	100.0
Causes amenable to preventive action and treatment	5,542	29.3	1,514	56.5	1,823	35.7	2,205	19.8
Infective and parasitic diseases	1,233	6.5	454	16.9	425	8.3	354	3.2
Alcoholism, cirrhosis of liver, and external causes	1,772	9.4	550	20.5	600	11.8	622	5.6
Bronchitis and cancer of lung	474	2.5	14	.5	87	1.7	373	3.3
Maternal deaths and cancer of cervix uteri	1,414	7.5	480	17.9	592	11.6	342	3.1
Diabetes mellitus	649	3.4	16	.6	119	2.3	514	4.6
Other causes								
Other malignant neoplasms	3,556	18.8	215	8.0	1,063	20.8	2,278	20.4
Cardiovascular diseases	6,214	32.8	308	11.5	1,215	23.8	4,691	42.1
Other	3,620	19.1	643	24.0	999	19.6	1,978	17.7

[a]Source: Puffer and Griffith (1967).

tected and treated through multiphasic screening programs. A comprehensive approach to disease prevention requires both "life-style reform" and changes in institutional behavior.

It lies beyond the scope of this chapter to set out detailed strategies for specific preventive interventions in urban societies. This has been done for the United States in a recent review (Nightingale, Cureton, Kalmer, &

Trudeau, 1978). The United States model may not be appropriate for those countries where infectious diseases are still the main problem. Even where these have been reduced, less developed countries cannot devote the same resources to prevention as the affluent ones. Under these conditions, economics becomes a key tool in the wise allocation of resources. To assure that economic wisdom is translated into effective program implementation, the planning, economic, and budgetary functions of the urban health authorities should be placed under a single administrative umbrella.

The obstacles that lie in the way of disease prevention are formidable. Economic constraints have already been mentioned. In some areas, there is a lack of professional infractucture and technical expertise. In others, the expertise is there but health funds have been allocated preferentially to the hospital system, which is burdened with the expensive task of treating, sometimes without success, cheaply preventable diseases. Administrative fragmentation of preventive services can be a serious problem, with ad hoc efforts by dozens of public and private agencies creating duplications in some areas and lack of services in others. Influential interest groups, such as producers of tobacco and sweetened milk, may oppose needed changes. Finally, low-income groups may be discriminated against in the provision of such basic services as clean water, public education, mother/child services, and the like.

The solution to these problems is clearly not restricted to the technical and administrative side. Where social, medical, and commercial elites are actively opposed to preventive interventions, political change is an indispensable prelude to effective preventive measures. Where the external environment is more sympathetic to public health, preventive campaigns can move forward.

Curative Services

Both developed and less developed countries spend a lot of money of providing curative services, especially through hospitals. The existing animus in the international health community against location of curative services in large cities can lead one to overlook problems of location, distribution, and access that limit the ability of the urban poor to use existing services. As England (1978) has pointed out:

> The urban services that tend to absorb the vast proportion of resources and return few benefits are largely those hospital-based treatments at the disposal of higher incomes which offer advantageous remunerative opportunities of providers. They are inappropriate because they are the wrong kinds of services, not because they are in the wrong place. There is no reason why urban health services cannot be extremely cost-effective and reach large numbers of urban

populations with needed maternal and child health and family planning programs and there is every reason why they should be doing so.

The fact that quality medical services are generally *available* in most cities should not mask the fact that they are not always *accessible* to the populations living in them. Even in the United States, a relatively wealthy country, 5,000 of the 25,000 census tracts are medically underserved, as measured by a composite index reflecting the ratio of primary-care physicians to total population, the infant mortality rate, the percentage of the population aged 65 and over, and the percentage of population with family incomes below the poverty line (U.S. Department of Health, Education and Welfare, 1975).

In rich countries and in poor ones, the bottlenecks to access can be physical (long distances to facilities), economic (services that cannot be afforded), temporal (because facilities are closed outside wage earners' working hours), or psychological (because of social distance between consumers and providers of medical care). Salkever (1975) has found that in four urbanized settings in developed countries, higher family income was associated with greater access to pediatric care, regardless of level of need. In the United States, the "near poor," with incomes too high for Medicaid eligibility and not high enough to buy private insurance, constitute a group with limited access. In less developed countries, the urban poor, like their rural counterparts, form part of a large pool of the unskilled underemployed, with few prospects for stable earnings, for sick leave, for health insurance, or for other forms of medical protection. The poor working-class urbanite is worse off than his rural counterpart in that the former has no extended family or community support mechanisms to take care of him when he is ill. Moreover, he does not produce his own food, and must bear the brunt of food price inflation. Even the poor farm worker, in contrast, is often paid in kind, so that his medical needs need not compete for his resources with the need to eat.

The inequities in access to quality medical care are in part due to structural inequities in urban settings as a whole. There are, however, other, specific influences that serve to promote inequity. One such influence is the imitation of unsuitable models from Western countries. Facilities planning is usually in the hands of ministry-level physicians, largely Western-trained. They have little sympathy for indigenous or folk medicine, less sympathy for the poor than for the rich, and a firm commitment to the ad hoc acquisition of high technology equipment, without regard to regional needs or the elimination of gaps and overlaps. The influence of foreign donors has often distorted or augmented indigenous preferences. As Donaldson (1976) has stated, reviewing Rockefeller Foundation aid to Thai medical education, "the shortcoming of these programs is not that they create the inequality associated with professional services throughout the developing world, but that they so neatly serve those who maintain it." Medical curricula, with their heavy clinical emphasis, have tended to neglect the problems of epidemiology, ecology, economics, and health care organization. The naive medical graduate of today becomes the resource misallocator of tomorrow, often lacking any background in the principles of assessment, resource allocation, and regionalization that form the groundwork of solid planning.

Equitable financing systems for personal health services are part of the answer, but equal access to a fragmented system is not an adequate solution to the problems cited above. The importance of a regionalized health system, which is self-evident in rural areas, has been overlooked in many cities. The tertiary teaching hospital should not exist in splendid isolation but as part of a system with referral, consultation, and training links at every level. The successful regionalization of urban health services in Cuba and China (Tejeiro Fernandez, 1975; Sidel, 1974) is illustrative of how the echelons of the health system can be tied together to the benefit of the system and of the patient alike. No doubt centralization of authority in these two countries has helped them direct their manpower in this fashion. The concept, however, could be adapted to democracies, given the vast reservoirs of unemployed manpower in the developing countries.

The Role of Health Planning

Health planning assesses situations, describes goals and objectives, and designs programs to meet them, with a view to cost-effectiveness and consideration of alternate approaches to goal attainment. It is not widely practiced in the developed or the less developed world, where the health sector functions in a profession-oriented, not a goal-oriented way (Bryant, 1969). In many health ministries, each program, such as the hospital, malaria, or tuberculosis department, functions separately from the others, following its own internal logic and meeting its own agenda without reference to well-defined ministry objectives. This lack of focus is often due to the absence of system and goals within the ministry. Departments cannot follow a ministry that does not lead. In recent years the situation has changed. Health plans are more common, goals are more defined, and the direction comes both from the ministries of health and from the planning commissions. Many of the plans are still on paper and are not acted upon by the ministries.

Ideally, a ministry that takes a leadership position will do so with an eye to social and economic equity. This means, for example, planning and execution of programs to correct maldistribution of resources between town and village, to install a community-based system of regionalized health care stressing health center care where possible in preference to hospital care, and to assure better access to the health system for all levels of society. Since politics play an important role in planning, the political system of a country may frustrate achievement of plan goals. For example, India's progressive health plans, which have been produced for 28 years as part of a national process, have thus far failed to achieve an equitable distribution of resources between classes and geographical areas. What India's current draft plan says about land redistribution is equally applicable to health and other resources: "critical for the success of all redistributive laws, policies and programmes, is that the poor be organized and made conscious of the benefits intended for them" (Chopra, 1978).

India has long experience in planning for health, but other countries' health planning is still in the embryonic stages. Recent efforts by international agencies have tried to help nationals shape well-defined goals. The USAID has supported a health planning project in Ghana and is now likely to support another in Somalia. The World Health Organization, through its country representatives, has provided planning and programming expertise to ministries of health. The World Bank has required reorganization of management functions in the areas of bank support and has done country analyses itself. The urban poor may yet get recognition if health planning data are collected and subjected to intelligent analysis and follow-through. Analyses of service utilization data in urban areas will point to system inequities; economic analyses will point to the feasibility of such low-cost preventive services as provision of potable water, immunization, and the like. None of the foregoing is likely to happen, however, in the absence of political representation and political widsom.

Conclusions

The urban health care system does not exist separately from the society of which it is a part. In the developing countries, particularly, urban society is complex, stratified, and fragmented; so, too, is the health care system. Not only are there large traditional and nontraditional private sectors, but the public sector is fragmented and stratified among various agencies and levels within agencies. Gaps and overlaps in health services are inevitable in such a system, and only regional planning, encompassing whole metropolitan areas, can reduce its unfortunate consequences. The most useful model of regional planning is one administered by a single authority.

The concept of regionalization, indispensible to coverage of all classes and neighborhoods in a city, is hard to realize in societies where vast areas of inequity persist. To achieve penetration of health services into unserved and underserved populations, political will is as necessary as money. Community participation is indispensible to politically responsible decision making. The questions of resource allocation are not purely technical ones, since in rich countries and poor ones proposals of equal technical merit compete for scarce resources. Questions of public spending become questions of public policy, and mechanisms of political responsibility are necessary to assure that public funds are spent so as to assure the greatest benefit to the greatest number.

No need in the constellation of urban health needs should obscure the overriding need to eradicate poverty. As long as the issues of income distribution, access to opportunity, and employment for all who seek it are left unresolved, health services in the city, whatever their preventive and curative components, will fall short of the objectives. Health for all will remain a frustrated ideal until proper attention is paid to the nonsystemic determinants of health.

References

Boesch, E. E. *Communication between doctors and patients in Thailand. Part I: Survey of the problem and analysis of the consultations.* Saarbruckën: Socio-Psychological Research Centre on Development Planning, University of the Saar, 1972.

Bryant, J. *Health and the developing world.* Ithaca and London: Cornell University Press, 1969.

Chopra, P. A brave new plan—But will it work? *International Development Review,* 1978, *3/4,* 18.

Clark, M. *Health in the Mexican-American culture.* Berkeley: University of California Press, 1970.

Coelho, G. V., & Stein, J. J. Coping with stresses of an urban planet. In *Trends in mental health.* DHEW Publication No. ADM 78-609. National Institute of Mental Health, 1978.

Donaldson, P. J. Foreign intervention in medical education: A case study of the Rockefeller Foundation's involvement in a Thai medical school. *International Journal of Health Services,* 1976, *6,* 251–270.

England, R. More myths in international health planning. *American Journal of Public Health,* 1978, *68,* 153–159.

Faris, R. E., & Dunham, J. W. *Mental Disorders in Urban Areas.* Chicago: University of Chicago Press, 1939.

Federici, N., de Sarno Prignano, A., Pasquali, P., Cariani, G., & Natale, M. Urban/rural differences in mortality, 1950-1970. *World Health Statistics Report,* 1976, *29,* 249–378.

Holmes, T. H. Multidiscipline studies of tuberculosis. In P. J. Sparer (Ed.), *Personality, stress, and tuberculosis.* New York: International Universities Press, 1956, pp. 65–152.

Illich, I. *Medical nemesis.* Toronto, New York, and London: Bantam, 1977.

Manning, P. K., & Fabrega, H., Jr. The experience of self and body. In G. Psathas (Ed.), *Phenomenological sociology.* New York: Wiley, 1973, pp. 251–301.

Nightingale, E. O., Cureton, M., Kalmar, V., & Trudeau, M. B. *Perspectives on health promotion and disease prevention in the United States.* Washington: Institute of Medicine, National Academy of Sciences, 1978. Urban illness: Physicians, curers and dual use in Bogota. *Journal Health and Social Behavior,* 1969, *10,* 209–218.

Press, I. Urban folk medicine: A functional overview. *American Anthropologist*, 1978, *80*, 71–84.

Puffer, R. R., & Griffith, G. W. *Patterns of urban mortality*. PAHO Scientific Publication 151. Washington: Pan American Health Organization, 1967.

Salkever, D. S. Economic class and differential access to care: Comparisons among health care systems. *International Journal of Health Services*, 1975, *5*, 373–395.

Sidel, R. Urban neighborhood health and social services. In J. R. Quinn (Ed.), *China medicine as we saw it*. Bethesda: John E. Fogarty International Center for Advanced Study in the Health Sciences, National Institutes of Health, 1974.

Tejeiro Fernandez, A. F. The national health system in Cuba. In K. W. Newell (Ed.), *Health by the people*. Geneva: World Health Organization, 1975.

Tyroler, H. A., & Cassel, J. Health consequences of culture change: The effect of urbanization on coronary heart mortality in rural residents. *Journal of Chronic Diseases*, 1964, *17*, 167–177.

U.S. Department of Health, Education and Welfare. *Forward planning for health*. Washington: DHEW, 1975.

Wray, J. D. Population pressure on families: Family size and child spacing. In *Rapid population growth: Consequences and policy implications*. Baltimore and London: Johns Hopkins University Press, 1971, pp. 403–461.

IV

Methodology for Health Analysis

Introduction

Until this point we have emphasized the need for awareness of the socioenvironmental, psychological, and cultural dimensions of health and illness.
But awareness alone is not enough, of course; it is merely the first step
toward action. Health planners and practitioners have long attempted to
develop, and to improve, methodologies for measuring and evaluating these
dimensions and for incorporating them into the health delivery process. The
three chapters in this section deal with such methodologies. These articles
should be viewed as providing examples rather than constituting a comprehensive overview. The first two chapters discuss some issues raised by the
ecological perspective in program design and evaluation. The third chapter
describes the goals, design, and pitfalls of a methodology used for international health planning.

In the first chapter, Moos emphasizes the socioecological perspective in
treatment and evaluation. He reports some provocative results of his own
efforts to develop scales for measuring the socioecological environment.
These scales are the Family Environment Scale (FES), measuring the social
climate of families, and the Work Environment Scale (WES), measuring the
social climate of work settings. The FES, like the WES, encompasses three
broad categories of dimensions: (1) the Relationship dimensions, which
refer to cohesion or supportiveness, expressiveness (the open and direct
expression of feelings), and the degree of conflict-laden interactions; (2) the
Personal Growth or Goal Orientation dimensions, which include independence, achievement orientation, intellectual-cultural orientation, active-rec-
reational orientation, and moral-religious emphasis; (3) the System Maintenance and System Change dimensions, which assess "the extent to which

the environment is orderly, clear in its expectations, maintains control, and is responsive to change."

Using the FES dimensions, the author and his colleagues have identified six distinctive types of families: expression-oriented, structure-oriented, independence-oriented, achievement-oriented, moral/religious-oriented, and conflict-oriented. Summarizing his own research and that of others, the author cites some evidence that the type of family environment is related to the incidence of drug abuse and alcoholism, as well as to the successful or unsuccessful outcome of institutional treatment.

The author then calls attention to further research problems arising from the measurement of family and work environment. These include the relationship of environmental dimensions to stress and to illness-related variables, and the development of coping mechanisms that protect some individuals, but not others, from the deleterious effects of the environment. He calls for incorporating into the treatment process systematic information about the patient's family and work settings, so that the proper intervention —one with the greatest chances of success—may be undertaken. The chapter ends with a renewed emphasis on the need for a socioecological perspective in analyzing and changing social settings and in promoting better mental health.

The second chapter, by O'Connor, Klassen, and O'Connor, emphasizes the need for program evaluation that incorporates the perspective of the the client as well as that of the community into the evaluation process. This contrasts with the tendency of many evaluation studies today to focus solely on the therapeutic techniques. The authors note the need to study the interactive effect of the characteristics of the client (psychological and demographic variables and, in particular, patterns of social participation) plus the characteristics of his environment as they affect the outcome of treatment. In addition, they note the need to study interaction of the client with his environment. Most evaluation research today, by contrast, concentrates primarily on the comparison of several modalities of treatment, while either ignoring, randomizing, or holding constant the characteristics of clients and of their environments.

The evaluation method proposed in this article is based on an ecological perspective. It regards the characteristics of the ecounit—the interaction of the individual with his environment—as both independent variables, affecting the course of treatment, and dependent variables, indicating the effectiveness of treatment. To accomplish the evaluation, the authors assert, it is necessary to collect data on the patient's pretreatment and posttreatment behavioral and environmental characteristics, including his patterns of family and occupational participation. The authors compare several statistical techniques for data analysis and offer a format for data collection that is comprehensive, simple, and flexible enough to apply to the diverse needs of clients and staff in different settings.

In the third chapter, Ahmed and Kolker turn our attention to some broad issues involved in international health planning. This article presents a brief overview of the objectives, design, and limitations of Health Sector Assessment, a health planning methodology used by the United States Agency for International Development (AID) since 1972. As they state it, Health Sector Assessment (HSA) involves "gathering, organizing, and analyzing data on the health policies and resources of a developing country for the identification of possible solutions" and for developing "a strategy or a set of strategies for health improvement." The Health Sector Assessment may vary in the scope of its goals from preparing a program-planning document for an AID-supported project in the host country to preparing the groundwork for a comprehensive national health plan for the country. The intermediate processes involve collecting data on the country's demographic, economic, political, and health conditions; identifying existing health services and areas of special need; and developing a set of policy alternatives and possible projects. The HSA calls for a team effort, with maximal involvement of the host country's officials in both analysis and planning. On the basis of the HSA, future joint projects or plans may be negotiated between AID and the host country.

The article calls attention to several limitations of the HSA. These include possibly the lack of consensus about the goals of the effort, insufficient attention to building up the host country's capabilities in health planning and analysis, inadequate involvement of the host country's officials, and inadequate dissemination of the results of the HSA. The authors conclude that the HSA is a potentially powerful tool for health planning, whose usefulness could be enhanced by a greater clarification of its objectives and priorities and by a more careful tailoring of the scope and cost of the effort to fit the projected benefits.

16

Evaluating Family and Work Settings

Rudolf H. Moos

A physician advises a harried executive with hypertension to switch to a job with fewer deadlines and less work pressure. A vocational counselor recommends that a shy, introverted student apply for a job in a company in which co-workers are friendly and managers are supportive. A pediatrician suggests that an underdeveloped, neglected child be sent to a foster home. A social worker attempts to place a mildly hyperactive child with structured rather than unstructured adoptive parents.

Each of these people is responding to the belief that the social environment has important effects on health and health-related behavior. Their search for information and their recommendations reflect the assumption that one can distinguish different types or dimensions of environmental stimuli, that these dimensions can have distinctive influences on psychophysiological processes and health, and that their effects may differ widely from one individual to another. I believe that these assumptions are valid. In this chapter I illustrate the concept and assessment of social climate, discuss the underlying social climate patterns of family and work settings, describe the utility of the social climate concept by drawing on examples from our program of research, summarize evidence indicating that the social environments of family and work settings have important effects,

Rudolf H. Moos • Social Ecology Laboratory, Department of Psychiatry, Stanford University School of Medicine, Palo Alto, California 94305. Preparation of this chapter and the work reported herein was supported by NIAAA Grant AA02863, NIMH Grant MH28177, and Veterans Administration Medical Research Funds.

and focus on some practical applications that follow from the foregoing material.

Our work has been carried out within a social-ecological perspective, which provides a distinctive framework by which the transactions between people and their environments, and the impacts of these transactions on human functioning, can be conceptualized. This perspective, which is being integrated into clinical and community psychology (Holahan, 1978), developmental psychology (Bronfenbrenner, 1977), and gerontology (Lawton & Nahemow, 1973), is relevant to health psychology and behavioral medicine (Moos, 1979a). Although I focus primarily on social-environmental (e.g., social climate) variables here, our work is also concerned with physical-environmental (i.e., ecological) variables such as architectural and building design characteristics (Moos, 1976a).

Defining and Measuring the Social Climate of Family Settings

Although many people agree that the family environment is implicated in the onset, development, and course of illness, in the utilization of medical care, and in the outcome of treatment (Litman, 1974; Pattison & Anderson, 1978), relatively few attempts have been made to evaluate systematically the social climate of families. Pless and Satterwhite (1973) developed an instrument for assessing the overall adequacy of family functioning from semistructured interview data. Factor analysis of the responses resulted in five dimensions labeled communication, togetherness, closeness, decision making, and child orientation.

Deykin (1972) presented a model for assessing life functioning in families of delinquent or predelinquent boys. The technique provides for the quantification of six major areas of family life functioning: decision making, marital interaction, child-rearing, emotional gratification, perception of and response to crisis, and perception of and response to community. Deykin found that families with better functioning scores were more likely to have children who displayed passive antisocial behavior, whereas families with poorer life functioning scores were more likely to have children who displayed aggressive antisocial behavior. Children in the latter families tended to show no change or even deterioration after intensive treatment, suggesting that the family environment may influence both the specific characteristics of a delinquency problem and the outcome of treatment for that problem.

Some examples may serve to clarify the manner in which the family environment can affect health status and health-related behavior. Many studies have shown that delinquency rates are higher in crowded neighborhoods. High population density conditions affect the pattern of social relationships in the family, and adolescents' responses to the stressful social relationships that housing conditions have helped to create. Crowded families are more likely to inhibit expressiveness, are often forced into close social relationships with neighboring families, show more conflict and strain, and so on (e.g., Mitchell, 1971). To reduce the consequences arising from high density, children are given greater freedom to leave the home, thereby weakening the control the family has over them. This increase in conflict and decrease in support and control may facilitate the development of the kinds of delinquency and drug abuse problems that are characteristic of high density communities.

Another important aspect of the family environment is the attitude toward the institutionalized individual once he or she returns home. For example, in homes in which family members have high expectations of patients (e.g., achievement orientation), patients may expect more of themselves. These greater pressures for success, for a return to normal living, and for the fulfillment of work and school functions are likely to be translated into better postinstitutional performance (e.g., Manino & Shore, 1974). Family support has also been shown to be important in affecting posthospital adjustment after treatment for mental illness (Myers & Bean, 1968). These studies suggest that aspects of the family environment such as cohesion, support, expressiveness, conflict, achievement expectations, and control may influence health status and health-related behavior.

Constructing the Family Environment Scale (FES)

The foregoing considerations led us to develop a Family Environment Scale (FES), which assesses the social climate of different types of families. The FES focuses on the interpersonal relationships among family members, on the directions of personal growth emphasized in the family, and on the organizational structure of the family.

The steps involved in the construction of the FES illustrate the logic underlying the measurement of social climate. Several methods were employed to gain a naturalistic understanding of family social environments and to obtain an initial pool of questionnaire items. Many individuals were interviewed to determine the characteristics of their families. Several people were involved in writing a broad range of potential items. Possible dimensions and additional items were adapted from the other Social Climate Scales. Alternative initial forms were constructed on which preliminary information was gathered. After the original pool of items was developed, items were assigned to dimensions by two naive raters on the basis of independent agreement that they "belonged" to a particular dimension. These procedures resulted in a 200-item questionnaire, representing 12 conceptual dimensions.

This initial 200-item form of the FES was administered to more than 1,000 individuals in a sample of 285 families. Data were collected from a wide range of families to ensure that the resulting scale would be applicable to a variety of family situations. This was accomplished by sampling families from diverse sources, e.g., church groups, newspaper advertisements, local high school students, and so on. An ethnic minority sample was recruited from these sources and by having black and Mexican-American research assistants obtain data from samples of black and Mexican-American families. A disturbed or "clinic" family sample was collected from two sources—a psychiatrically oriented family clinic and a probation and parole department affiliated with a local correctional facility.

Various criteria were used to select items for inclusion in the revised form. Each item had to relate highly to its own subscale. The subscales had to show only low to moderate interrelationships. Each item had to discriminate among different families. Each subscale had to have an approximately equal number of items scored true and scored false to control for acquiescence response set. These criteria resulted in the current 90 true/false item FES Form R grouped into 10 subscales.

The development of the FES is more fully discussed elsewhere (Moos, 1974a). In brief, the 10 subscales have adequate internal consistency (ranging from .64 to .79), show good 8-week test-retest reliability (ranging from .68 to .86), and have average intercorrelations of around .20, indicating that they measure distinct though somewhat related aspects of family social environments. All 10 of the subscales significantly discriminate among families. (The Work Environment Scale [WES], which is also composed of 90 true/false items representing 10 dimensions, was derived in an analogous manner using data obtained from employees and supervisors in 44 work groups [Moos & Insel, 1974]).

There are three parallel forms of the FES: (1) The Real Form (Form R) asks family members (or observers, such as social workers and family therapists) how they perceive the current family social environment; (2) the Ideal Form (Form I) asks people how they conceive of an ideal family environment; (3) the Expectations Form (Form E) asks people what they think the social milieu of a family is like. (The WES also has three parallel forms, as do each of the other Social Climate Scales; see Moos, 1974b).

Underlying Patterns of Family and Work Settings

Recent research has shown that vastly different social environments can be described by common or similar sets of dimensions. I have conceptualized these dimensions in three broad categories: Relationship dimensions, Personal Growth or Goal Orientation dimensions, and System Main-

Table I. Underlying Patterns of Family and Work Settings

Setting	Relationship dimensions	Personal growth or goal orientation dimensions	System maintenance and system change dimensions
Family	Cohesion	Independence	Organization
	Expressiveness	Achievement orientation	Control
	Conflict	Intellectual-cultural orientation	
		Active recreational orientation	
		Moral-religious emphasis	
Work	Involvement	Autonomy	Work pressure
	Peer cohesion	Task orientation	Clarity
	Staff support		Control
			Innovation
			Physical comfort

tenance and System Change dimensions. These categories of dimensions are similar across many environments, although vastly different settings may impose unique variations within the general categories. The dimensions identified in family and work settings are listed in Table I.

Relationship dimensions assess the extent to which people are involved in the environment, the extent to which they support and help one another, and the extent of spontaneity and free and open expression among them. For example, cohesion in families measures the degree to which family members are committed to the family and are helpful and supportive of one another. Expressiveness in families reflects the degree to which family members act openly and express their feelings directly, whereas conflict assesses the extent to which the expression of anger and aggression and conflict-laden interactions are characteristic of the family. Involvement in work settings measures the extent to which employees are concerned with and committed to their jobs, whereas staff support and peer cohesion assess the extent to which management is supportive of employees and employees are friendly and supportive of each other.

Personal Growth or Goal Orientation dimensions assess the basic directions along which personal development and self-enhancement tend to occur in an environment. The exact nature of these dimensions varies somewhat among different environments depending on their underlying purposes and goals. In families these dimensions are independence (the emphasis on being assertive and self-sufficient), achievement orientation (the degree to which activities are cast into an achievement-oriented or competitive framework), intellectual-cultural orientation (the emphasis on political, social, and cultural activities), active recreational orientation (the degree to which family members participate in recreational and sporting activities), and moral-religious emphasis (the degree of concern with ethical and religious issues). In work settings the Personal Growth dimensions are autonomy (the extent to which employees are encouraged to be self-sufficient and to make their own decisions) and task orientation (the emphasis on planning, efficiency, and "getting the job done").

System Maintenance and System Change dimensions assess the extent to which the environment is orderly, is clear in its expectations, maintains control, and is responsive to change. The relevant dimensions in family environments are organization (the emphasis on structuring of activities, financial planning, and explicitness and clarity in regard to rules and responsibilities) and control (the degree to which the family is organized in a hierarchical manner, and the rigidity of family rules and procedures). The relevant dimensions in work settings are work pressure (the extent to which the press of work and time-urgency dominate the job milieu), clarity (the explicitness of rules and policies), control (the extent to which management uses rules and pressures to keep employees under control), innovation (the emphasis on variety and change), and physical comfort (the extent to which the physical surroundings contribute to a pleasant work environment).

My colleagues and I have completed work in eight other types of social environments: hospital-based and community-based psychiatric treatment programs, correctional institutions, military basic traning companies, junior high and high school classrooms, university student living groups, social and task-oriented groups, and, most recently, sheltered care settings for the elderly. We have developed Social Climate Scales for each of these environments. Each of the dimensions (subscales) on each of these scales was empirically derived from independent data obtained from respondents in that particular environment.

Our studies have shown that the above three broad categories of dimensions are relevant to each of these environments, and are useful in characterizing the social and organizational climates of a variety of groups and institutions (Moos, 1974b, 1976a). Other investigators have found conceptually similar dimensions using other types of assessment devices (see Moos, 1974c; Walberg, 1976). Formulating three broad categories of dimensions gives us a convenient framework within which to provide an overview of the utility of the concept of social climate.

Describing and Classifying Family and Work Settings

One of the most important uses of information about social climate is to provide a detailed description of how people perceive an environment. For example, the FES and WES can be used to compare the perceptions of different groups of people (e.g., parents and children in families, employees and supervisors in work settings) and to monitor fluctuations in the social climate of an environment over time. The degree of agreement among employees and between employees and supervisors about the social environment is an important descriptive characteristic of their work setting.

A more complete description of an environment may be obtained when the Ideal Form of the relevant Social Climate Scale is used. In what areas are parents' goals similar? In what areas do children agree with parents? In what areas do they basically disagree? To what extent do personal growth goals vary from family to family? To what extent do parents in high-socioeconomic-level families have different views of ideal families? To what extent do ethnic minority families have different value orientations with regard to family climate? In what areas are employees', managers', and executives' goals similar with respect to their work setting?

The FES and WES can also be completed by observers or other individuals who are not participants in a setting. For example, therapists can fill out the FES on the basis of their expectations (Form E) and/or observations (Form R) of a family in therapy. A social worker can fill out the FES on the basis of a home visit to a family. Prospective employees can fill out the WES on the basis of their observations of a work setting. Although the Social Climate Scales assess people's perceptions of an environment, their applicability is not limited to those who are currently participating in that environment.

Constructing a Typology of Family Settings

A more comprehensive approach to description is to construct general classification schemes of family or work settings. The need for this approach is apparent from research that indicates that different dimensions of family environments are related to differential family outcomes. We therefore attempted to develop an empirical typology of the social environments of family settings from FES data obtained from a sample of 100 families. The 10 FES mean scores for each of the 100 families were subjected to an empirical cluster analysis, and six distinctive types of families were identified: expression-oriented, structure-oriented, independence-oriented, achievement-oriented, moral/religious-oriented, and conflict-oriented.

The 24 families in the independence-oriented cluster emphasize being assertive and self-sufficient, making their own decisions, and thinking things out for themselves. Three distinct subclusters of independence-oriented families were identified. The 11 families in the expressive independence subcluster are above average on all three Relationship dimensions (see Figure 1). There is substantial cohesion and unity in these families, and they encourage the open expression of feelings (including anger and conflict). These families emphasize the Personal Growth dimensions of intellectual-cultural and active recreational orientation, but have little emphasis on organization and control.

The 10 families in the structured independence subcluster are particularly high on independence (almost two standard deviations above average; see Figure 1). They are slightly above average on cohesion and expressiveness, and somewhat below average on conflict. In terms of other Personal Growth goals these families show slightly above-average emphasis on achievement orientation and intellectual-cultural orientation. They are also somewhat above average on organization. (The third subtype, labeled apathetic independence and composed of only three families, emphasized independence in the context of below-average emphasis on all three Relationship and on most of the other Personal Growth dimensions).

The 19 families in the achievement-oriented cluster are characterized by a strong emphasis on placing different types of activities (i.e., school

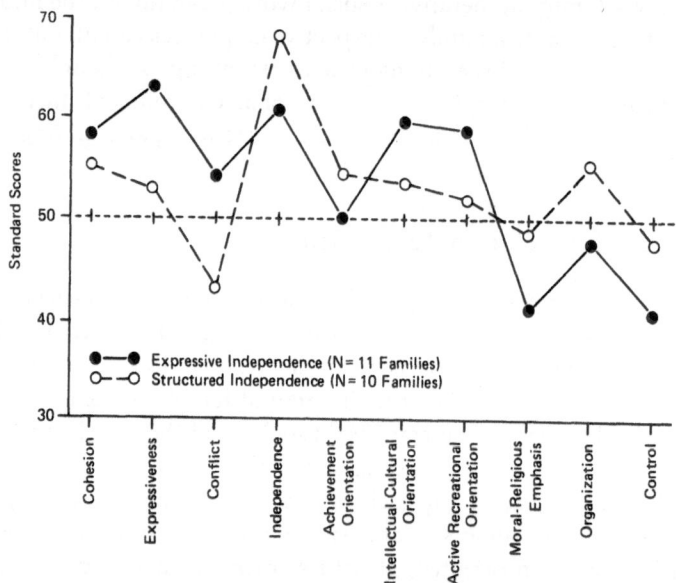

Figure 1.   Mean Family Environment Scale profiles for two independence-oriented subclusters.

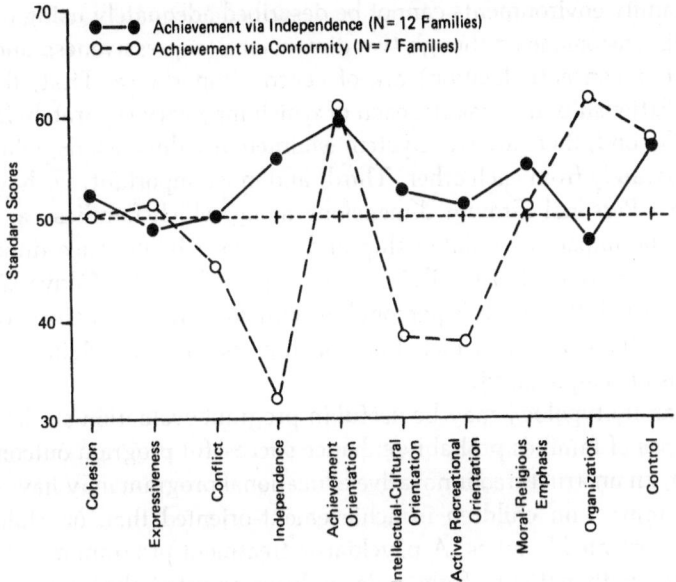

Figure 2. Mean Family Environment Scale profiles for two achievement-oriented subclusters.

and work) into an achievement-oriented or competitive framework. Family members are particularly interested in working hard and getting ahead. The 19 families fell into two subclusters, as shown in Figure 2. The 12 families in the achievement-via-independence subcluster emphasize achievement, but do so within a framework of independence (i.e., being assertive, self-sufficient, and autonomous). This emphasis on independence is focused mainly on activities outside the family, since hierarchical organization (control) in these families is substantially above average.

The seven families in the achievement via conformity subcluster also show a strong emphasis on achievement orientation, but within a quite different context. These families emphasize conformity (as indicated by their low scores on independence) and are not concerned with intellectual and cultural or with recreational and sporting activities. They show well-above-average emphasis on organization and control (see Moos & Moos, 1976, for methodological details, for a description of the other four clusters, and for a discussion of the fact that there are a variety of possible empirical solutions for any clustering problem).

The results indicate that prior conceptualizations of family environments have been oversimplified. Family environments are often measured by two major parental attitudes: acceptance versus rejection (a Relationship dimension) and high versus low control (a System Maintenance dimension). Family environments cannot be described adequately using only two major dimensions, even though two dimensions (expressiveness and structure in our conceptualization) are of central importance. First, there are three Relationship dimensions, each of which may vary separately from the others. Second, there are two System Maintenance dimensions, which may vary separately from each other. Third, and most important, we have identified five Personal Growth dimensions along which families can be oriented. The impact of Relationship and System Maintenance dimensions depends in part on the family's personal growth goals. Conversely, the extent to which the family's personal growth goals will be realized depends in part on the extent to which Relationship and System Maintenance dimensions are emphasized.

A family typology may be useful in program evaluation studies, since some types of families probably enhance successful program outcome. For example, an unstructured innovative educational program may have greater positive impact on children in achievement-oriented than on children in structure-oriented families. A psychiatric treatment program may be more successful with patients from independence-oriented than with patients from conflict-oriented families. The development of typologies of other social environments, such as those of junior high and high school classrooms (Moos, 1978) and of hospital-based and community-based psychiatric treatment programs (Moos, 1975), raises the possibility of studying the interactive effects of different types of settings.

Although less empirical work has as yet been completed, the foregoing considerations are relevant to the description and classification of work settings. For example, the WES has been used to describe the work environments of radio stations (Simek, 1975), of community mental health centers (Amante & Van Houton, 1976), and of work groups in various educational, medical, and other settings (see Moos & Insel, 1974, for examples).

Comparing and Contrasting Family and Work Settings

Another major use of information about social environments is to make comparisons among family and work settings. How do several work groups in the same organization differ? How do work settings supervised by more experienced managers differ from those supervised by less experienced ones? Do large work settings have more emphasis on supervisor control and less emphasis on innovation than small work settings? How do the social environments of families with an alcoholic member differ from matched control families?

This type of research is illustrated by a comparison of the social environments of families receiving counseling in a university clinic with "non-clinic" families selected from those who enrolled a child in a university preschool facility. The families who were seeking help scored significantly lower on the FES cohesion, expressiveness, and organization subscales, whereas they scored significantly higher on the conflict subscale (Scoresby & Christensen, 1976). In a comparison of 42 clinic and 42 matched (on family size and composition) "normal" families, we found the clinic families to obtain significantly lower scores on cohesion, intellectual-cultural orientation, and active recreational orientation, whereas they obtained higher scores on conflict and control (Moos, 1974a).

In more recent work, we have characterized the social environments of 122 families in which one family member had been treated for alcoholism in a residential alcoholism program. The data on the family environment were obtained 6 to 9 months after the patients were discharged from the program. The mean scores of the alcoholic families resembled closely those of the families in our normative sample on 7 of the 10 FES dimensions. The three exceptions were conflict, intellectual-cultural, and active recreational orientation, with the alcoholic families perceiving significantly less emphasis than the normative group on all three dimensions. (Results from our recently completed second follow-up show that these three FES differences still hold after about 24 months have elapsed since treatment.) The results for conflict are consistent with the notion that families of recovered alcoholics are careful to avoid conflicts and tension for fear of triggering renewed drinking (see Bromet & Moos, 1977; Moos, Bromet, Tsu, & Moos, 1979).

In another relevant study, Jones and Jones (1977) used the FES to compare the family environments of 276 long-distance runners to our normative sample. The joggers perceived their family environments to be higher in cohesion and active recreational orientation, and lower in conflict and control than the normative sample. The authors suggest that a serious physical exercise regimen may operate to release tension and frustration, and to change physiological, psychological, and sociological functioning to produce a decrease in the propensity for conflict. These notions are intriguing, but speculative, since the jogging and control families were not matched on relevant sociodemographic characteristics, and since the level of conflict perceived by the nonjogging spouse was not assessed.

In an interesting use of the FES, Penk, Robinowitz, Kidd, and Nisle (1979) found that heroin users' retrospective perceptions of their family of origin differed significantly from the norms provided by our 285 families describing their current family environments. Specifically, herion users remembered their family environments as stressing achievement and adherence to moral and religious norms, while de-emphasizing family relationships, independence, and intellectual-cultural orientation. The authors suggest that heroin addicts typically come from families that stress high achievement while inhibiting expression, and that the addict may have turned to heroin as a result of his failure to achieve the high goals expected from him. (See Penk *et al.*, 1979 for additional analyses that focus on ethnic differences in heroin users' past and present family environments.)

In related work on this issue, Pringle (1976) used the FES to compare the perceptions of the family of origin of alcoholic patients who had an alcoholic parent with those of alcoholic patients who came from nonalcoholic family backgrounds. Families of origin were generally seen as emphasizing control and as de-emphasizing expressiveness, independence, and intellectual-cultural and active recreational orientation. The patients who came from an alcoholic family background, in contrast to their counterparts who did not, perceived their family of origin as emphasizing high achievement levels, independence, and the expression of feelings, but doing so within a highly conflict-oriented milieu.

FES data on these patients' perceptions of their conjugal families indicated that they believed their current family environments to be substantially different from their memories of their families of origin (but see Penk *et al.*, 1979, for data suggesting that heroin users' conjugal family environments "recreate" their past family milieu). Information about how other family members (e.g., the nonalcoholic spouse) perceive the current family environment would constitute useful information on this point. Although one cannot assume that retrospective perceptions of families are "accurate," they provide fascinating data about the relationships between the perceived conjugal family, the family of origin, and the currently preferred and/or expected future family environment.

The WES has also been used to compare and contrast work settings. Amante and Van Houten (1976) gave the WES to 108 staff members of a community mental health center (CMHC). Staff members in different units in the CMHC perceived their work settings differently. For example, the outpatient units were seen as more involving, cohesive, supportive, autonomous, and physically comfortable than the inpatient units. Workers in nonmanual positions felt more involved, friendly, and supportive toward fellow employees, whereas those in manual positions felt that job clarity and physical comfort were higher. The authors concluded that the CMHC had a stratified social system, and that mental health personnel should evaluate the environment they create for their employees before trying to help the larger community (see Simek, 1975, for a comparison of the work environments of different types of radio stations).

Two related uses of information about perceived climate involve testing theoretical predictions regarding the ways in which social environments should differ from one another (see Hearn & Moos, 1976, for an example), and monitoring the degree to which the implementation of a program of organizational or individual change actually affects the social climate of a setting. Although there are no completed studies as yet of this type of use of the FES or WES, relevant studies in related areas have shown that the treatment environments of hospital-based psychiatric programs are affected by the development of token economy (Curtiss, 1976; Gripp & Magaro, 1971) and group psychotherapy (Leviege, 1970) programs, and that the social environments of correctional programs run under a behavior modification orientation are different from those run under a transactional analysis orientation (Jesness, De Risi, McCormick, & Wedge, 1972).

Evaluating the Impact of Family and Work Settings

As noted above, several investigators have emphasized the importance of family functioning in contributing to a more differentiated understanding of the reasons for postinstitutional success or failure. Community environments, particularly family and work settings, have long been known to affect the outcome of institutional release (e.g., Brown, Birley, & Wing, 1972; Davies & Sinclair, 1977; Maluccio & Marlow, 1972).

Family Environment and Alcoholism Treatment Outcome

The general issue of environmental contingencies is of special importance in studies of alcoholics and in the outcome of treatment for alcoholism. Cahalan (1970) found that environmental support for heavy drinking was related to the degree of an individual's current drinking problem, and concluded that external environmental factors determine whether the individual is encouraged to drink heavily. Specific social setting influences implicated in the development and maintenance of problem-drinking behavior include the general drinking environment and choice of drinking companions, the psychosocial equilibrium between an individual and his environment, the degree to which family models favor alcohol use for problem solving, and occupational and social group influences.

In our recent study, we focused on the relationship between family environment and the outcome of treatment for alcoholism. Four outcome criteria were selected to provide data on the major dimensions of functioning:

1. *Alcohol consumption,* ounces of ethanol from beer, wine, and hard liquor consumed on a typical drinking day.

2. *Subjective rating of drinking problem* (1 = no problem, 5 = quite often a problem).

3. *Physical impairment,* a subscale derived from patients' responses to the question: How often did you experience the following during the past month—with regard to the following symptoms: DTs or shakes, memory

lapses or blackouts, dry heaves or cold sweats, difficulty sleeping, hallucinations or vague fears, severe hangover, nervous or tense, upset stomach,
headaches, dizzy spells?

4. *Psychological well-being,* a subscale for patients' self-descriptions
on the following items: pleased about accomplishing something, relaxed
and comfortable, in control of your life, knowing where you want to go in
life, getting all that you want out of life, and feeling on top of the world.

In general, alcoholic patients who functioned more poorly at follow-up
(that is, consumed relatively more alcohol, rated their drinking problem as
more severe, had a higher degree of physical impairment due to drinking,
and reported poorer psychological functioning) came from families showing
more emphasis on cohesion, expressiveness, and active recreational orientation. Intellectual-cultural orientation and moral-religious emphasis were
also positively related to the functioning of the family member who had
been treated for alcoholism.

A stepwise discriminant function analysis was conducted to relate the
FES subscales to an overall index of treatment outcome. Two groups of
families differing in the treatment outcome of the alcoholic member were
defined. In order to be considered "highly improved," five separate criteria
had to be met: (a) no rehospitalization for alcoholism, (b) either abstaining
or drinking no more than 2 ounces of alcohol per day, (c) self-rating of
drinking problem as either "not at all" or "rarely a problem," (d) essentially no complaints of physical symptoms related to drinking, and (e)
satisfactory psychological functioning. Alcoholic patients who did not meet
these criteria were classified into a "slightly improved" outcome group.
Almost all the 122 alcoholic patients were functioning better at follow-up
than at intake, and, in general, they showed better treatment outcome than
their counterparts who were not living in families (See Bromet & Moos,
1977; Moos *et al.,* 1979).

Results indicated that the combination of cohesion and active recreational orientation provided the best discrimination between the two outcome
groups, correctively classifying 68% of the cases. An exploratory analysis
was conducted to identify family functioning variables that differentiated
between the two groups of misclassified cases. Fourteen highly improved
alcoholic patients were predicted to be only slightly improved, whereas 17
slightly improved patients were predicted to be highly improved. The families of the 17 patients who did more poorly than "expected" were higher
than their counterparts who had "better-than-expected" outcome on cohesion and active recreational orientation, as well as on expressiveness, independence, and intellectual-cultural orientation. These families were also
higher on reported religious attendance, and lower on physical ailments,
total disagreements, and disagreement over alcohol. In fact, their pattern of
results was strongly suggestive of excellent treatment outcome, except that

they experienced more negative life-change events than their better-than-expected treatment outcome counterparts.

In evaluating these findings, it is important to note that the results linking treatment outcome to the family environment were generally similar regardless of which family member's perceptions were used in the analysis. In addition, some of the FES subscales that differentiated between the two alcoholism treatment groups have been related to disturbed versus normal family status (Janes & Hesselbrock, 1976; Scoresby & Christensen, 1976) and to treatment outcome in other areas such as multiple family therapy workshops (Bader, 1976) and behaviorally oriented parent training groups (Rosenthal, 1975).

Work Environment and Alcoholism Treatment Outcome

There are very few studies relating the work environment to the outcome of treatment for alcoholism. Mayer and Meyerson (1970) found an association between improved relations with fellow workers and improved drinking behavior among a group of stably employed alcoholics. Although we found no other direct evidence in the literature on this issue, several studies have related different aspects of the work environment to employees' mental health. From his review of these studies, Kasl (1974) concluded that poorer mental health was associated with factors such as repetitious and uninvolving jobs, low levels of social interaction, poorer relationships with supervisors, lack of autonomy, unclear or conflicting job demands, and undesirable working conditions.

Our sample included 68 working alcoholics living with their families who completed the WES. Fifty-five working alcoholics not living in family settings also completed the WES. Correlations between patients' perceptions of their work environments and outcome criteria were relatively strong and consistent for the nonfamily alcoholics in three of the four performance areas (all but alcohol consumption), whereas they were relatively weak for the alcoholics living in family settings. For example, perceived work involvement, peer cohesion, and supervisor support were each significantly related to three of the four outcome criteria for the nonfamily alcoholic sample, whereas only two of the analogous nine correlations were significant for the family alcoholic sample. In addition, alcoholic patients not in families, who perceived their work environment as emphasizing more task orientation, clarity, innovation, and physical comfort, tended to show better social and psychological functioning. These results generally held for residualized treatment outcome, that is, after sociodemographic and initial alcohol functioning characteristics were controlled (Bromet & Moos, 1977).

One explanation for these results is the "buffer hypothesis." Clum (1975) contended that the marital situation acts as a "buffer to improve the likelihood of a patient's making a good adjustment" (p. 422). Dissatisfaction with a job may be viewed with greater detachment by alcoholics with families to cushion any adverse impact. More negatively perceived work environments may also have less overall import for alcoholics during the "reorganization" phase when a great deal of emotional energy is focused on the family. Unmarried patients have fewer "significant others" to buffer or relieve the tensions produced by an unsatisfactory work situation. It may thus take on greater significance for their overall treatment outcome.

Other Related Research Foci

There are several salient research issues in this area, three of which I mention here briefly. One issue derives from the fact that most people who are exposed to "high-risk" family, work, and other settings do not break down or develop illness. We need to identify the coping processes these individuals use, and their relationship to particular socioenvironmental conditions.

Many treated alcoholic patients resume drinking to excess when they encounter environmental stress, but some patients do not. In our study of the treatment outcome of alcoholic patients we hope to identify differences among groups of patients who react differently (in terms of their drinking behavior) to high- and low-"risk" settings. The most interesting group is that of the environmentally resistant patients who remain abstainers or controlled drinkers during the follow-up period, even though they are under considerable environmental stress (as defined by negative life-change events). The study of "environmental-resistant" or "invulnerable" people may help to identify personal and environmental characteristics associated with the ability to transcend environmental pressure (e.g., see Garmezy, 1974; Zubin & Spring, 1977).

A related approach is to focus on the coping mechanisms people use to handle environmental stress. In the second follow-up of our families, patients and spouses were asked to focus on a major life-change event and to identify the coping techniques they used to handle the event. Cluster analyses of 17 coping items identified five types of coping skills: active behavioral coping (e.g., tried to find out more about the situation), active cognitive coping (e.g., considered several alternatives), avoidance (e.g., got busy with other things), tension reduction (e.g., drank, ate, smoked, or exercised more), and resignation-acceptance (e.g., prepared for the worst).

The frequency of reported use of the techniques of active behavioral and cognitive coping did not differentiate between alcoholics and spouses. However, a higher proportion of the alcoholic patients reported using tension-reduction coping techniques such as taking their frustrations out on others, and smoking and drinking (specifically, 37% of alcoholic patients stated that they smoked more and 35% that they drank more, compared to 22% and 13%, respectively, of their spouses). Although these results are preliminary, they suggest that the systematic study of coping mechanisms may help to further understand individual differences in treatment outcome.

A second area involves delineating the relationship between the family environment and stress- and illness-related variables. For example, we obtained data on the number of positive and negative life-change events experienced by our 122 families during the preceeding 12 months. Families with more negative life-change events placed more emphasis on conflict and control. However, there were no significant relationships between the number of positive life-change events and the family social milieu.

Families in which members had more physical and emotional ailments were higher on conflict and lower on cohesion and organization. The number of medical conditions was not related to the family environment, with the exception that families in which one or more members had a serious medical condition had significantly higher scores on moral-religious emphasis. A reasonable interpretation is that moral-religious orientation is a coping mechanism that families use to help handle serious illnesses. Since the ability of family members to help the patient and each other strongly affects the choice of coping strategies and the ultimate outcome of all types of illness, these and related issues need to be studied in relation to the onset, treatment, and rehabilitation of physical illness (Moos, 1977).

Third, the contemporary family is being asked to assume a formidable array of health functions (Pratt, 1972). The family is used as a therapeutic resource by medical personnel, and families are expected to assume a major role in the care and rehabilitation of disabled, mentally ill, chronically ill, alcoholic, and aged members. We need to focus on some of the unanticipated effects of these expectations. Grad and Sainsbury (1968) found the social costs of psychiatric care to be higher if the patient was treated in a community care than in a hospital-based service. They raised the question of whether the continued presence of the patient in the home ultimately leads to the production of more mental illness in the community. The degree to which unanticipated personal and social costs occur needs to be specified and its relationship to environmental resources and preferred coping mechanisms to be systematically investigated.

Some Promising Practical Applications

Two major sets of suggestions for practical intervention have been developed from the literature in this area; one focuses primarily on the individual, the other on the environment (Cowen, 1977). Since the social milieu has an important mediating influence on the effects of other environmental variables, several investigators have focused on the desirability of changing the social climate, particularly developing cohesion and support (e.g., Hinkle & Loring, 1977). Cohen, Class, and Phillips (1977) have suggested that feelings of helplessness and an inability to control environmental stimuli may be more important than the actual characteristics of the environment itself. My own work has led me to identify several related areas in which a focus on social environments may be useful for evaluating and changing individuals and community settings, and thus, potentially, for enhancing health and well-being (Moos, 1976b).

Formulating Ecologically Relevant Clinical Case Descriptions

Systematic information about patients' environments, such as their work and family settings, can be used in clinical case descriptions and in overall treatment planning. Such information can help health care professionals to better understand a patient's life situation and to plan more rationally his or her treatment (see Renshaw, 1976, for an informative discussion of how a person's family and work settings may interact).

For example, the usual patient focus in treatment may work well when a relatively high level of marital cohesion exists, but it is unlikely to be successful when cohesion is low. In the latter instance, elements of cohesion may have to be developed before symptom- or individual-focused treatment can be successful. The findings that cohesion and support are related to the outcome of treatment for alcoholism and that expressiveness is related to the outcome of treatment for schizophrenia have related implications. These results indicate that it would be useful to assess the family environment of patients before release from hospital to identify those families in which preventive intervention and aftercare services might be most beneficial. Similar considerations apply in the treatment and rehabilitation of major physical illnesses such as severe burns, heart attacks, strokes, and organ transplants.

Robert Fuhr and I (Fuhr & Moos, 1977) used the FES and the WES, as well as the Classroom Environment Scale and a Health and Daily Living Questionnaire in an attempt to construct an ecologically relevent family case description. The family had come to an outpatient clinic primarily because the 15-year-old daughter (Beth) had dropped out of school. The therapist found it difficult to obtain specific information about school from Beth, and the extent to which her problems were academic or social was unclear. The therapist also wanted to know more about Beth's life outside the classroom. How did she actually spend her time? What type of family did she live in? Were her parents contributing to the problem?

A clear picture of the family emerged from the information we obtained in two 2-hour sessions with the family at their home. The FES and WES results indicated that the parents described their relationships at home relatively favorably and that they were highly committed to and satisfied with their jobs. Both worked hard, enjoyed a good deal of responsibility, and felt that their co-workers were friendly and supportive.

In contrast, Beth gave a highly critical assessment of her family on the FES, rating it very low on cohesion, active recreational orientation, and control, and relatively high on conflict. Although the family status quo was satisfactory for her parents in view of their demanding and rewarding work environments, this resulted in a lack of focus and energy on family activities, and Beth's feeling that her parents did not care about her (e.g., they did not even institute strict controls she could rebel against). This and our other data led us to conclude that Beth's school problems probably had their roots in the family social environment (see Panio, 1977, for some brief clinical interpretations of the FES profiles of drug abusers and their families).

Social-ecological assessment techniques should have broad clinical utility in that the information obtained can be used to organize the discussion of issues in treatment, to teach clients to break down problems into small, clearly defined units that can be handled in an organized step-by-step fashion, to gain a heightened awareness of some of the powerful, yet controllable, influences of the physical and social environment, and to take an active part in shaping the nature of their goals and to track their progress in therapy. The semistructured, easily understandable format of the procedures makes it possible to collect a great deal of information very quickly. Also, although it may be preferable in some instances, the clinician need not be present for all phases of the assessment; a paraprofessional can be trained to obtain the information and to answer typical questions.

Facilitating Environmental and Individual Change

Feedback and utilization of findings regarding social and physical environments can facilitate environmental change. The methods we use involve four simple steps: (1) a systematic assessment of the environment, (2) feedback to participating groups with particular stress on real–ideal setting differences, (3) planning and instituting specific changes in the setting, and (4) reassessment. Since there is no specific "end point" to this process, continual change and continual monitoring and reassessment may occur (see Moos, 1979b for a review of relevant studies).

Information about the social environment can be used to identify settings in which preventive intervention might be particularly useful. Studies conducted in quite different social settings (i.e., high school classrooms, student living groups, psychiatric treatment wards, and military basic training companies) have shown that settings seen as low in involvement, autonomy, and/or student influence and high in competition, strictness, and control tend to be characterized by high rates of "dysfunctional" behavior such as complaints of physical symptoms, sick call, dropout and absenteeism rates, and the like (Moos, 1979a). Health psychologists might focus their consultation and preventive intervention attempts on these "high-risk" environments. Since the work environments of health care staff (e.g., intensive care units, terminal cancer wards) are often highly stressful, health psychologists might also consider attempts to evaluate and change these settings.

In a relevant demonstration study on families, Robert Fuhr, Norman Dishotsky, and I (Fuhr, Moos, and Dishotsky, 1978) administered the Real and Ideal Forms of the FES to a couple at the beginning of therapy and again 3 months later. Our purpose was to compare the picture of the family provided by the FES with that developed by the therapist in his assessment sessions, and to explore how feedback of information derived from the FES to the family could facilitate the ongoing therapeutic process.

The FES results generally confirmed the descriptions of the family given by the therapist, although they also raised some additional hypotheses that had not been considered previously. The couple was given information about their FES profile, about their individual perceptions, and about their real–ideal discrepancies. The therapist then focused on salient areas by carrying out an item-by-item analysis and discussion of pivotal dimensions. For example, in one session, the couple compared their Real and Ideal scores on cohesion, and discussed each question on this dimension, in an attempt to clarify and reconcile their perceptions and values.

Some of the advantages of this procedure included (a) structuring and focusing each therapy session, thereby ensuring that the discussion did not wander aimlessly and unproductively; (b) enhancing the probability of a more balanced discussion, since each person's views were explicitly represented by the FES data and thus the more forceful partner would not easily dominate the formulation of goals or speak for the other person to gloss over real differences; and (c) identifying similarities of perceptions and ideals leading to a feeling that the couple had many things in common and to an additional incentive to work productively on shared areas of dissatisfaction. The progress shown in therapy was confirmed by the results of the FES given at follow-up.

The results of this demonstration project suggest that information about family functioning can be used systematically and productively in ongoing therapy and counseling. This is important since there is increasing emphasis on the family as a focus of intervention (Benjamin, 1977; Caplan, 1976). For example, Klein, Alexander, and Parsons (1977) evaluated the effects of a family systems intervention on recidivism and sibling delinquency, and concluded that the most efficacious focus was on changing family interaction patterns in the direction of increased clarity, precision, and reciprocity of communication.

Enhancing Environmental Competence

From a broader perspective, we need to develop health care professionals who understand environments, who understand the kinds of reactions people have in them, and who understand the environmental dimensions and mediating mechanisms involved. When this information is combined with additional information, much of which still must be developed, about how people generally cope with and adapt to different types of environments, then a new role of environmental educator can be implemented. We have some examples of the use of information about social environments as an aid in teaching people who may become environmental educators (e.g., the Ward Atmosphere Scale has been used to teach residents and interns about the functioning of psychiatric wards, and the Family Environment Scale has been used as a teaching aid in a course on marriage and family living); however, the general utility of this area remains largely unexplored.

In this connection, some of the foregoing ideas may be applicable to the development of environmental consultation programs. An environmental consultant could be responsible for regularly assessing a work setting and communicating the results of the assessments to managers and employees in an understandable and usable form. The consultant could perform several functions: evaluating the environment, discussing and interpreting the environmental evaluations, identifying areas for change, and advocating change.

For example, Work Environment Scale data obtained in health care facilities could provide the basis for staff discussions in which it would be possible to focus on a comparison between administrators' and staff perceptions, to compare a facility with itself over time, or to compare it with other similar facilities. In addition, administrators' and staff's ideal environments could be assessed, providing information about the discrepancies between the real and ideal environment and between staff and administrative objectives. This information could be used to develop more accurate perceptions of staff problems, and as an impetus for changes in individual behaviors or for group level changes in policies and procedures (see Kish, 1971, for a discussion of how this type of assessment and feedback could become a regular service provided by a hospital psychology department).

A social-ecological perspective can sensitize us about what to look for in analyzing social settings. For example, the three types of social climate dimensions (Relationship dimensions, Personal Growth or Development dimensions, and System Maintenance and System Change dimensions) provide a useful way of understanding the confusing complexity of social settings. Understanding these dimensions may help individuals select a wide range of environments in which to participate in their everyday lives. In addition, those responsible for selecting or changing the environments of others (such as children or the elderly) can do so with a better awareness of the personal traits alternative environments may foster. Cassel (1976) has suggested that preventive health services might identify families and groups at high risk by virtue of lack of fit with their environment, and determine the nature and form of social supports that should be strengthened if such people are to be protected from disease outcome. I believe that the systematic evaluation of social environments can be useful in furthering these aims, and, thus, in promoting health and well-being.

References

Amante, D., & Van Houten, V. *Social climate measurement in a community mental health center.* Muskegon, Mich.: West Shore Mental Health Clinic, Muskegon County Community Mental Health Services, 1976.

Bader, E. *Redecisions in family therapy: A study of change in an intensive family therapy workshop.* Doctoral dissertation, California School of Professional Psychology, 1976.

Benjamin, L. Structural analysis of a family in therapy. *Journal of Consulting and Clinical Psychology,* 1977, *45,* 391–406.

Bromet, E., & Moos, R. H. Environmental resources and the posttreatment functioning of alcoholic patients. *Journal of Health and Social Behavior,* 1977, *18,* 326–338.

Bronfenbrenner, U. Toward an experimental ecology of human development. *American Psychologist,* 1977, *32,* 513–531.

Brown, G., Birley, J., & Wing, J. Influence of family life in the course of schizophrenic disorders: A replication. *British Journal of Psychiatry,* 1972, *121,* 241–258.

Cahalan, D. *Problem drinkers: A national survey.* San Francisco: Jossey-Bass, 1970.

Caplan, G. The family as a support system. In G. Caplan & M. Killilea (Eds.), *Support systems and mutual help.* New York: Grune and Stratton, 1976.

Cassel, J. The contribution of the social environment to host resistance. *American Journal of Epidemiology,* 1976, *104,* 197–123.

Clum, G. Intra-psychic variables and the patient's environment as factors in prognosis. *Psychological Bulletin,* 1975, *82,* 413–431.

Cohen, S., Glass, D., & Phillips, S. Environment and health. In H. Freeman, S. Levine, & L. Reeder (Eds.), *Handbook of medical sociology.* Englewood Cliffs, N.J.: Prentice-Hall, 1977.

Cowen, E. Baby-steps toward primary prevention. *American Journal of Community Psychology,* 1977, *5,* 1–22.

Curtiss, S. The compatibility of humanistic and behavioral approaches in a state mental hospital. In A. Wandersman, P. Poppen, & D. Ricks (Eds.), *Humanism and behaviorism: Dialogue and growth.* New York: Pergamon, 1976.

Davies, M., & Sinclair, I. Families, hostels and delinquents: An attempt to assess cause and effect. *British Journal of Criminology,* 1971, *11,* 213–229.

Deykin, E. Life functioning in families of delinquent boys: An assessment model. *Social Service Review,* 1972, *46,* 90–102.

Fuhr, R., & Moos, R. H. *The clinical use of ecological concepts: A family case description.*

Paper presented at the American Psychological Association Convention, San Francisco, August 1977.

Fuhr, R., Moos, R. H., & Dishotsky, N. *The clinical utility of the Family Environment Scale in ongoing family therapy.* Stanford: Social Ecology Laboratory, Department of Psychiatry, Stanford University, 1978.

Garmezy, N. Children at risk: The search for the antecedents of schizophrenia. *Schizophrenia Bulletin, 1974, 8, 13–90.*

Grad, J., & Sainsbury, P. The effects that patients have on their families in a community care and a control psychiatric service—A two-year follow-up. *British Journal of Psychiatry, 1968, 114, 265–278.*

Gripp, R., & Magaro, P. A token economy program evaluation with untreated control ward comparisons. *Behaviour Research and Therapy, 1971, 9, 137–139.*

Hearn, J., & Moos, R. H. Social climate and major choice: A test of Holland's theory in university student living groups. *Journal of Vocational Behavior, 1976, 8, 293–305.*

Hinkle, L., & Loring W. *The effects of the man-made environment on health and behavior.* Washington, D.C.: U.S. Government Printing Office, 1977.

Holahan, C. *Environment and behavior: A synthesis.* New York: Plenum, 1978.

Janes, C., & Hesselbrock, V. *Perceived family environment and school adjustment of children of schizophrenics.* Paper presented at the American Psychological Association Convention, Washington, D.C., September 1976.

Jesness, C., De Risi, W., McCormick, P., & Wedge, R. *The Youth Center Research Project.* Sacramento: American Justice Institute and California Youth Authority, 1972.

Jones, S., & Jones, D. *Serious jogging and family life: Marathon and submarathon running.* Paper presented at the American Sociological Association Convention, Chicago, 1977.

Kasl, S. Work and mental health. In J. O'Toole (Ed.), *Work and the quality of life.* Cambridge, Mass.: M.I.T. Press, 1974.

Kish, G. Evaluation of ward atmosphere. *Hospital and Community Psychiatry, 1971, 22, 159–161.*

Klein, N., Alexander, J., & Parsons, B. Impact of family-systems intervention on recidivism and sibling delinquency: A model of primary prevention and program evaluation. *Journal of Consulting and Clinical Psychology, 1977, 45, 469–474.*

Lawton, P., & Nahemow, L. Ecology and the aging process. In C. Eisdorfer & P. Lawton (Eds.), *The psychology of adult development and aging.* Washington, D.C.: American Psychological Association, 1973.

Leviege, V. Group relations: Group therapy with mentally ill offenders. *Corrective Psychiatry and Journal of Social Therapy, 1970, 16, 15–25.*

Litman, T. The family as a basic unit in health and medical care: A social-behavioral overview. *Social Science and Medicine, 1974, 8, 495–519.*

Maluccio, A., & Marlow, W. Residential treatment of emotionally disturbed children: A review of the literature. *Social Service Review, 1972, 46, 230–250.*

Manino, F., & Shore, M. Family structure, after-care, and posthospital adjustment. *American Journal of Orthopsychiatry, 1974, 44, 76–85.*

Mayer, J., & Myerson, D. Characteristics of out-patient alcoholics in relation to change in drinking, work and marital status during treatment. *Quarterly Journal of Studies on Alcohol, 1970, 31, 889–897.*

Mitchell, R. Some social implications of high density housing. *American Sociological Review, 1971, 36, 18–29.*

Moos, R. H. *Family Environment Scale preliminary manual.* Palo Alto: Consulting Psychologists Press, 1974. (a)

Moos, R. H. *The Social Climate Scales: An overview.* Palo Alto: Consulting Psychologists Press, 1974. (b).

Moos, R. H. *Evaluating treatment environments: A social ecological approach.* New York: Wiley-Interscience, 1974. (c)

Moos, R. H. *Evaluating correctional and community settings.* New York: Wiley-Interscience, 1975.

Moos, R. H. *The human context: Environmental determinants of behavior.* New York: Wiley-Interscience, 1976. (a)

Moos, R. H. Evaluating and changing community settings. *American Journal of Community Psychology,* 1976, *4,* 313–326. (b)

Moos, R. H. *Coping with physical illness.* New York: Plenum, 1977.

Moos, R. H. A typology of junior high and high school classrooms. *American Educational Research Journal,* 1978, *15,* 53–66.

Moos, R. H. A social-ecological perspective on health. In G. Stone, F. Cohen, & N. Adler (Eds.), *Health psychology.* San Francisco: Jossey-Bass, 1979. (a)

Moos, R. H. Social climate feedback and the development of environmental competence. In R. Munoz, L. Snowden, & J. Kelly (Eds.), *Research in social contexts: Bringing about change.* San Francisco: Jossey-Bass, 1979. (b)

Moos, R. H., & Insel, P. *Work Environment Scale preliminary manual.* Palo Alto: Consulting Psychologists Press, 1974.

Moos, R. H., & Moos, B. A typology of family social environments. *Family Process,* 1976, *15,* 357–372.

Moos, R. H., Bromet, E., Tsu, V., & Moos, B. Family characteristics and the outcome of treatment for alcoholism. *Journal of Studies on Alcohol,* 1979, *40,* 78–88.

Myers, J., & Bean, L. *A decade later: A follow-up of social class and mental illness.* New York: Wiley, 1968.

Panio, A. *Assessing the families of drug abusers utilizing the Family Environment Scale.* Paper presented at the National Drug Abuse Conference, San Francisco, 1977.

Pattison, E., & Anderson, R. Family health care, with special emphasis on the U.S.A. *International Public Health Review,* 1978, *7* (1–2), 83–134.

Penk, W., Robinowitz, R., Kidd, R., & Nisle, A. Perceived family environments among ethnic groups of compulsive heroin users. *Addictive Behaviors,* in press.

Pless, I., & Satterwhite, B. A measure of family functioning and its application. *Social Science and Medicine,* 1973, *7,* 613–621.

Pratt, L. Conjugal organization and health. *Journal of Marriage and the Family,* 1972, *34,* 85–94.

Pringle, W. *The alcoholic family environment: The influence of the alcoholic and non-alcoholic family of origin on present coping styles.* Doctoral dissertation, California School of Professional Psychology, 1976.

Renshaw, J. An exploration of the dynamics of the overlapping worlds of work and family. *Family Process,* 1976, *15,* 143–165.

Rosenthal, M. *Effects of parent training groups in behavior change in target children: Durability, generalization and patterns of family interaction.* Doctoral dissertation, University of Cincinnati, 1975.

Scoresby, A., & Christensen, B. Differences in interaction and environmental conditions of clinic and non-clinic families: Implications for counselors. *Journal of Marriage and Family Counselling,* 1976, *2,* 63–71.

Simek, M. *An analysis of psychosocial work environments in radio broadcast stations of a single market.* Master's thesis, University of Oregon, Eugene, 1975.

Walberg, H. Psychology of learning environments: Behavioral, structural or perceptual? In L. Shulman (Ed.), *Review of research in education* (Vol. 5). Itasca, Ill.: Peacock, 1976.

Zubin, J., & Spring, B. Vulnerability—A new view of schizophrenia. *Journal of Abnormal Psychology,* 1977, *86,* 103–126.

17

Evaluating Human Service Programs: Psychosocial Methods

William A. O'Connor, Deidre S. Klassen, and Karen S. O'Connor

Program Evaluation: Trends in the Seventies

Over the last decade, program evaluation has assumed greatly increased importance, as reflected in the development of highly sophisticated systems approaches and the development of a wide variety of new instruments and procedures (Attkinson, 1976; Streuning & Guttentag, 1975; Weiss, 1972). Levels of evaluative activity range from the relatively narrow internal focus reflected in system resource management to the broad community impact focus; informational capability ranges from natural systems data to highly specialized data collection capability, and the functional role of the evaluator extends from simple statistical functions to a leadership role involving coordinative decision making (McIntyre, 1977).

Specific techniques range across all these dimensions, but the basic issues that have been identified in mental health research are also reflected in the broader program evaluation area (Beigel, 1976; Fox & Rappaport, 1972): the complexity of the natural situation; assessment of both clients

William A. O'Connor • Department of Psychiatry, University of Missouri; Kansas City; Missouri 64110. Deidre S. Klassen • The Greater Kansas City Mental Health Foundation, Kansas City, Missouri 64108. Karen S. O'Connor, • Rainbow Health Center, Kansas City, Kansas 66103.

and situations across the pretreatment, treatment, and follow-up phases; the relative contributions of interactive variables; and finally, designs where clients with multiple problems are assigned to complex combinations of treatment modalities and continuity of care systems.

Techniques for the evaluation of large sample data have been developed; mental health assessment and broader social functioning may be seen, for example, in Missouri's use of the Community Adjustment Profile Scale (Evenson, 1976), the California Five County Cost Effectiveness Study utilizing the PARS III, the VA cooperative study conducted by Ellsworth (1965), the North Carolina Evaluative Research Section follow-up studies (Stephens, 1976), and the application of the Denver Community Mental Health Questionnaire developed by Ciarlo and Reihman (1974).

Health service delivery systems in general are experiencing growing pressures for accountability to consumers and the community at large. Requirements for program evaluation make necessary the acquisition of acceptable, utilizable systems with appropriate records/documentation components to meet such requirements. These requirements include defining and measuring client outcomes, fulfilling the need of clinical staff and administrators for feedback that can be used effectively to modify therapeutic intervention, and documenting the need for proposed changes in the health care delivery system.

Health Service Standards as a Basis of Recent Trends

Admirable professional standards exist in the health field. At one extreme, health professionals are committed to the delivery of comprehensive services that benefit and contribute to the health of the community as a whole in an economical fashion; at the other extreme, clinicians are committed to the uniqueness of the individual and the integrity of each specific professional–client interaction (Holden, 1972). These commitments generate hard choices in the evaluation arena (Huber & Ullman, 1973). At the most general level, systems resource management and health service utilization data provide critical information with which the total delivery system can maintain its commitment to the community as a whole (Chapman, 1976; Windle & Volkman, 1973). At the other extreme, the outcome of interventions that extend into the consumer's participation in the community provide data that are of central concern to consumer and professional; the treatment contract implies outcome that is relevant to the individual's stated problems and that individual's capacity to function in the normal role (Erickson, 1975; Lick, 1973).

The difficulties in designing a fully comprehensive system are seen clearly in the stated goals of existing approaches (Weiss, 1973). Management information systems are designed to characterize the population at risk, measure patient movement through the system, make effective census control possible for a variety of agencies, and facilitate resource allocation in and among agencies. Recent developments in the field have attempted to coordinate such data with the evaluation of program effectiveness, development of new programs, implementation of basic research, and an ability of the system to identify and respond to exceptions (Schainblatt, 1977). But, as Lick (1973) has indicated, consumers are interested in specific changes of a highly subjective nature. From this perspective, the only defensible set of outcome measures are those that assess the patient's functioning in the community at follow-up: such measures as personal satisfaction, symptoms, and total health functioning.

To some degree, most management systems and specific outcome instruments attempt to define both individual client characteristics and the complex interaction between treatment and community situations in which treatment is embedded (Fiske, 1974; Luborsky, 1974; Weissman, 1975). Some instruments focus primarily on individual psychosocial symptomatology, such as the SCL–90 (Derogatis, 1974), Global Assessment Scale (E.ndicott, 1976), or Menninger Health–Sickness Rating Scale (Luborsky, 1974). Many instruments attempt to assess social role behavior in addition to personal distress or symptomatology, for example, the KAS (Katz & Lyerly, 1963), PARS (Ellsworth, 1975), Psychiatric Status Schedule (Spitzer, 1970), and Social Adjustment Scale (Weissman & Paykel, 1974).

Some recent attempts have extended well beyond the addition of social and personal subscales. For example, Goal Attainment Scaling has been designed to be compatible with at least two major points of view (Kiresuk, 1973; Cline, 1973). The approach is compatible with management-by-objective systems but also assesses a wide variety of consumer and professional goals. The goals may include relatively subjective or dynamic aspects of a particular therapeutic interaction, but may also include posthospital social functioning as reflected by objective outcome measures. In terms of its range of applicability, Goal Attainment Scaling attempts the difficult range of extension from the idiographic to the nomathetic.

Beginning at the other end of the client-versus-the-situation dilemma, such comprehensive efforts as Streuning and Guttentag's (1975) review of evaluation research allow the integration of a variety of existing methods. Contributions by Lehmann, Streuning, and Cassel suggest a broad ecological model in which service delivery can be considered from a psychosocial process point of view.

While program evaluation research has wrestled with the difficult range of individual clients through broad system measures, yet another dilemma has been confronted. While both health professional and client come into contact within the treatment system, the perspective both of the community at large and of the client begin and end outside the treatment situation itself (Bloom, 1968). To evaluate effectively both clients and situations, informational systems would theoretically require data regarding the client's behavior before initial contact and clearly require extended information regarding the congruence of the client's needs and satisfactions with the demands of the community (Blum, 1974).

The perspective of health facilities is often focused on the symptoms of the client between admission and discharge. Further, the communication and evaluation systems of the facility can limit the view of system managers with respect to the actual experiences of individual patients, and may also limit clinical staff to a view of therapeutic activities that seem embedded only within the service delivery structure.

Focus on the pretreatment person and setting interaction can be seen most clearly in needs assessment techniques (Rosen, 1974). But needs assessment techniques are specific in their focus on the potential client population. In many cases, the specific variables involved in assessment of health service needs require a specialized taxonomy that is tailored to the characteristics of the community as a whole and is difficult to coordinate with data collected in treatment evaluation terms (Gabbay & Windle, 1975).

For the posttreatment community and client interaction, there are neither precise measures of service impact nor accepted definitions of the scope of service activities (McIntyre, 1977). Attempts to define expectations from both recipients and funders of services have presented major difficulties (Diamond, 1973). Again, the dilemma has at times been temporarily resolved by focusing specifically on the characteristics of the posttreatment community involvement. POMR systems, for example, begin with the definition of admitting problems and can be adapted to "track" resolution through the follow-up or the continuity of care phases (Ciarlo & Reihman, 1974). But again, community involvement from the point of view of the client makes the assessment of treatment impact difficult for the lack of clear knowledge of pretreatment situations and client participation patterns. On an individual client basis, a Goal Attainment Scaling technique can begin at the point of the client's pretreatment functioning. But it does not create a uniform taxonomy of both client and situation that is readily interpreted on an interactive level; that is, the problem of assessing the relative contribution of various pretreatment and posttreatment situational factors remains difficult.

The problem of client and situation taxonomies has been most obvious in the context of recent developments in clinical mental health research: the application of such approaches to program evaluation has been lacking. The primary reason for this difficulty is that careful identification of the source of various outcome events has required careful controls (K. S. O'Connor,

1977). If both pretreatment and treatment, client and situational variables contribute to outcome, then a consistent taxonomy of these variables is required. Further, until the most recent data reduction techniques, statistical programs required a particular sample size and an essentially matched or randomly assigned comparison groups design. To apply such an approach to the natural situation, measures must first be reduced (Fleiss & Zubin, 1969). Specific clusters are then identified. Essentially, to adapt such techniques to a program evaluation approach, the evaluation system itself must describe and classify both clients and situations, since the treatment delivery system itself is not subject to total manipulation and random assignment (Wilkinson & O'Connor, 1977a; W. A. O'Connor, 1977).

Thus, the current focus in health system evaluation depends on application of technical advances in once basic clinical research. The assessment of complex person–setting interactions in social psychological research, for example, appears to be impacting psychosocial program assessment and may well be predictive of trends and developments over the next several years.

Current and Future Trends: Psychosocial Assessment

One of the longest debates in social sciences has focused on whether personal or situational variables serve as primary determinants of behavior. Trait theory, emphasizing behavior and personality consistency, has dominated psychological research for much of the early part of this century (Allport, 1966). In the last decade, however, proponents of a situational specificity theory of behavior have amassed a substantial body of supporting data (Mischel, 1968).

But the traditional person versus situation debate appears to be giving way to an integrative theoretical framework emphasizing the interactive process between persons and situations (Ekehammer, 1974). In this context, behavior is viewed as a continuous interaction between person and situation (Endler, 1976). Moos and Houts (1968) have suggested that ultimately the contribution of social atmospheres as opposed to the contribution of individual behavior is an open question; no doubt this will vary depending on the environment, environmental dimensions, subclasses of organizations, and subcategories of individual studies. However, the potential importance of interaction between person and setting has been demonstrated clearly.

The development of this perspective in the area of personality research has been closely paralleled by interactive studies in the psychotherapy literature. Psychotherapy has often been evaluated in reference to a particular strategy's effectiveness across a wide range of populations or in relation to a particular therapeutic problem (Luborsky, Chandler, Auerbach, Cohen, & Bachrach, 1971). However, researchers are currently suggesting that the effectiveness of various psychotherapeutic techniques may be influenced by the particular population of individuals exposed to them (Strupp & Bergin, 1969). Support has been found for the effects of broad treatment system delivery variables and community conditions, such as system utilization style, initial contact variables, treatment assignment agreements, and a host of demographic, social, and economic factors (Hornstra, Lubin, Lewis, & Willis, 1972; Lubin, Hornstra, Lewis, & Bechtel, 1973; Udell & Hornstra, 1975).

What is most essential and most important to the conflicting theoretical positions, however, is the effect that these assumptions have on basic methodology and design. It is becoming evident that the methodology employed in clinical research may focus on a particular aspect of the interactive system so that the design itself has a major impact on the results (Wilkinson & O'Connor, 1977b). At a methodological level, many of the studies to date may be categorized in terms of the specific focus of the study. The design itself may measure variables and compare groups at four levels: individual subject characteristics, interpersonal behavioral events, situational events, or systems interactions between populations and environments (O'Connor & Ramchandani, 1970). A number of examples may be given for each basic frame of reference.

Psychopathology research, for example, has often attempted to describe the characteristics of particular personality types or diagnostic groups by comparison with the normal population (Handel, 1965). Although the contribution of personality types or well-defined psychopathological variables may be quite significant, the relative contribution of situations is impossible to determine where such situational variables are held constant, randomized, or simply ignored (Golding, 1975). Psychotherapy research, by contrast, has faced the necessity of dealing with the psychotherapeutic situation or interaction itself. Often, however, such research has proceeded in one of two directions. Either the treatment variable has been assessed across a wide range of individuals in an attempt to isolate the situational component (Luborsky *et al.*, 1971) or the treatment situation has been approached on an essentially interpersonal basis—the interaction of specific therapist-client diads (K.S. O'Connor, 1977). Again, the contribution of the therapist variables, treatment modalities, and specific therapist-client interactions should not be dismissed; however, the isolation of these variables makes their relative contribution in the actual clinical setting difficult to assess (Bowers, 1973; Searle, 1971).

Most recently, an attempt has been made to approach the design and analysis of studies in a manner that made the relative contribution of person, setting, and interaction open to interpretation. For example, Hodges

(1968) found an interactive relationship between manifest anxiety and situational conditions of ego threat. Person–situation interactions have also been found in relation to college course outcome (Domino, 1971), anxiety (Ekehammer, Magnusson, & Ricklander, 1974), and honesty (Bishop & Witt, 1970). In terms of therapeutic interventions, Anchor, Vojtisek, and Patterson (1973) reported that a self-disclosure technique was more successful with high trait-anxious patients. Sarason (1968) found that high trait-anxious patients tended to view evaluative comments by a therapist as more threatening, when compared to less anxious clients. Similar interactive relationships have been reported between speech anxiety and desensitization (Meichenbaum, Gilmore, & Fedoravicius, 1971), authoritarianism and therapy structure (Canter, 1971), as well as smoking behavior in relation to several therapy techniques (Best, 1975). Most recently, Mariotto and Paul (1975), in a study of the behaviors of severely disabled psychiatric patients across two dimensions of situations in two treatment environments, found that behavioral consistency was a complex function of type of behavior, psychological demand in the situation, and overall situational characteristics.

The major difficulty encountered in such applications to psychotherapy, however, lies in developing an effective descriptive system or taxonomy of clinical situations. Several systems have been attempted (e.g., Ellsworth, 1965; Findikyan & Sells, 1966; Pace & Stern, 1958; Stern, 1963, 1965). But interactional approaches have largely required either assignment to a predefined condition or assessment of general atmosphere on a scale limited to specific item ratings. The major thrust in describing complex natural environments has come from environmental psychology (Wohlwill, 1970). Ecological psychologists, in particular, have extensively explored situational variables that impact individual behavior.

Essentially, ecological studies have viewed behavior as being greatly regulated by the existing milieu (Barker, 1968). Support for this position exists not only in ecological research but also in studies of institutional or organizational variables as they influence a variety of behaviors (Barker, 1963a, b; Engel & Moos, 1967; Gump, Schoggen, & Redl, 1957; Miller, 1965; Sells, 1963; Willems, 1964; Zinner, 1963).

The methodology and general orientation utilized by ecological psychologists and by researchers of social atmosphere heavily emphasize molar unit characteristics and structure. In addition to the relevance of individual characteristics pointed out by Moos (1967), such a systems approach provides additional emphasis on the importance of interaction and participation in the total environment. The comprehensive character of such assessment approaches has particular significance. Handel (1965) has pointed out that limited results may arise from a study of part, but not all, of the relationships in an interpersonal system.

Psychosocial Assessment: Initial Applications to Program Evaluation

The initial application of psychosocial methods in a program evaluation model has been made only recently. Klassen (1977) has described the evaluation of 16 drug treatment programs that constituted the treatment delivery system of a large metropolitan area. In many cases, the characteristics of pretreatment or posttreatment community environments played a more significant role in outcome than did the treatment situation itself. Further, in a number of instances the type of outcome was unrelated to both the identified problem of the client and the stated goal of treatment (e.g., minimal effects on drug use patterns with significant effects on such areas as employment, social interaction, or housing and transportation patterns). In some cases it appeared that interaction of client type and treatment approach was not the major determinant of outcome; for certain types of treatment modalities a broad range of effects was noted across many client types, whereas for a few distinctive client types consistent outcome was obtained with a variety of modalities. The approach provided data that extended beyond the limits of the institution to present the patient in the context of life-style and community interaction before and after the formal treatment career. Furthermore, both patient-contact staff and administration were provided a comprehensive view of clients and their movement through the treatment delivery system. The basic design used by Klassen has been described as applicable to a wide range of health delivery systems (K.S. O'Connor, 1977).

Basic Design in Psychosocial Health Assessment

Psychosocial research is based on the assumption that there are relationships between populations and environments. Methodology is therefore appropriate to the extent that it identifies sources of variance most relevant to the investigator's hypothesis. Figure 1 illustrates the design alternatives that confront the health evaluator.

If an investigator samples from a restricted population (that is, a population in which the distribution of the dependent measure is too narrow relative to its distribution in other populations), then variance will inevitably be derived from variations in the environments that the restricted sample occupies. The design is essentially a single-population/multiple-environment design. Barker and Gump's (1964) study of large and small schools, for example, involved a population of adolescent high school students. The differences identified were between the large and small school

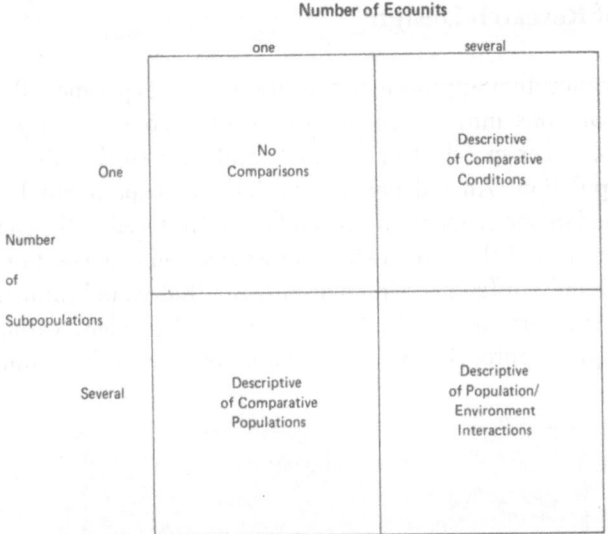

Figure 1. Ecosystems design: comparisons.

environments. This type of design, in which the population is regarded as homogeneous, is typical of the research of ecological psychologists: Barker indicated that motivation stems from the environment, not the individual; his entire theoretical formulation rests on the assumption that variance in behavior is caused by environmental variables.

On the other hand, research design may involve several populations in a single environment or environments that are assumed to be equivalent. Social competence theorists such as Smith (1966) and White (1960) have observed and measured variations in individual performance under uniform or random experimental conditions. Their classic study of Peace Corps training was clearly designed to identify individual characteristics that would contribute to success in the varied environments to which Peace Corps volunteers might be assigned.

The clinician in a health setting faces a similar situation in preparing his client to handle living in the community, with all its demands and varied experiences. Clinical research has therefore focused on the characteristics of persons. But health-oriented services have been directly slighted in the process. Clinical methodology tends to ignore the environment and the individual's interaction with the environment. The prevention specialist may wish to intervene in the environment of the community itself to influence the epidemiology of illness; he may wish to identify environmental conditions that interact with an at-risk population to produce health problems.

Effects of Research Design

The conceptual approach classically used in experimental research divides populations into experimental or control comparison groups; these groups are either matched or selected randomly so that they represent a single population. An independent variable or experimental condition is then applied to one or more groups and not introduced in the control group; the environment of the experiment is otherwise held constant or equivalent, so that the only differences in environments that would influence the outcome measure are those introduced by the independent variable. Such a design is quite appropriate for the isolation of relationships among specific

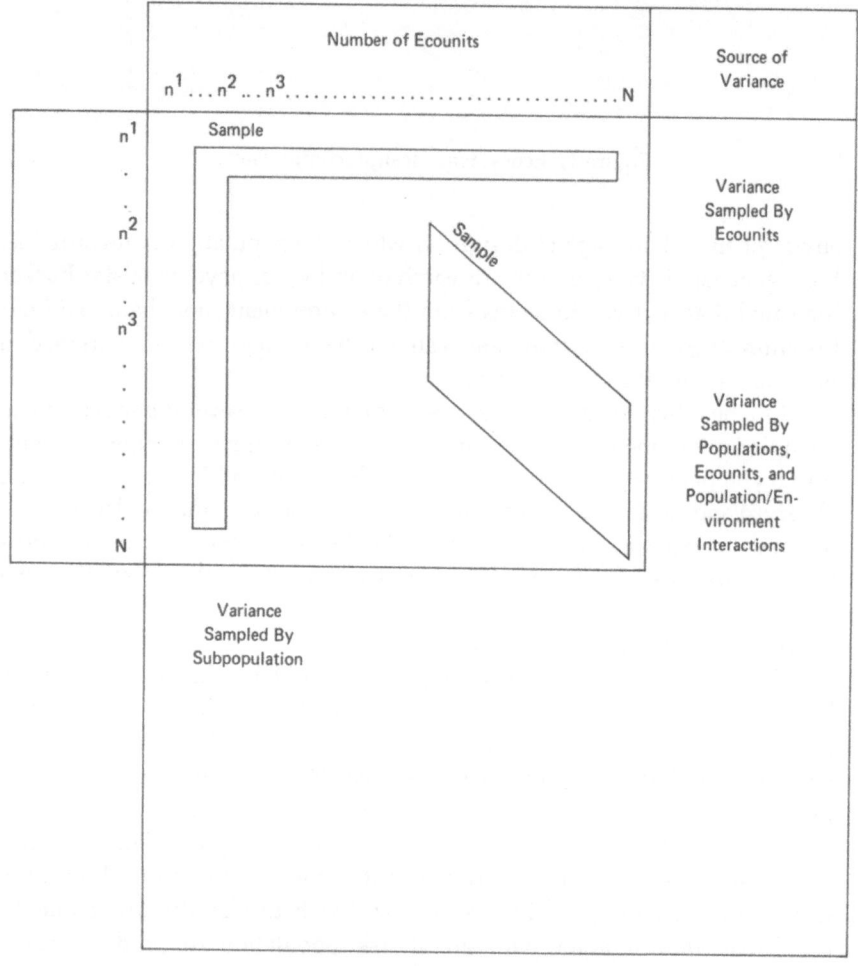

Figure 2. Ecosystems design: sampling.

variables. However, to determine the magnitude of effect of such variables relative to the total natural situation in which individuals function requires comparison of a number of variables under a number of conditions. With only one environment and several population differences, variance is inevitably population-derived.

By contrast, a researcher may choose to focus on a specific ecounit defined by environmental properties and may study population differences within that unit. In this case, the interaction of populations or individuals in the specific ecounit will be unclear; no comparison environment exists. The investigator may draw inferences with regard to the population but does not know the interactive mechanisms involved. The investigator may also choose to define the ecounits involved in the total ecosystem of a particular population. If the population is not subdivided with regard to some characteristics, variance will be noted from environmental sources. Again, inferences must be limited to those environmental variables that were observed.

If a research design involves multiple populations and multiple environments, outcome possibilities are more varied. For example, Moos (1967) studied several state hospital wards with measurable differences in ward social atmosphere; Moos's subjects were divided into distinctly different groups based on psychopathology and demographic differences. The results indicated that a substantial proportion of the variance in outcome was accounted for by the *interaction* of persons and settings. Similarly, Wicker (1973) studied subpopulations of high school students in schools of varying size. With multiple population and environmental categories, Wicker found an interaction between subject variables and setting variables. The design itself allowed consideration of all sources of variance: person, setting, and interaction (see Figure 2).

Data Analysis

Data analysis in psychosocial ecosystems research presents the same problems as those encountered with respect to measurement and design. That is, the analysis of data must reflect the investigator's intent, focus, and hypotheses with regard to interaction of populations and environments.

The most frequently used statistical technique in behavioral research is the analysis of variance. In ecosystems designs, ANOVA can identify the relative contributions of different independent variables, an often-neglected feature of the technique. When ANOVA is utilized, a significant probability level can be misleading where sources of variance are not specified. A variable that reliably produces a measurable difference of two units, but accounts for only 5% of all the differences obtained among persons on the measure, may be difficult to interpret. In such cases, ANOVA only tests the probability that a relationship exists rather than specifying several sources of variance. The advantage of ANOVA in ecosystems research is its capacity to describe several population characteristics under several conditions, as in Endler (1973), Endler and Hunt (1966, 1968, 1969), Endler, Hunt, and Rosenstein (1962), Medley and Mitzel (1963), and Medley, Mitzel, and Doi (1956). Analysis of variance is performed and the obtained mean squares are solved for all obtainable variance estimate components as omega-squared ratios. The size of these variance components for persons and situations is compared.

Golding (1975) has stated that omega-squared ratios are inappropriate and that the coefficient of generalizability (Cronbach, Gleser, Naja, & Rajaratnam, 1972) is the appropriate measure when the person-situation components are of central concern. He argues that omega-squared ratios almost never equal coefficients of generalizability, that the inferential value of omega-squared ratios in person–situation formulations cannot be interpreted unambiguously with reference to size alone. These represent only some of the techniques for estimating the components of variance. Searle (1971) has written an extensive review of variance components. He describes the models underlying variance component estimates for fixed-effects models, random-effects models, mixed models, and fixed or random. A major section is devoted to the analysis of variance method for use with balanced data. For unbalanced data, nine methods of variance component estimates are given: general quadratic forms, Henderson's method 1, Henderson's method 2, the fitting constants method, analysis of means method, symmetric sums method, infinitely many quadratics, maximum likelihood method, and best quadratic unbiased estimation.

Searle (1971) also argues for the importance of designing experiments to estimate variance components. An extensive review of experimental design by Helzberg and Cox (1969) led them to conclude that relatively little work had been done on designing experiments for the purpose of estimating variance components. Optimal designs have been presented by Anderson (1960), Bainbridge (1963), and Anderson and Crump (1967).

More recently developed multiple analysis of variance techniques (MANOVA) can also be utilized to specify variance from dependent measures. This capacity to deal with multiple dependent measures may be important in certain designs. It is possible that no univariate F would yield significance on several measures, but MANOVA would indicate significance on the *set* of measures as a whole.

In the area of applied research there is an obvious need for techniques that identify subgroups in the natural environment, because such research cannot predefine control groups and conditions. Zubin (1938) first proposed a technique for organizing a heterogeneous collection of data into homogeneous "clusters" of individuals. Numerous extensions and improvements have been developed since that time, such as Tryon (1939), Rao (1966), McQuitty (1954), Zubin (1955), Sawrey, Keller, and Conger (1960), Sokal and Sneath (1963), and Edwards and Cavalli-Sforza (1965).

Clustering techniques have also been used to test hypotheses, as in Kendall (1968), who applied clustering to the problem of the nature of depression as a unimodel or bimodel phenomenon. Cluster analysis has been applied widely, particularly in the field of psychopathology (Gerard & Mattsson, 1964; Guertin, 1952; Katz & Cole, 1962; Lorr, 1966; Monro, 1955). However, limitations have been described in detail by Zubin and Fleiss (1965), Bailey (1967), and Fleiss and Zubin (1969); Fleiss and Zubin (1969) quite rightly state that a major problem in clustering is the lack of means of testing a goodness of fit and that clustering techniques will mechanically produce subgroups even if the sample is homogeneous.

A combination of factor analysis and cluster analysis has been shown to be a highly useful and appropriate technique with psychosocial data (Klassen, 1977; K. S. O'Connor, 1977). In factor analysis complex data were reduced to factor-loading scores; that is, data that were essentially classification data or descriptive data were weighted on particular factors, giving the data a numerical score for each subject relative to the factors. This technique identified a limited number of population types (factors) extracted from a large number of demographic and personal variables, and a limited number of varieties of settings (factors) extracted from complex environmental data. Changes in factor scores or differences among populations may then be evaluated.

Cluster analysis has also been used to transform data describing populations into discrete groups. Using a quasi-experimental design, these discrete groupings by subject and by situational participation were treated as comparison groups in an analysis of variance. Such a procedure may be used with raw data or with more complex data. The measures may be first reduced to factor-loading scores for each subject, with factor-loading scores cluster-analyzed to produce comparison groups and either raw scores or factor-loading scores as criterion scores (O'Connor & Klassen, in press; O'Connor, Wilkinson, & Daniels, in press).

A large number of useful analyses can be performed on this information. For example, it is possible to analyze individuals' changes in a treatment program over time by comparing their distances as computed from a cluster centroid. The analysis would suggest convergence or divergence as a result of treatment exposure for the client population or for selected subpopulations of clients.

Finally, it is not necessary to utilize exclusively parametric statistics in order to analyze psychosocial data. Nonparametric techniques, even those as simple as a Chi-square, can be used where the taxonomies or classifications reflect those population and environmental variables that the investigator has separated or selected for study. Nonparametric statistics assume that subjects can be assigned to categories that are discrete or mutually exclusive; these may be either subject categories, such as males and females, or environmental categories, such as those who did and did not receive an experimental condition. More importantly, nonparametric statistics do not assume that individuals have continuously distributed scores; that is, it is not necessary to have a numerical score for each subject relative to a particular variable, because calculation does not require mathematical treatment of separate scores for each subject. In a Chi-square, for example, a 2×2 table might be used with subjects above or below the median on one variable, compared with condition or environment A or B. Nonparametric statistics are often not used because they are described as less "powerful" than parametric techniques. However, the investigator may prefer a nonparametric technique if the hypothesis suggests a strong relationship between a small number of conditions (e.g., Hume, O'Connor, & Lowery, 1977). For a great deal of research, for example, mean differences may not be of practical importance; what may be important are individuals that do or do not become readmissions or individuals who do or do not survive a particular illness. A very small but statistically significant difference obtained by analysis of variance may not tell the clinician what is important in a real-world situation. The nature of the question asked may be such that subtle differences are irrelevant and only the most powerful and categorical relationships desirable.

Practical Application of Psychosocial Methods in Service Settings

Although effective program evaluation is obviously desirable, it may easily be slighted in the day-to-day pressures created by client load, budget, allocation of staff, time, and the like. The system proposed is designed to survive such competition in several respects. It is intended to be as economical as possible, to be routinely implemented, and to blend with existing records rather than presenting a "special research project" adding to the existing work load. In this respect the instruments themselves are designed to meet the existing standards for documentation and accreditation. The results of evaluation, as well, are designed to be functional: the automatic production of reports in simple text form does not require special evaluation by a research committee but is consistently available in the daily decision-making process of the service unit.

An evaluation system as a product must have at least four key characteristics. First of all, it must be needed (Canter, 1971). In these terms, the instruments must anticipate problems and future trends (Glaser & Taylor,

1969): more comprehensive and systematic program evaluation is increasingly required of human service facilities, and the growing community and consumer role in such evaluation demands specific and nontechnical information (Weiss, 1971). Concrete patterns of community participation and involvement provide a response to this need.

At the same time, the actual users of the system demand simplicity, a wide level of applicability from administrative through staff levels, and a set of basic instruments that have face validity for all groups (Chesler & Flanders, 1967; Joly, 1967; Rosenblatt, 1968). In this sense, the forms themselves should allow the professional to use his or her individual experience to directly interpret the data, but at the same time, the types of data collected and the output of the system should answer the obvious questions raised by administrators and system managers. The effectiveness of the product depends on involvement at all levels, from professional staff through administrative and managerial (Klein, 1968).

The product must also have a combination of economy, robustness, ease, and ready integration with the existing system. On a practical level, any evaluation system must absorb inaccuracy, incomplete data, and errors; for this reason, the measurement proposed must be relatively molar, that is, not subject to disruption by minor errors. For administrative purposes, the system must also be low cost, both in terms of the instrumentation and analysis and in terms of the administrative and organizational changes necessary to implement the system. Thus, it must integrate well with existing processes (Mackie & Christensen, 1967; Weiss, 1971).

Finally, the "kit" itself must be easily adaptable and maximally flexible. A product that requires total implementation in precise terms is not likely to be used in a variety of settings. Rather, it must be subject to modification by each institution and be capable of introduction on a practical basis. If each part of a comprehensive system can be modified easily and applied in clinical settings, its more extended use is likely to follow (Glaser & Taylor, 1969; Shartel, 1961).

Design of the System

The following sections describe in more specific detail the components that must be developed in order to implement program evaluation utilizing a psychosocial ecosystems approach.

System Manuals

A comprehensive evaluation program will necessarily interface with a variety of staff members employed in many different capacities within a service agency. It will nearly always be advisable to allocate some time initially for staff development and training in regard to the new system and the roles staff will be expected to play both in providing the needed input and in making effective use of the results. It is essential that policies, definitions, and procedures be presented clearly to staff at the beginning of the implementation period, and also that staff have access to an indexed reference document whenever questions about the system arise. For both of these uses, it is essential to provide written documentation describing every component of the system. Obviously, the system manual should include samples of the data-collection instruments; procedures for interviewing clients and for coding, editing, and keying the data; definitions of all data items and code categories; flow charts of data-processing operations; and descriptions of output reports. In addition, the manual will be more useful if it contains summary sections oriented toward specific positions such as top management, data-processing personnel, staff members involved in data collection, and professional staff who will utilize the outputs. Ideally, the manual will include a comprehensive index, and will be distributed in a format that facilitates periodic updating.

Types of Measures

The measures to be adopted should be those that contributed most heavily in prior research to interactive client, treatment, and community data clusters, forming critical item subsets. The variables are generally of the following types:

Demographic Data. These measures consist of specific category ranges for variables such as sex, age, economic status, occupational background, education, marital status, treatment contact and entry mechanism, means of support and subsistence conditions, prior health system involvements, and current medical status.

Problem/Diagnostic Data. These measures are selected from items in the existing data base and client classification system at each site. The measures do not depend on a fixed set of categories but are developed for each site using cluster programs to identify subgroups. Either a diagnostic or a problem list format is acceptable raw data; multiproblem diagnostic systems are thus accommodated.

Community Participation Data. These measures are identified by the individual's interaction with various types of settings in the community: proportion of time, level of participation, and type of setting are assessed. The taxonomy of community settings reflecting the client's total ecosystem or life-style pattern, is collected for the pretreatment, intreatment, and posttreatment phases. Thus, major life-style and community participation patterns can be plotted over time, and the effect of variables outside of the formal treatment context (particularly applicable in partial hospitalization and outpatient modalities) is assessed. The most critical subsystems ordinarily identified are employment, education, social interaction, recreational and stress-reducing activities, commercial settings, transportation, health, and family (Klassen, 1977).

Treatment System Variables. Treatment system variables are primarily hours per day in treatment and length of stay. Using these two variables, system typologies are derived—for example, short-term outpatient, short-term inpatient, long-term outpatient, long-term inpatient. These patterns have proven consistent across widely divergent treatment systems studied thus far. In order to report periodically on new clients or other specific subpopulations, the date of admission and dates of changes in admission status should be recorded. Optionally, additional treatment system variables such as assignment to specific treatment programs, or selection of specific crisis intervention techniques, may be incorporated in the data analysis.

Treatment Activity Data. In addition to treatment system variables, treatment modalities in which clients participate are classified according to the same basic system used to assess community participation patterns. Based on each institution's record of patient activities, a catalog of basic treatments is developed. Actual patient activity data from each subject may then be collected to identify the specific activity patterns of each subject in terms that are comparable to community participation assessment.

Other Program Data. The community participation, treatment system, and treatment activities variables reflect broad system participation patterns. If, in addition, specific institutions wish to incorporate specialized analyses into the system, they may easily add, for example, unit cost, classification of staff, direct patient contact, or other variables of interest.

Format of the Assessment Package

Each of the six types of data described above corresponds to one data-collection instrument or procedure. The preferred format for these instruments or procedures will vary from one facility to another, depending on which data items are already available in an existing information system, the nature of data-processing services available, and other related characteristics. It is probable that most facilities already record all the relevant demographic variables, and that they also maintain either a problem list or a diagnosis for each client. Decisions concerning the best procedure for accessing these data for program evaluation must be made on the basis of the individual circumstances in each facility. For each type of data, it will be necessary to develop an interview schedule to elicit the data from the client, a procedure for staff to observe and record the relevant data, or a procedure to retrieve the data from an existing manual or automated record system.

The following considerations are relevant to the design of forms to be used for collecting data items not recorded previously. First, the overall organization and appearance of the document should facilitate use by the professional staff and other relevant persons. It should be possible to select quickly from a list of precoded categories the correct response to each question. Since the form will usually become a permanent part of the client's file, it should incorporate spaces for writing verbatim observations—as frequently desired by the clinical staff—in addition to the required precoded variables. Second, the form should be organized to facilitate the data entry procedures available to each individual facility. Where data will be entered by keypunch or keytape operators, formatting information such as column and deck numbers should be printed on the form, arranged in such a manner that the response code for each column is readily apparent, preferably along one margin of each page. Some facilities may choose to design a form compatible with optical scanners, mark–sense readers, or other data input devices that may be available. Third, the forms should be compatible with existing record systems at the facility. This system should be coordinated with established working procedures for interviewing, record keeping, and data processing to an extent that minimizes disruption to the facility during implementation.

Data-Collection Schedule

The types of data described above, obtained by whichever procedure is most appropriate in each facility, should be organized into three basic data-collection operations: an intake interview, an intreatment interview, and a follow-up interview. The collection schedule, showing which types of data should be collected at each time, is suggested as follows:

1. *Intake*—within 48 hours after admission.
   Demographic data
   Problem/diagnosis data
   Community participation data (pretreatment pattern)
2. *Intreatment*—first treatment contact after admission. Subsequent intreatment interviews through date of discharge, with a final interview 3 months after the last treatment activity recorded.
   Treatment system variables
   Treatment activities
   Other program data

      Problem/diagnosis data

      Community participation

3. *Follow-up interview*—3 months after the final interview indicated above (i.e., 6 months after the last treatment).

      Problem/diagnosis data

      Community participation

This proposed data-collection procedure repeatedly provides measurements of the client's status at an initial time, measurements of interventions or treatments assigned to the client during a subsequent time period, and repeated measures of the client's status at the end of the time period. The interview process is illustrated in the flow chart in Figure 3.

Analysis Techniques

A wide variety of analyses are possible using the data set described above. The proposed minimal analysis would follow generally the steps described in the methods section. Briefly, clients can be separated empirically into clusters that categorize them according to their demographic characteristics, their community participation patterns, and their problem/diagnosis status. The impact of different treatments upon each type of client can be measured as sufficient cases are entered into the system over time, and predictions regarding outcomes for new clients can be made based upon the observed outcomes of former clients. In modifying the research design to create a continuing process for program evaluation, several significant changes are proposed. First, many human service facilities often admit clients for treatment who have just experienced or who are in the process of experiencing a significant crisis in some aspect of their lives. This circumstance frequently results in application of a crisis intervention, short-term form of immediate treatment, usually followed by other longer-term treatments designed to impact the underlying conditions that contributed to the crisis. Therefore, in anticipation of rapid changes in both treatment modality and problem/diagnosis status within a few days following admission, the data-collection schedule specifies the second interview to take place only 1 week following admission. The first interview, which takes place as soon as feasible after admission, collects pretreatment patterns and problem status, including a description of the immediate crisis, if any. The second interview records the interventions and treatments of the 1st week, and updates the problem status to indicate the postcrisis diagnosis or problem list. These distinctive features of the 1st week in treatment imply that analysis of change during that week should be performed separately from

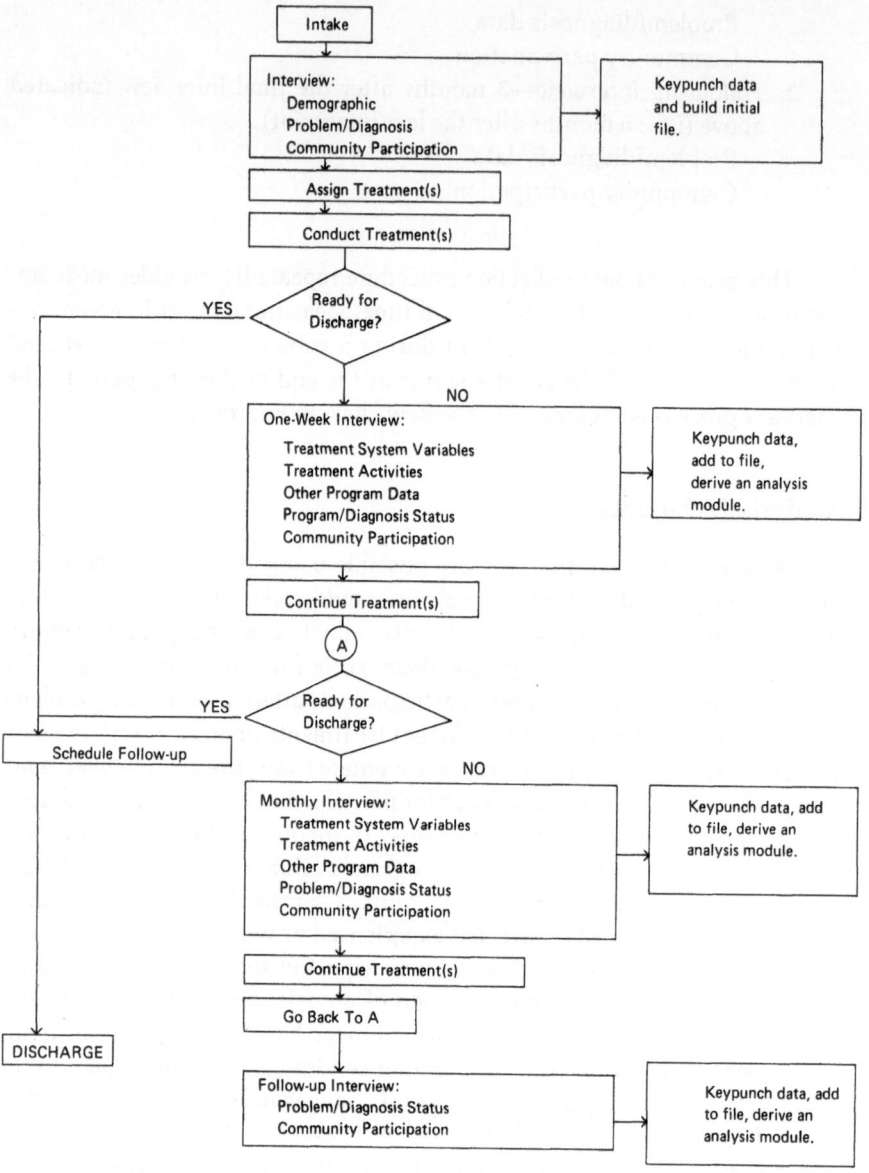

Figure 3. Flow of clients through system, showing points of data collection for initial sample.

other specified analyses. The analysis techniques, however, remain the same.

Particularly in facilities that provide treatment over a period of months, the repeated monthly interviews will provide multiple opportunities to test the impact of treatment upon each client. Any two interviews describing the same client can be taken jointly to form an "analysis module," or set of data amenable to evaluation. An analysis module is here defined as a set of data providing measurements upon one client at two distinct times, including measures of the client's problem/diagnosis status and the client's community participation pattern at both times, and measures of the client's treatment assignments and activities during the intervening time period. Thus, the joining of two successive monthly interviews together provides one analysis module client per month, and each treatment can be evaluated in terms of the amount of change observed (as measured by both problem/diagnosis status and community participation) taking place over these monthly intervals. Of course, as soon as the system has been in operation long enough to provide the requisite data, it is highly significant to form analysis modules consisting of the initial problem/diagnosis status and pretreatment community participation pattern, combined with the final follow-up measures of these same items, and using measures of treatment derived from adding together all the treatment assignments and activities reported in the intervening interviews. Findings derived from these modules will indicate the total impact of the treatment experience by comparing pretreatment measures of patterns and problems to postreatment measures of the same patterns and problems, with both sets of measurements relating to the client's ability to function in the community.

The additional varieties of analysis that may be conducted upon these data include comparisons of specific treatment modalities, comparisons of clients assigned to different staff members, comparisons from one year to the next or one month to the next, comparisons of outcomes before and after adopting changes ranging from new policies to new staff members to new or expanded physical plant.

Types of Reports

Reports developed from this data set can be tailored to the needs of individual facilities. Certain types of reports, however, are basic to the design of the system and would always be generated. These include a periodic report showing the impact of different treatments upon the various client types. Such a report can be produced separately for the 1st week in treatment, for month-long intervals of treatment, and for total episodes of treatment. This same basic report can be generated for other subpopulations of the clients in order to accomplish specific evaluations, as suggested above.

The second basic type of report, available only after sufficient data have accumulated, consists of predictions of outcome for new clients, based upon the client's pretreatment characteristics and each potential treatment assignment. These predictions are derived from the assessment of similar previous clients who were assigned to each of the possible treatment modalities.

As the system continues to function over time, different facilities may find different subsets of the data items consistently accounting for the greatest share of the explained variance, while other data items may have little impact in a particular facility. Such observations may lead to modifications in which some data items are deleted from analysis, while the pattern of results may suggest additional relevant variables. The general system described here can be applied without conceptual modification to such modified data sets. Addition of new variables could expand the system to produce reports related to expenditures, to the percent of utilization of various facilities or pieces of equipment, or to the utilization of staff in various activities. In short, this system is designed to respond flexibly to the needs of the service facility.

The practical results of the psychosocial ecosystems approach allow both clinical utilization and programmatic application. The techniques and measurements allow identification of a relatively broad spectrum of treatment approaches, of client types who are likely or unlikely to benefit from a variety of approaches, and, most significantly, to identify the appropriate combinations of client and treatment approach that lead to a broad range of specified outcomes. The clinical application of such a model involves not only treatment approaches but also the identification of community variables that may lead to effective preventive illness and health support programs in specific community settings.

References

Allport, G. W. Traits revisited. *American Psychologist,* 1966, *21,* 1–10.

Anchor, K. N., Vojtisek, J. E., & Patterson, R. L. Trait anxiety, initial structuring, and self-disclosure in groups of schizophrenic patients. *Psychotherapy: Theory, Research and Practice,* 1973, *10,* 155–158.

Anderson, R. L. Uses of variance components analysis in the interpretation of biological experiments. *Bulletin of International Statistics,* 1960, *37,* 71–90.

Anderson, R. L., & Crump, P. P. Comparisons of designs and estimation procedures for estimating parameters in a two-stage nested process. *Technometrics,* 1967, *9,* 499–516.

Attkinson, C. C. *Evaluation of human service programs.* New York: Academic, 1976.

Bailey, N. T. J. *The mathematical approach to biology and medicine.* New York: Wiley, 1967.

Bainbridge, T. R. Staggered, nested designs for estimating variance components. *American Society of Quality Control 17th Annual Conference Transcript,* 1963, 93–103.

Barker, R. G. *Stream of behavior.* New York: Appleton-Century-Crofts, 1963. (a)

Barker, R. G. On the nature of the environment. *Journal of Social Issues,* 1963, *18,* 17–38. (b)

Barker, R. G. *Ecological psychology.* Stanford: Stanford University Press, 1968.

Barker, R. G., & Gump, P. *Big school, small school.* Stanford: Stanford University Press, 1964.

Beigel, A. Evaluation on a shoestring: A suggested methodology for the evaluation of community mental health services without budgetary and staffing support. Chapter 3, Resource Materials for Community Mental Health Program Evaluating. National Institute of Mental Health, 1976.

Best, J. S. Tailoring smoking withdrawal procedures to personality and motivational differences. *Journal of Consulting and Clinical Psychology*, 1975, *43*, 1–8.

Bishop, D. W., & Witt, P. A. Sources of behavioral variance during leisure time. *Journal of Personality and Social Psychology*, 1970, *16*, 352–360.

Bloom, B. L. An ecological analysis of psychiatric hospitalization. *Multivariate Behavior Research*, 1968, *3*, 423–463.

Blum, H. *Planning for health*. New York: Human Sciences Press, 1974.

Bowers, K. S. Situationalism in psychology: An analysis and a critique. *Psychological Review*, 1973, *80*, 307–336.

Canter, F. M. Authoritarian attitudes, degree of pathology, and preference for structured vs.unstructured psychotherapy in hospitalized mental patients. *Psychological Reports*, 1971, *28*, 231–234.

Chapman, R. L. *The design of management information systems for mental health organization: A primer.* Rockville, Md.: National Institute of Mental Health, 1976.

Chesler, M., & Flanders, M. Resistance to research and research utilization. *Journal of Applied Behavioral Science*, 1967, *3*, 387–469.

Ciarlo, J. A., & Reihman, J. *The Denver Community Mental Health Questionnaire: Development of a multidimensional program evaluation instrument.* Unpublished, 1974. (Available from the Mental Health Systems Evaluation Project, Denver, Colorado.)

Cline, D. W. Goal-attainment scaling as a method for evaluating mental health programs. *American Journal of Psychiatry*, 1973, *130*, 105–108.

Cronbach, L. J., Gleser, G. C., Nanda, H., & Rajaratnam, N. *The dependability of behavioral measurements: Theory of generalizability for scores and profiles.* New York: Wiley, 1972.

Derogatis, L. R. The Hopkins Symptom Check List (HSCL): A self-report symptom inventory. *Behavioral Science*, 1974, *19*, 1–15.

Diamond, H. Consultation, education, and training perspectives from an urban community mental health center: The context of dilemma. *American Journal of Public Health*, 1973, *62*, 1602–1605.

Domino, G. Interactive effects of achievement orientation and teaching style on academic achievement. *Journal of Educational Psychology*, 1971, *62*, 427–431.

Edwards, A. W. F., & Cavalli-Sforza, L. L. A method for cluster analysis. *Biometrics*, 1965, *21*, 362–375.

Ekehammer, B. Interactionalism in personality from a historical perspective. *Psychological Bulletin*, 1974, *81*, 1026–1048.

Ekehammer, B., Magnusson, D., & Ricklander, L. An interactionist approach to the study of anxiety. *Scandinavian Journal of Psychology*, 1974, *15*, 4–14.

Ellsworth, R. *Effective and ineffective psychiatric training programs.* Unpublished manuscript, Roseburg Veterans Administration Hospital, Roseburg, Oregon, 1965.

Ellsworth, R. Consumer feedback in measuring the effectiveness of mental health programs. In M. Guttentag and E. Streuning (Eds.), *Handbook of evaluative research* (Vol. 2). Beverly Hills: Sage Publications, 1975.

Endicott, J. The Global Assessment Scale: A procedure for measuring overall severity of psychiatric disturbance. *Archives of General Psychiatry*, 1976, *33*, 766–771.

Endler, N. S. The person versus the situation—A pseudo issue? A response to Alker. *Journal of Personality*, 1973, *41*, 287–303.

Endler, N. S. The role of person by situation interactions in personality. In F. Weitzman & I. C. Uzgiris (Eds.), *The structuring of experience*. New York: Plenum, 1976.

Endler, N. S., & Hunt, J. McV. Sources of behavioral variance as measured by the S-R Inventory of Anxiousness. *Psychological Bulletin, 1966, 65,* 287–303.

Endler, N. S., & Hunt, J. McV. S-R Inventories of hostility and comparisons of the proportions of variance from persons, responses, and situations for hostility and anxiousness. *Journal of Personality and Social Psychology, 1968, 9,* 309–315.

Endler, N. S., & Hunt, J. McV. Generalizability of contributions from sources of variance in S-R Inventories of Anxiousness. *Journal of Personality, 1969, 37,* 1–24.

Endler, N. S., Hunt, J. McV., & Rosenstein, D. J. An S-R Inventory of Anxiousness. *Psychological Monographs, 1962, 76*(17, Whole No. 537).

Engel, B. T., & Moos, R. H. The generality of specificity. *Archives of General Psychiatry, 1967, 16,* 574–581.

Erickson, R. Outcome studies in mental hospitals: A review. *Psychological Bulletin, 1975, 82,* 519–545.

Evenson, R. C. *Community Adjustment Profile Scale* (Rev.). Columbia: Missouri Institute of Psychiatry, June 1976.

Findikyan, N. S., & Sells, S. B. Organizational structure and similarity of campus student organizations. *Organizational Behavior and Human Performance, 1966, 13,* 169–190.

Fiske, D. W. The use of significant others in assessing the outcome of psychotherapy. In I. Waskow & M. Parlaff (Eds.), *Psychotherapy change measures.* DHEW Pub. No. (ADM) 74–120. Rockville, Md.: National Institute of Mental Health, 1974.

Fleiss, J. L., & Zubin, J. On methods and theory of clustering. *Biometrics Research,* New York State Department of Mental Hygiene and Columbia University, 1969. (Abstract)

Fox, P. D., & Rappaport, M. Some approaches to evaluating community mental health services. *Archives of General Psychiatry, 1972, 26,* 172–178.

Gabbay, M., & Windle, C. *Demographic data to improve services: A sampler of mental health applications.* MHDPS, Working Paper No. 33. Rockville, Md.: National Institute of Mental Health, 1975.

Gerard, R. W., & Mattsson, N. The identification of schizophrenia. In J. A. Jacquez (Ed.), *The diagnostic process.* Ann Arbor: University of Michigan, 1964, pp. 81–99.

Glaser, E. M., & Taylor, S. *Factors influencing the success of applied research.* Washington, D.C.: National Institute of Mental Health, Department of Health, Education and Welfare. Final Report on Contract No. 43–67–1365, January 1969.

Golding, S. L. Flies in the ointment: Methodological problems in the analysis of the percentage of variance due to persons and situations. *Psychological Bulletin, 1975, 82,* 278–288.

Guertin, W. H. An inverted factor analytic study of schizophrenics. *Journal of Consulting Psychology, 1952, 16,* 371–375.

Gump, P., Schoggen, P., & Redl, F. The camp milieu and its immediate effects. *Journal of Social Issues, 1957, 13,* 40–46.

Handel, G. Psychological studies of whole families. *Psychological Bulletin, 1965, 63,* 19–41.

Helzberg, A. M., & Cox, D. R. Recent work on the design of experiments: A bibliography and a review. *Journal of the Royal Statistical Society, 1964, A132,* 29–67.

Hodges, W. F. Effects of ego threat and threat of pain on state anxiety. *Journal of Personality and Social Psychology, 1968, 8,* 364–378.

Holden, C. N. On mental health centers: A movement that got bogged down. *Science, 1972, 177,* 413–415.

Hornstra, R. K., Lubin, B., Lewis, R., & Willis, B. S. Worlds apart: Patients and professionals. *Archives of General Psychiatry, 1972, 27,* 553–557.

Huber, G. P., & Ullman, J. C. *Effect of feedback on program performance on program administrators.* Unpublished manuscript, 1973.

Hume, N., O'Connor, W., & Lowery, C. Family, adjustment, and the psychosocial ecosystem. *Psychiatric Annals, 1977, 7,* 32–49.

Joly, J. Research and innovation: Two solitudes? *Canadian Education and Research Digest*, 1967, *2*, 184–194.

Katz, M. M., & Cole, J. O. A phenomenological approach to the classification of schizophrenic disorders. *Diseases of the Nervous System*, 1962, *24*, 147–154.

Katz, M. M., & Lyerly, S. B. Methods for measuring adjustment and social behavior in the community: I. Rationale, description, discriminative validity, and scale development. *Psychological Reports*, 1963, *13*, 503–535.

Kendall, R. E. *Declassification of depressive illnesses.* London: Oxford University Press, 1968.

Kiresuk, T. J. Goal attainment scaling at a country mental health service. *Evaluation*, 1973, Special Monograph No. 1, 12–18.

Klassen, D. Person, setting, and outcome in a drug abuse treatment program. *Psychiatric Annals*, 1977, *7*, 80–104.

Klein, H. D. *The Missouri story: A chronicle of research utilization and program planning.* Paper presented at the National Conference of Social Workers, May 1968.

Lick, J. Statistical vs. clinical significance in research on the outcome of psychotherapy. *International Journal of Mental Health*, 1973, *2*, 130.

Lorr, M. (Ed.). *Explorations in typing psychotics.* Oxford: Pergamon, 1966.

Luborsky, L. Assessment of outcome of psychotherapy by independent clinical evaluators: A review of the most highly recommended research measures. In I. Waskow & M. Parloff (Eds.), *Psychotherapy change measures.* DHEW Pub. No. (ADM) 75–120. Rockville, Md.: National Institute of Mental Health, 1974.

Lubin, B., Hornstra, R. K., Lewis, R. V., & Bechtel, B. S. Correlates of initial treatment assignments in a comprehensive community mental health center. *Archives of General Psychiatry*, 1973, *29*, 497–500.

Luborsky, L., Chandler, M., Auerbach, A., Cohen, J., & Bachrach, H. Factors influencing the outcome of psychotherapy: A review of quantitative research. *Psychological Bulletin*, 1971, *75*, 145–185.

Mackie, R. R., & Christensen, P. R. *Translation and application of psychological research.* Technical Report 716–1. Goleta, Calif.: Santa Barbara Research Park, Human Factors Research, Inc., 1967.

Mariotto, M. J., & Paul, G. L. Persons versus situations in the real-life functioning of chronically institutionalized mental patients. *Journal of Abnormal Psychology*, 1975, *84*, 483–493.

McIntyre, J. Components of program evaluation capability in community mental health centers. *Resource materials for community mental health program evaluation.* National Institute of Mental Health, 1977.

McQuitty, L. L. Pattern analysis illustrated in classifying patients and normals. *Educational and Psychological Measurement*, 1954, *14*, 598–604.

Medley, D. M., & Mitzel, H. E. Measuring classroom behavior by systematic observation. In N. L. Gage (Ed.), *Handbook of research on teaching.* Chicago: Rand McNally, 1963.

Medley, D. M., Mitzel, H. E., & Doi, A. N. Analysis of variance models and their use in a three-way design without replication. *Journal of Experimental Education*, 1956, *24*, 221–229.

Meichenbaum, D. H., Gilmore, J. B., & Fedoravicius, A. A group insight vs. group desensitization in treating speech anxiety. *Journal of Consulting and Clinical Psychology*, 1971, *36*, 410–421.

Miller, R. *Human ecosystems.* New York: Appleton-Century-Crofts, 1965.

Mischel, W. *Personality and assessment.* New York: Wiley, 1968.

Monro, A. B. Psychiatric types: A Q-technique study of 200 patients. *Journal of Mental Science*, 1955, *101*, 330–343.

Moos, R. H. Differential effects of ward settings on psychiatric patients. *Journal of Nervous and Mental Disease,* 1967, *145,* 272–283.

Moos, R. H., & Houts, P. Assessment of the social atmospheres of psychiatric wards. *Journal of Abnormal Psychology,* 1968, *93,* 595–604.

O'Connor, K. S. Methods and problems in psychosocial ecosystem research, *Psychiatric Annals,* 1977, *7,* 16–32.

O'Connor, W. A. Ecosystems theory and clinical mental health. *Psychiatric Annals,* 1977, *7,* 63–77.

O'Connor, W. A., & Klassen, D. Person, setting, and outcome in drug abuse treatment. *Journal of Clinical and Consulting Psychology,* in press.

O'Connor, W. A., & Ramchandani, K. Community mental health: Training for innovation. *International Journal of Social Psychiatry,* 1970, *16*(3), 194–200.

O'Connor, W. A., Wilkinson, C. B., & Daniels, S. The relationship of aspirations to competence and lifestyle variables in black adolescent males from single parent families. *Black Scholar,* in press.

Pace, C. R., & Stern, G. G. *A criterion study of college environment.* Syracuse: Syracuse University Psychological Resource, 1958, p. 29.

Rao, S. Literacy and mental hospital admissions. *Psychologia: An International Journal of Psychology in the Orient,* 1966, *9,* 232–235.

Rosen, B. M. *A model for estimating mental health needs using 1970 census socioeconomic data.* DHEW Pub. No. (ADM) 74–63. Rockville, Md.: National Institute of Mental Health, 1974.

Rosenblatt, A. The practitioner's use and evaluation of research. *Social Work,* 1968, *13,* 53–59.

Sarason, I. G. Verbal learning, modeling, and juvenile delinquency. *American Psychologist,* 1968, *23,* 254–266.

Sawrey, W. L. Keller, L., & Conger, J. J. An objective method of grouping profiles by distance functions and its relation to factor analysis. *Educational and Psychological Measurement,* 1960, *20,* 651–673.

Schainblatt, A. H. *Monitoring the outcomes of state mental health treatment programs: Some initial suggestions.* Washington, D.C.: Urban Institute, 1977.

Searle, S. R. Topics in variance components estimation. *Biometrics,* 1971, *27,* 1–76.

Sells, S. B. *Stimulus determinants of behavior.* New York: Ronald, 1963.

Shartle, C. L. The occupational research program: An example of research utilization: In *Case studies in bringing behavioral science into use: Studies in the utilization of behavioral science* (Vol. 1). Stanford: Institute for Communication Research, Stanford University, 1961, pp. 59–72.

Smith, M. B. *Competence and mental health: Problems in conceptualizing human effectiveness.* An address to the National Symposium—The Definition and Measurement of Mental Health, National Center for Health Statistics, Washington, D.C., May 1966, p. 39.

Sokal, R. R., & Sneath, P. H. A. *Principles of numerical taxonomy.* San Francisco: W. H. Freeman, 1963.

Spitzer, R. L. The psychiatric status schedule: A technique for evaluating psychopathology and impairment of role functioning. *Archives of General Psychiatry,* 1970, *23,* 41–55.

Stephens, C. D. *A follow-up study of child and adolescent clients served by the state's residential treatment facilities: Introductory report.* Raleigh, N.C.: Department of Human Resources, Division of Mental Health Planning and Evaluation Services (draft report), July 1976.

Stern, E. *Scoring instructions and college norms—Activities index, college characteristics index.* Syracuse: Syracuse University, Psychological Research Center, 1963.

Stern, G. Student ecology and the college environment. *Journal of Modern Education,* 1965, *40,* 132–154.

Streuning, E. L., & Guttentag, M. (Eds.). *Handbook of evaluative research* (Vol. 1). Beverly Hills: Sage Publications, 1975.

Strupp, H. H., & Bergin, A. Some empirical and conceptual bases for coordinated research in psychotherapy: A critical review of issues, trends, and evidence. *International Journal of Psychiatry*, 1969, *7*, 18–90.

Tryon, R. C. *Cluster analysis: Correlations profile and orthometric (factor) analysis for the isolation of unities in mind and personality*. Ann Arbor: Edwards, 1939.

Udell, B., & Hornstra, R. K. Good patients and bad. *Archives of General Psychiatry*, 1975, *32*, 1533–1537.

Weiss, C. H. *Organizational constraints on evaluation research*. Report to NIMH. Contract No. 46–69–82, Bureau of Applied Social Research, Columbia University, New York, May 1971.

Weiss, C. H. *Evaluating action programs: Readings in social action and education*. Boston: Allyn and Bacon, 1972.

Weiss, C. H. Between the cup and the lip. *Evaluation*, 1973, *1*, 49–55.

Weissman, M. M. Assessment of social adjustment. *Archives of General Psychiatry*, 1975, *23*, 357–365.

Weissman, M. M., & Paykel, E. S. *The depressed woman: A study of social relationships*. Chicago: University of Chicago Press, 1974.

White, R. W. Competence and psychosexual stages of development. In M. Jones (Ed.), *Nebraska symposium on motivation*. Lincoln: University of Nebraska Press, 1960, pp. 97–141.

Wicker, A. Undermanning theory and research: Implications for the study of psychological and behavioral effects of excess human populations. *Representative Research in Social Psychology*, 1973, *4*, 185–206.

Wilkinson, C. B., & O'Connor, W. A. Introduction and overview: An ecologic approach to mental health. *Psychiatric Annals*, 1977, *7*, 10–15. (a)

Wilkinson, C. B., & O'Connor, W. A. Growing up male in a black single parent family. *Psychiatric Annals*, 1977, *7*, 50–59. (b)

Willems, E. Review of research. In R. Barker & P. Gump, *Big school, small school*. Stanford: Stanford University Press, 1964, pp. 29–37.

Windle, C., & Volkman, E. M. Evaluation in the centers program. *Evaluation*, 1973, *1*, 69–70.

Wohlwill, J. The emerging discipline of environmental psychology. *American Psychologist*, 1970, *25*, 303–312.

Zinner, L. *The consistency of human behavior in various situations: A methodological application of functional ecology*. Unpublished doctoral dissertation, University of Houston, 1963.

Zubin, J. A technique for measuring likemindness. *Journal of Abnormal and Social Psychology*, 1938, *33*, 508–516.

Zubin, J. Clinical vs. actuarial prediction: A pseudo-problem. In *Invitational conference on testing problems*. Princeton: Educational Testing Service, 1955, pp. 107–128.

Zubin, J., & Fleiss, J. L. Taxonomy in the mental disorders: A historical perspective. In *Symposium on explorations in typology with special reference to psychotics*. New York: Human Ecology Fund, 1965, pp. 1–12.

18

Health Sector Assessment

Paul I. Ahmed and Aliza Kolker

Introduction

The decades since World War II have witnessed growing concern in developing countries about upgrading their health services, and a reciprocal desire among developed countries and international donor agencies to provide technical and financial assistance for that purpose. A growing recognition of the inefficiency and waste resulting from haphazard programming and from uncoordinated aid has led to the development of several methodologies for assessing the health needs of developing countries and for developing rational, integrated health programming.

In this chapter we analyze a major methodology for health planning, Health Sector Assessment (HSA), employed principally by the United States Agency for International Development (AID). Although health-planning techniques have been used by international agencies and national governments for at least two decades, the concept of health sector assessment as a specific methodology is relatively recent (for other methodologies see, for example, Chasse, 1975; Farr, 1975; PAHO/WHO, 1965; Ahmed,

Paul I. Ahmed • Office of International Health, U.S. Department of Health, Education and Welfare, Rockville, Maryland 20857. Aliza Kolker • Department of Sociology, George Mason University, Fairfax, Virginia 22030. This chapter reflects the professional opinions of the writers and does not represent the policy of the U.S. Department of Health, Education and Welfare. An earlier version of this article was presented to a conference on Integration of Health in Economic Development, sponsored by USAID and HEW in San Diego, March 24–25, 1978.

1975; Gutierrez, 1975; IBRD, 1975). The purpose of this chapter is to describe briefly the goals and design of the Health Sector Assessment and to explore its uses and limitations as a tool for health planning. The discussion is based largely on the authors' personal familiarity with this and other health-planning methodologies, on internal papers and memos circulated by the Agency for International Development, and on informal interviews with health officials in international agencies.

Health sector assessment is conceptualized as a tool for coordinated and integrated planning directed toward improving health conditions in developing nations. It involves a process of gathering, organizing, and analyzing data on the health policies and resources of a developing country for the identification of possible solutions to its health problems. The purpose of a health sector assessment is to develop a strategy or set of strategies for health improvement in developing countries. As mentioned above, the concept of health sector assessments as a specific methodology is relativly recent; it has only been used in a few Latin American and Middle Eastern countries since 1972. The demand for health sector assessment arose from the need for long-term planning on the part of the donors, international financial committees, and the countries themselves.

Several factors have converged to create a need for integrated, long-term planning in the third world. These factors include (1) more demand for health services; (2) a scarcity of resources; (3) the transfer of new technology, vaccines, and drugs; and (4) strong donor interest in providing preventive health services. Congressional and administrative mandates in the United States have reflected these factors and have created the climate for this new approach. President Carter reemphasized the United States policy in his statement of May 2, 1978, announcing a program to strengthen United States participation in efforts to overcome disease and ill health. The president stated:

> Our efforts will be based on the following principles: a basic minimum level of health, nutrition and family planning services should be available to the world's poor, whether they live in rural areas or urban slums. Developing nations can eventually meet their own needs if we assist them in strengthening their institutions and building their own health systems. Community-based health care, including the use of community resources and the training of appropriate health personnel as near as possible to where they deliver services, is the most effective means of achieving the standard of health we desire for all people.

This affirmation of goals of United States international health policy by the president has led to active involvement of all United States international health agencies in long-term planning. This interest is also expressed in terms of development of new methodologies for health planning. Assessment is one of the tools that the USAID has used for long-term planning. In order to understand its usefulness to planning, we need to know its purposes, its methodology, and the nature of its final product.

The Concept of Health Sector Assessment

Health sector assessment, designed for efficiency and comprehensiveness, involves a team effort. It is important that members of the host country play a large part, since, ideally, the planning and design of future health programs will evolve out of the HSA.

The ultimate goals of health sector assessment are (1) to provide a data base for programming AID support to the health sector; (2) to contribute to the improvement of the country's institutional capability in health planning by (a) structurally analyzing health sector problems and alternative solutions, (b) assessing the country's health-planning requirements and developing estimates of the manpower and resource requirements needed to accomplish those requirements; and (3) to establish a basis for national and AID investments within the health sector.

In order to accomplish these goals certain intermediate objectives must be met. Most of these are accomplished in the host country in the process of the assessment. These are as follows:

1. Clarify the nature of existing health problems within the total social, economic, and political context. (In particular, the political climate and the human and technological resources of the country appear relevant to the HSA; see Westinghouse, 1978.)
2. Place in clear focus the important *interrelationships* of the health sector with the social and economic sectors.
3. Choose among several HSA models the one most appropriate to the host country's situation (more on the various models follows below).
4. Help to elaborate alternative health strategies in a format that constitutes a basis for choice and that is useful for decision-makers.
5. Promote and facilitate implementation of health development programs in high-priority areas.
6. Identify program areas requiring well-managed development projects. Such areas may include existing programs, possible revisions of those, and areas not yet addressed by existing or planned programs.
7. Strengthen national capabilities in health planning, in project formulation, and in program evaluation.
8. Identify program areas and projects for which foreign assistance may be forthcoming (e.g., from bilateral agencies, from the International Bank for Reconstruction and Development, from the United Nations Development Program, from the World Health Organization, or from the World Food Program).

It should also be noted that the idea of developing and implementing a health sector program that extends over several years and integrates multiple projects is another possible objective of a health sector assessment. Ideally, such a program should lead to more efficient utilization of resources in the service of national health goals. Long-term planning attempts to avoid the pitfalls of uncoordinated, haphazard health projects that in the past have sometimes diminished the effectiveness of foreign assistance programs.

The Initiation of an Assessment

The intricate processes that precede the assessment offer insight into both the function and the limitations of the method. What follows is a brief description of these processes.

The director of the USAID mission and his technical staff are responsible for the first step, which is a decision to provide assistance to a particular country. The kind or extent of health assistance that might be provided is determined on the basis of suggestions formulated by the country health ministry. With the aid of the technical staff's advice, the mission director develops a plan concept, or Project Identification Document (PID), for an aid program. The PID is then approved in Washington, after which the mission director can make a decision to implement the project on sites, provided the cost is below specified levels. If the costs exceed a specified level, the project plan is developed in detail, submitted to review committees in Washington, and approved again before implementation.

It is important to keep in mind that political interests of the United Stataes government and those of the government of the receiving country underlie and determine the total amount of assistance that can be given or absorbed at any time, the nature of the projects that might be undertaken, and the allocation of resources and sites of proposed projects within the receiving country. Following are a few of the factors that must be considered in determining what health projects are suggested:

1. What has the host government formally requested or indicated through informal discussions? Does it meet the AID mandate of helping the poor majority? Is it an area of AID priority, such as health services, integrated health delivery, or environmental sanitation?

2. What would be the receptiveness of the host government to the idea of any American influence over its health policies?

3. What is the attitude of the existing economic leadership toward partial support of potential projects in the initial stages of growth and full support for maintenance in future years?

4. What are the political or economic motivations of the central government? Has the government developed a sincere interest in the health of a segment of the population? Does the government believe that improved

health conditions of that segment will be advantageous to the economic development of the entire nation? What pressures are being brought to bear on the government to solve certain countrywide health problems? Does the government require help for a specific area of the country perceived as neglected for one reason or another and where the population is believed to bear a disproportionate burden of disease and poor environmental conditions?

5. What countries or organizations are now participating in joint health programs or are urging that new programs be undertaken? Do they clash with United States interests or use up valuable resources, or can they be coordinated to supplement or complement any American proposals?

6. What sizable existent programs that have demonstrated their benefit to the population are being phased out because of inadequate support?

7. How many American nationals will be involved in the project? Can the AID mission provide the necessary support?

8. What obvious budgetary, political, or other constraints would affect the initiation and continuation of any project?

The process of project selection is multifaceted. Sometimes projects are selected without long-term planning. Other times, planning aid is requested in the form of health sector assessments. Prior to the initiation of an assessment, the mission or the regional bureau of AID may request a preliminary background paper on the country. This "syncrisis" is based on secondary research and varies in format and scope. It is designed to present a summary of known geographic, demographic, economic, and health data about the country, as well as a statement of the major health problems and an estimate of the resources needed for a full-scale health sector assessment.

The Nature of a Health Sector Assessment

Several alternatives exist at this point, depending on AID policy considerations, on the interest and commitment of the host country, and on the constraint of available time, money, and manpower resources. First, it is possible that, for whatever reasons, no further action will be taken. If a decision is made to proceed with an HSA, several alternative models are available, ranging in scope from a very limited effort to a rather comprehensive one. The following alternative models, which a given HSA may adopt, were developed during a recent Westinghouse evaluation of three HSA (for a fuller discussion, see Westinghouse, 1978):

1. Preparation of AID program plan only. This plan is the least expensive and places the minimum burden on the mission and on the host country's government. Prepared entirely by AID staff or by consultants, it is

tied to the AID funding cycle and addresses the HSA objectives as discrete projects rather than as components of the program-planning process.

2. Preparation of an AID program plan with selected additional objectives. This model is essentially similar to the first, except that a limited number of additional objectives may be included (e.g., formal training or a survey of nutritional conditions). The objectives, as well as the degree of involvement of the host country's staff, are decided on the basis of detailed negotiations with the host country's representatives. As in the first model, primary responsibility for program planning rests with AID.

3. Preparation of an AID program plan, with a parallel multiobjective health-planning effort. This model is designed to reconcile AID's need for a program-planning document tied to the funding cycle with the host country's interests in broader or longer-range objectives. Such objectives may include extended training or otherwise expanding the health-planning capability of the country. This model calls for much greater commitment on the part of the host country, and is partly independent of the AID funding cycle.

4. Preparation of a national health plan, with other HSA objectives, followed by preparation of an AID program plan. This model aims primarily at producing "a comprehensive national health plan, from which the AID program plan would derive, and it would be carried out independently of the AID funding cycle" (Westinghouse, 1978, p. 8). This model requires the largest investment in resources and the most extensive commitment on the part of the host country.

If a decision has been reached to proceed with a "full-scale" HSA a multidisciplinary team is put together. Team members come from the AID staff, from the U.S. Public Health Service, consulting firms under contract with AID, and from the host country. Strong emphasis is placed on participation of professionals from the host country, since the concept of a full partnership in development is perceived as a crucial element of the HSA philosophy and process. The actual composition of the team depends upon the specific objectives of the assessment, but may include any or all of the following professionals (of course, several specialties may be combined in the same person): (1) public health physician and primary care specialist, who may act as team leader; (2) maternal and child health physician and family planning specialist; (3) health manpower and training specialist; (4) nurse/midwife, nursing education specialist; (5) epidemiologist/environmental health specialist; (6) pharmaceutical, medical supply, and logistics specialist; (7) health development economist/financial analyst; (8) social anthropologist; (9) program design specialist; (10) vital statistics specialist; and (11) sanitary engineering specialist. Although team members usually have extensive overseas experience as advisors to AID missions, it is desirable that they have 2 or 3 weeks to collect and digest background materials before they assemble in Washington for briefings and departure.

The team may be aided by methodological and technical tools such as the *Guidelines for Health Sector Analysis,* a series of manuals published by AID and the Office of International Health of the U.S. Public Health Service. These manuals, which are also intended to be used by the host country's officials as well as by their American counterparts in planning or administering projects, cover such areas as financing the health sector; economic appraisal of health projects; planning for environmental health; controlling communicable diseases; planning for health services facilities and manpower; and cultural, social, and behavioral aspects of health planning.

The assessment team's visit to the host country varies in length, depending on the scope of the HSA. Typically, it may last 3 to 4 weeks. In advance of the visit, AID officials in the host country make certain preparations to facilitate the work of the team. These include briefings of officials in the Ministry of Health, in international health organizations in the country, and, ideally, in other governmental minstries relevant to health. Also briefed are staff members who are expected to work with and to host the visiting team. In addition, logistical preparations and work schedules are laid out as far in advance as possible.

The Health Sector Assessment

Depending on the model followed, the HSA will vary in length, format, and substance. The following are examples of elements that may be included:

1. Demographic data and forecasts. Information may typically include the age structure of the population, its rural/urban distribution, crude birth and death rates and fertility rates, infant mortality rates, and as many of the vital statistics as are available. Existing sources of data are used; usually no new data are collected. The purpose of assembling demographic data is to produce the best possible set of population (and population composition) forecasts. This is necessary not only for assistance in setting health targets but also for developing strategies.

2. Economic data. The data may include, as a minimum, existing and projected health budgets and estimates of new program costs. Other data may include projections of the Gross National Product or of the growth of revenues and expenditures in the public sector. There are many uses for economic data of this kind, but the basic ones are (a) to fit some boundaries on potential growth of the national health budget; (b) to take into account the likely impact of general development policy on the setting of health

priorities, targets, and strategies; and (c) to estimate recurrent cost implications of new health investments.

3. Health status data. The data may usefully include a good national picture of the incidence and prevalence of disease by age, sex, location, etc. Possible tables presented may include ones showing mortality rates and morbidity rates by disease class. It is most useful for these tables to include relevant intercountry or intracountry comparisons. These tables are used by the team to assist in the setting of health priorities and in the identification of targets for the program period.

4. and 5. Health services and environmental health services. Summary tables are presented of existing health establishments, environmental health services, and health manpower categories. The tables, showing the distribution of health services and environmental health services in different geographic regions, should provide an estimation of the extent to which the population in rural and urban areas has access to or utilizes such services.

6. Unit cost data. After determining the appropriate units of output (e.g., vaccinations performed, hospital bed days, health clinic visits), an attempt is made to calculate the cost per unit. These data, if available, are used in analyzing the feasibility of alternative strategies and programs.

7. Policy data. The team collects relevant data on (a) national development policies, goals, and objectives; (b) national health policies; (c) the extent of understanding of health planning and health policy analysis and of commitment to them.

The Impact of the HSA on Health Programs

The suggestions resulting from the team's efforts are discussed within AID and in negotiations with the host country. These negotiations may (it is hoped) lead to the development of objectives and projects agreed upon by all sides—objectives and projects arising from, and supported by, the HSA. If AID is to partake in future projects, it may need to recruit long-term advisors and/or short-term consultants for assignment to the project.

An important part of the agreement concerns the organizational framework for carrying out the project. This framework may be the use of counterparts, the use of a joint organization for planning and administration, or the so-called "liaison approach."

The counterpart relationship, the one most frequently encountered in AID overseas missions, involves the appointment of local partners from the Ministry of Health to work with each senior American technician for the purpose of coordinating the work and of exchanging information. In practice, this system works well only when the counterpart is actually the head of a department and the American is acting as his advisor.

The joint plan is a small temporary organization composed of "technicians" from both sides led by "administrators" of equal authority. Ideally, all work together with a clear common interest and mutual confidence and make decisions jointly. For this plan to work, the joint group must have a sizable degree of authority.

The liaison approach implies a separation between the two countries in both technical and policy-making functions. AID provides the funds, the commodity support, and the approval of the project. The host government plans and executes the project. This approach, although inefficient, may be used out of political necessity when a country does not desire foreign technicians, or when AID does not deem it advisable for American technicians to be involved directly in field operations.

Finally, it should be noted, if only for the sake of completeness, that no joint projects or planning at all may result from the HSA. This may be due to reasons explored below.

Criticisms and Limitations of Health Sector Assessment

Having briefly described the purposes and process of health sector assessment, we will now discuss a number of problems and issues raised by the implementation of HSA in several Latin American and Mideastern countries. The following issues were highlighted by the 1978 report of Westinghouse Health Systems to AID:

1. Conflicting HSA objectives. The HSA was designed to accomplish multiple objectives that often may turn out to be incompatible. These include a program-planning document for AID, a comprehensive health plan for the host country, and building up institutional capabilities in the host country (the latter will be discussed below). AID requires a program-planning document tied to its funding cycle. This is a short-term effort that must be met in a timely and efficient manner. The host country's need for a comprehensive health plan is a long-term goal that requires considerable resources. An attempt to meet both of these goals impedes the achievement of both goals and strains resources heavily. Of the alternative models outlined above, only one addresses this dilemma; yet the relative weight assigned to the different objectives needs to be clarified further, and the distinct endeavors separated more clearly.

2. Inadequate fulfillment of the institution-building goal. If a major objective of the HSA is to enhance the host country's institutional capabilities in health planning and management, different resources and commitments are called for. Not only formal training of personnel but reorganization of the health sector is required. Yet this is rarely achieved. One reason is the pressure of time; another is the failure to institutionalize the new

skills on a permanent basis, since after the HSA is completed the host country's participants may return to their previous jobs or may even be transferred outside the health sector. A further reason is outlined below.

3. Inadequate involvement of host country nationals. Whether because of lack of skills, lack of time for training, scarcity of manpower, or the pressures to produce a timely and efficient planning document, a discrepancy often arises between the roles of visiting team members and those of the host country nationals. The latter commonly contribute little to the endeavor beyond descriptive statistics, while the former perform the high-powered analysis and eventually write the document. This undermines the value of the HSA as an educational or institution-building tool.

4. Conflicting AID and host country objectives. Whereas AID is concerned with producing a program-planning document, the host country may have longer-range goals, such as preparing a comprehensive national health plan or building up institutional capabilities. The host country may view the HSA effort as a "donor project," a bureaucratic requirement unrelated to its own real needs, or duplicating already existing efforts. The need to withdraw scarce, highly skilled manpower from other areas of the already strained health sector presents further problems.

5. Inadequate follow-up. On several occasions, the HSA has turned out to be a one-shot effort, instead of the hoped-for basis for future planning for cooperative projects. This has resulted from AID's failure to translate the documents into Spanish and, in some cases, from the host government's reluctance to disseminate a document perceived as harmful to its image.

6. Policy limitations. The HSA must operate within the framework of AID's changing policy constraints as well as those of the host country. Consequently, it may neglect to look at the total health picture from an open-minded point of view and to offer fresh policy options. One example is the current policy of AID not to build new hospitals. This policy obviously limits the options that may be considered. Similarly, current AID priorities do not include several important areas of health, such as mental health. The HSA will therefore not address itself to these problems. These constraints limit the utility of the HSA as a comprehensive health-planning document.

7. Cost effectiveness. HSAs have ranged in effort from two man-years in one country to several dozen man-years in another. Given the limited uses of the HSA, it is difficult to justify such variation in expended resources. A more realistic appraisal of the different possible outcomes of the HSA may help to tailor the expenditure of resources more closely to the expected benefits. As it stands now, the HSA has proved to be more useful as a short-term program-planning document than as an ongoing, comprehensive effort to reorganize the health sector of a country. As an educational tool, the HSA has proved more useful in increasing the awareness of the

host country's personnel of the significance of health problems than in upgrading institutional capabilities in analysis and planning or in significantly redirecting health policies. As in the case of any attempt to reorganize major sectors of government on a more rational and efficient basis, political, economic, and bureaucratic forces combine to limit the impact of the change. This is the case not only in developing countries but in Western countries, too, of course. This does not call for abandoning the efforts to apply scientific analysis and planning techniques to social problems. But it should lead us to appraise realistically both the objectives and the priorities of such techniques, to consider the limitations of resources and of external factors, and to direct our efforts to where they will produce the most good.

ACKNOWLEDGMENTS

The authors are deeply grateful to Joseph Hacket of FDA, who shared a communication on the description of Health Sector Assessment. They are also grateful to Dr. Joseph Davis for an internal memo entitled "Guidelines for Health Sector Assessment." Both documents have been amply used in the development of this article. In addition, they are grateful to Nicholas Frisco of Westinghouse Health Systems and to Dr. Kenneth Farr for reviewing and commenting on earlier drafts of this chapter.

References

Ahmed, P. I. WHO methodology for country health programming. 1975. (Mimeo)

Chasse, J. D. World Bank health sector assessment process. 1975. (Mimeo)

Farr. K. PAHO methodology. 1975. (Mimeo)

Gutierrez, J. L. G. Health planning in Latin America. *American Journal of Public Health,* 1975, *65,* 1046–1059.

IBRD. *The assault on world poverty.* Baltmore: Johns Hopkins University Press, 1975.

PAHO/WHO. Health planning: Problems of concept and method. Scientific Publication No. III, April 1965.

Westinghouse Health Systems. *Reports for the evaluation of health sector assessments.* Submitted to Office of Health, Agency for International Development, Washington, D.C., 1978.

V

Implications for Practitioners and Policy Planners

Introduction

A wise statesman once remarked, "There are no easy problems left; all the easy ones have already been solved." It is well to remember this as we pause to assess the state of the world's health in the last quarter of the 20th century. As Margaret Mead remarked in the introduction to this book, the progress already made in both developed and developing countries is awesome. By any scale, the achievements, products of modern science and technology, greatly outweigh the failures.

It is clear, however, that future improvements in the state of health will call for new directions in both research and policy. A scanning of the chapters in this volume, as well as of other writings on health policy, reveals a bewildering variety of proposals, ranging from minor modifications of the health delivery system to major restructuring. Among the proposed changes are (1) replacing the present disease-specific model of medical care with "comprehensive care." Comprehensive care, which stresses advisory, preventive, and rehabilitative activities, is viewed as more personalized and more compassionate than the present segmented care (see, for example, Stevens, 1971); (2) "deprofessionalizing" medical care by shifting responsibility for major aspects of it to paraprofessionals (see, for example, Maxman, 1976); (3) decentralizing health care by shifting resources away from hospital-based care to neighborhood health centers or village clinics (see New & Hessler, 1972); (4) putting greater emphasis on the patient's own involvement in the health care process (see Stokes, 1978); (5) reordering societal priorities away from curative care and toward environmental and social prevention (see Eckholm, 1977).

Even if we ignore the inevitable resistance of the established health professions to the radical restructuring envisioned by many reformers, it is clear that the proposals disagree on specific policy recommendations. Although there is little consensus on concrete changes, a unified underlying perspective emerges: Health services must be designed to serve the healthy and to improve the health of societies rather than to cure the disease, and the focus of health care must be on the whole person in his physical and social environment. These points are echoed in the final section of this book.

The articles presented in this section examine several specific and general issues that illustrate the policy alternatives and perspectives outlined above. The first two chapters, by Carter and by Gordon, respectively, address problems in mental health services; the third, by Ahmed and Fraser, emphasizes the importance of psychosocial factors in health planning in developing countries; and the fourth, by Bourne, deals with ethical and political issues that will affect the future of health care in developing and industrial nations alike.

In the first chapter, Rosalynn Carter, in her capacity as chairperson of the President's Commission for Mental Health, presents an address delivered to the Congress of the World Federation for Mental Health in 1977. With her characteristic compassion and insight, she expounds on the stigma attached to the label of mental illness, the stigma documented and analyzed by Robitscher in Part II. She decries the stigmatizing attitude of the patient, of his family, and of the public, an attitude that causes society to discriminate against the ex-mental patient and that prevents many people from seeking professional help. She emphasizes that until mental illness "comes out of the closet" and is accepted for what it is, it will be impossible to bring professional treatment to those who need it, to reintegrate ex-patients into the community, and to allocate the necessary societal sources to fighting the problem.

Gordon, in the second chapter, calls for a restructuring of mental health services, with less emphasis on conventional mental health services and more emphasis on alternative human services. The latter refer to the institutions that grew out of the 1960s—runaway houses, crisis hot lines, drug and alcohol counseling programs, rape crisis centers, and shelters for battered women. Conventional, professionally staffed mental health services, Gordon argues, suffer from the limitations of the biomedical paradigm discussed in Part I, i.e., they focus on eliminating a specific defect or curing a specific disease. Alternative services, on the other hand, serve a broad range of human needs, using a "holistic" or "humanistic" approach, and attempting to "strengthen the whole person in his total environment." In order to achieve this, they de-emphasize professionally centered and drug-based care. They emphasize self-therapy, the use of nonprofessional staff, and alternative therapies such as meditation and biofeedback. Furthermore, they approach mental health in its entire ecological context, by counseling the patient's family and by helping the patient to change his circumstances (e.g., to combat bureaucratic abuses or to leave an intolerable marriage) rather than changing himself through tranquilizers or psychotherapy.

The third chapter, by Ahmed and Fraser, discusses the limitations of Western medical knowledge and Western technology in developing countries. The authors argue that to improve health conditions in the developing countries, medical knowledge and technology must be supplemented by both cultural understanding and social action. To illustrate the importance of sociocultural factors in defining illness and in promoting health, the authors cite several examples, ranging from the belief of Latin-American Indians that disease is caused by ritual contamination or by undue exposure to heat and cold, to the contemporary Western belief that heart disease and hypertension are caused partially by psychosocial factors. The authors contend that a purely biomedical definition of disease and purely somatic treatment leave out large dimensions of illness and health, and that this gap is even larger in developing countries than in the Western world.

As an alternative to the biomedical model, the authors suggest the ethnomedical model, developed by Fabrega and others, which incorporates culturally determined beliefs about illness and cure as well as "objective" biomedical data. They call for greater sensitivity to the cultural needs and beliefs of the people receiving Western aid. Such rapport, they assert, may be achieved by incorporating the recipient community both into the health planning and into the health delivery processes.

In the last chapter in the book, Peter Bourne extrapolates from present trends in health care into the future. He points out that as developing nations industrialize, improve their public health measures, and bring their levels of mortality and morbidity closer to those of developed countries, their health problems will begin to resemble those of the latter. These will be the problems of an aging population: increasing demand for health care facilities and increasing incidence of chronic and degenerative diseases inherent in aging.

Bourne points out that the control of these diseases, unlike that of acute diseases, is not likely to come from scientific advances in combating microorganisms but rather from educational campaigns to change lifestyles. Thus, future advances in reducing the incidence of cancer, of cardiovascular disease, and of alcoholism depend on persuading large numbers of people to stop smoking, to change their dietary habits, and to increase their level of physical activity. Although the public is likely to resent excessive governmental interference in private lives (as in the case of resistance to the mandatory wearing of seat belts), there is evidence that the public will eventually accept these measures for its own good.

Another issue likely to rise in importance is the ethical dilemmas stemming from modern medicine's power to prolong life artificially beyond its meaningful span. Bourne sees hopeful trends in various executive and legislative efforts, particularly the Commission for the Protection of Human Subjects of Biomedical and Behavioral Research, to establish guidelines for such decisions.

If there is a single theme underlying the articles in this section, as well as the other chapters in the book, it is the humanizing of health care. The need for such humanizing has long been recognized and the process long begun. The recent contributions of medical, behavioral, and social sciences have made both the need and the potential for successful implementation greater than ever.

References

Eckholm, E. P. *The picture of health: Environmental sources of disease.* New York: W. W. Norton, 1977.

Maxman, J. S. *The post-physician era: Medicine in the twenty-first century.* New York: Wiley, 1976.

New, P. K. M., & Hessler, R. M. Neighborhood health centers: Traditional medical care at an outpost? *Inquiry,* 1972, *9,* 45–58.

Stevens, R. *American medicine and the public interest.* New Haven: Yale University Press, 1971.

Stokes, B. *Local responses to global problems: A key to meeting basic human needs.* Washington: Worldwatch Institute, 1978.

19

Toward a More Caring Society

Rosalynn Carter

Not long ago, Margaret Mead came to the White House to talk to me about my interest as a volunteer and citizen advocate for mental health and my job as honorary chairperson of the President's Commission on Mental Health. She has so much knowledge and so much feeling. I have admired her for years, and I was pleased to have the chance to benefit from her wisdom.

Dr. Mead told me she believes that if we select for first consideration the most vulnerable among us—the emotionally disturbed child, the institutionalized psychotic, the street addict—then our whole culture is humanized. She believes that our value as individuals, our success as a society, can be measured by our compassion for the vulnerable.

I think that all involved in the global mental health movement agree. And yet something is wrong. Something keeps holding us back.

What is holding us back is the stigma that is attached to mental illness. Negative public attitudes are holding back progress in our field. And this self-feeding cycle of fear, discrimination, and lack of understanding about mental illness is more than a vague uneasiness we detect from time to time. It is a troubling fact. For example, a study published a few years ago revealed that out of 21 groups of disabled persons, the ex-convicts, the retarded, the alcoholics were least preferred and were way down on the list, but the mentally ill were the last. Another survey of a community that undertook a massive public education program about mental illness showed

Rosalynn Carter • The President's Commission on Mental Health (1977–1978), The White House, Washington, D. C. 20500. This chapter originally was an address delivered to the World Federation for Mental Health Congress, Vancouver, B.C., Canada, August 24, 1977.

public prejudices actually deepened and were worse after the program than before.

The hardship that this stigma creates for the individual was expressed by Priscilla Allen, one of our 20 commissioners for mental health. She is a former mental patient, and this is what she said at our very first meeting at the White House. "I am half in the closet and half out," Priscilla said. "I am a former patient, and I intended to have everyone on the commission know that; but I did not want to announce it to the United States of America. With the press here, it was really difficult for me to identify myself. *There is definitely a great deal of stigma attached to mental illness.* I have been all over the United States—Florida, Pennsylvania, and I live in California—talking about mental health issues and about patients' rights issues. But the people in the place where I live do not know, most of them, that I am a former patient. I didn't tell the manager this when I filled out the form. When I told him later, he said he was glad he hadn't known because he would not have let me in."

This was the first time, but not the last, that the commission heard firsthand testimony from several hundred professionals and lay persons about the pain and difficulties that former mental patients encounter out in the real world.

Consider Priscilla's problem—and those of thousands of others—whose right it is to have a decent place to live. Where can they turn? In spite of all our efforts, many people are still afraid to live next door to an ex-patient. They think that crime will increase, their children will be harmed, their property values will be reduced.

And although we recognize the necessity to take patients out of back rooms and closets and into community-based treatment centers, the public worries that these might be dangerous and irresponsible members of society.

In many communities in the United States, sponsors of group homes have been forced to file suit in court when local zoning appeals boards have refused occupancy permits. In Massachusetts, New York, New Jersey, and California, however, judges have ruled that group homes can be established. Clearly, we must stop using zoning laws as weapons in the fight to keep ex-mental patients out of our communities. Never mind that almost every family in that community might be touched in some way by depression, marital problems, drug- and alcohol-related problems, the inability to cope as the result of a death or a serious accident, or simply low self-esteem.

The data our commission has gathered show that the public continues to be repelled by the notion of mental illness—although it is becoming less socially acceptable to say so!

And what about getting a job if you have been labeled a mental patient? During our commission hearings, a Philadelphia labor leader admitted publicly that mental health care affects job security and advancement. He said, "It's very, very difficult to bring mental health concerns directly into the workplace because of the stigma that is definitely attached to it."

The mother of a 28-year-old mentally ill son in San Francisco told us, "He could work, but the private enterprise is not going to give any jobs to the mentally ill. He could work and it would have done more to have built back his self-confidence, which is completely gone, and his ego, which is at zero level, than any drug, anything I could do, anything we can ever do for him."

It's almost impossible to determine the magnitude of this problem because good data on the employment of people with a history of mental illness just don't exist. Ex-mental patients who succeed in the job market usually do so because they hide their past history.

And what about the dilemma that is caused by the differences in cultural heritage that prevent so many from seeking the care and treatment they rightly deserve? Our commission learned quickly from Hispanic-Americans, Indians, and other minority groups that it is absolutely essential to develop within the mental health system a real sensitivity to their special needs.

We cannot impose the Euro-American standard of treatment on everyone, especially on those who are already alienated and excluded from the mainstream. We need to tailor services to ethnic and racial minorities, and we need to launch a broad attack against stigma in communities where these citizens live.

It is not going to be easy. In San Francisco, for example, an Asian psychiatrist told us that his people "reject the idea of having a mentally ill member of the family because of feelings of fear, rejection and/or ridicule. Asian Families tend to care for psychotics at home," he said, "postponing use of mental health services until an urgent situation arises."

Another witness in Tennessee told us about a woman in a migrant camp, whose name was never known, but who had been identified by a social worker as being in desperate need of help. When a staff member charged with Migrant Services tried to find and help her, he was told that no such woman existed and that the camp would not tolerate crazy people. Several days later her body was found by the side of the road, a victim of a hit-and-run driver.

Those of us here share a central mission to understand those things that bind people of different cultures together. Whether our traditions and heritage call for self-reliance, strength, working out one's own difficulties, not burdening others with one's pain—or whether we are moved by pride, fear, or superstitition—we share our human condition.

We need to care and to be cared for. But many people do not know how to reach out. They will—in order to avoid a label—seek alternatives to professional help. Studies show that the majority of persons do not go to professionals when they are bowed down with problems. They go to clergymen, family, friends, neighbors. They seek out a helper who is "safe" and will not brand them with disgrace.

The Institute for Social Research at the University of Michigan released research showing how Americans view their mental health. They have discovered that among people who seek help, slightly less than 70% do not go to mental health professionals. The single most important reason for not getting care is that people feel they should solve their problems by themselves. The second reason they stay away is because of overriding feelings of shame. And, significantly, this shame is twice as compelling as cost.

But even when the enlightened patient finally seeks out the mental health professional, there are attitudes that need to be scrutinized. In San Francisco, I was told by a former patient, "Mrs. Carter, at the risk of offending many professionals in this room, I have run into as much prejudice and fear in the therapist as I have in the many people who encounter my history."

Another former patient told me, "At this point, many members of the mental health profession are so condescending to their clients that it is impossible to even talk to them."

So stigma is a problem in getting people into treatment in the first place; it's a problem during treatment; and it's a problem in trying to get a patient reinvolved in the community.

In addressing himself to this subject at our first White House meeting, one of our distinguished commissioners spoke out forcefully about the need for the understanding and acceptance of mental illness. He told us he did not believe that we were out of the closet at all. If we were, he reminded us, we would be getting the necessary funds for research and services from the federal, state, and local governments. He says we aren't ever going to get that support until public attitudes change.

I think he is right. We must start talking to the public as much as we talk to each other. We must expand our ranks. Consider this: In the United States our Cancer Society has 2½ million volunteers; our Heart Association has 2 million; our Mental Health Association has only about 230,000.

Yet there is no rational basis for these figures. Twenty million Americans are in need of mental health care right now—roughly 10% of the population—whereas just over a million Americans died of heart attacks last year and more than 350,000 died of cancer.

So it is not that mental illness is less prevalent than other major diseases; it is that mental illness is simply not an acceptable condition people want to talk about or deal with. And we all know this state exists because of the misconceptions that prevail. We must work harder to replace each myth about mental illness with a reassuring truth. We must stop overintellectual- izing, stop worrying about our jargon, and speak in simple, direct language that people can understand.

Let me tell you how a state senator from New Jersey suggested to me that we approach the issue. He said that in the United States we need to try to create a national commitment, a national attitude, a national climate for the proper care and treatment of the mentally ill. Because if we do this, he says, the rest—the laws, the governmental reorganizations, the funding, the services—all will fall naturally into place.

I believe that. And I believe that is a message with global significance. Those of us around the world—in developing and developed nations—must commit ourselves to the creation of a caring society with global bonds. We must create a climate in which our most vulnerable are accepted. We must start first with them. Then the rest will fall naturally into place.

Mental Health Services: Alternatives Now and for the Future

James S. Gordon

The Problem

Recent estimates suggest that as many as 2 out of 10 Americans may be in "serious need" of mental health services (Bryant, 1977). Each year almost 1% of our population is admitted to mental hospitals. And each year we consume several billion doses of Valium and Librium. Millions of people are addicted—to barbiturates, heroin, methadone, and alcohol. Psychosomatic disease is endemic. We are a people sorely troubled, desperately looking for some answer to our problems or at least some relief from them.

Too often we forget that these problems have roots in the particular conditions of our society, that any attempts to achieve "mental health" must be inseparable from efforts to create a just, decent, and personally fulfilling society. We know that poverty predisposes people to psychosis and hospitalization; that fragmenting community structures and confused family relations promote depression, alcoholism, and "schizophrenia"; that pressured and alienating working conditions precipitate psychosomatic illness and drug use; that lack of employment opportunities and isolation and institutionalization depress older people. Yet we ignore this and focus our therapeutic attentions and our economic resources on individual sufferers.

James S. Gordon • Center for Studies of Child and Family Mental Health, National Institute of Mental Health, Rockville, Maryland 20857.

We call them "mentally ill," and all too often—as if their problems were simply analogous to a physical illness—treat them with drugs and electro-shock treatment. When they do not get "better," we lock them up in mental hospitals.

During the last several decades the mental health establishment has adopted two major approaches to the American people's problems in living: biomedical research and the establishment of community mental health centers. Neither of them has lived up to the enthusiasm with which it was heralded. Both have been flawed by the pervasive and narrowing influence of a "medical model of mental illness."

Biomedical researchers, ignoring the total ecological context—whole people in families and communities, workplaces and cities—have searched for the specific anatomic locations, the physiological and biochemical causes of schizophrenia, manic-depressive psychosis, depression, and anxiety. Similarly, they have experimented with medical and surgical cures—the right drug or the right operation, the right place in the brain to stimulate or depress—just as they might with treatments for diabetes or cancer of the lung.

The most dramatic product of early biomedical research was the development of the phenothiazine group of tranquilizers (Thorazine is the best known). Their history and their limitations are instructive. When phenothiazines were introduced in 1954, they were heralded as the "cure" for schizophrenia, the salvation of state hospital patients. An immediate exodus from state and county hospitals was followed over the years by a leveling-off process. Twenty-two years later, the percentage of the overall population in mental hospitals has decreased somewhat, as has the average length of stay, but the overall number of patients admitted has remained about the same.

Some of those who have been "maintained" on phenothiazines, or the other still more potent drugs that were soon developed, seemed to function well outside the hospital. But many of them have come to feel as constricted, as robbed of their full potential, by the stupefying and numbing effects of the chemicals as they had been by the hospital walls. They felt as embarrassed and degraded by their dependency on powerful drugs and authoritarian doctors as they had by their reliance on prisonlike institutions. And many of those who felt satisfied with the emotional level on which their medication kept them have found themselves experiencing severe physical side effects—impotence, extreme sensitivity to sunlight, chronic skin rashes, easy tiring, obesity.

The passage of the Community Mental Health Centers Act in 1963 was to be an even more important milestone. Hailed as a "bold new approach" by John F. Kennedy, it signaled a modification of the medical model, a growing sensitivity to the effects of poverty and social stress on the creation of "mental illness"; an increasing awareness of the possibilities of helping people to change by working with them, their families, and their communities to change their social situation. Community mental health centers were designed to help prevent institutionalization; to bring low-cost, readily available mental health services, including individual and group psychotherapy, to large numbers of people; and to make—through "consultation and education"—changes in families, schools, and communities that would forestall the development of mental illness in their members.

In fact, the community mental health centers have never resolved the contradiction between a social and a medical definition of "mental illness." Their legislative mandate depends on their responsiveness to community needs, on their capacity for helping people not to become chronic mental patients, and, ultimately, on their ability to change those conditions that make people "mentally ill." But the political power, social prestige, professional status, and high incomes of their leaders come from their roles as doctors and mental health professionals. Too many community mental health centers simply perpetuate the medical model and in so doing provide inappropriate services.

In outpatient clinics that are little more than an aggregation of private therapists' offices, they may insist that people fit into one or another diagnostic category and predetermined therapeutic experience. Instead of providing the services—economic and educational, vocational and counseling —that are necessary to help seriously disturbed people live successfully at home and in their community, they tend to obliterate anxiety about these problems with maintenance doses of antidepressants and phenothiazines. The consultation and education that they provide is often directed at strengthening the skills of other professionals—teachers, guidance counselors, etc.—rather than, say, changing the classroom conditions that frustrate students, teachers, and guidance counselors alike. Rarely do they provide services to people who, though needy, are unwilling to define and stigmatize themselves as mentally ill. Still more rarely do staff members spend substantial amounts of time in the community they are supposed to serve.

All during my medical and psychiatric training I was deeply troubled by the institutional condescension and coercion with which the medical model was compounded—enforced medication, electroshock treatment, locked doors, and seclusion rooms—and by the narrowness to which it urged its adherents.

Doing psychotherapy with poor people in a community mental health center, I became increasingly sensitive to the wrongheadedness of an ideology that emphasized talking about intrapsychic difficulties and largely ignored the day-to-day realities that confronted people when, after an hour, they left my office. I discovered how much faster some of the most troubled people would lose their "psychotic symptoms" if I devoted more of my energy to understanding the concrete and oppressive realities of their lives —and then helped them deal with those realities.

Driving one man to a welfare office, waiting with him, helping him prod its sluggish and indifferent bureaucracy into giving him emergency payments let him know more graphically than any words that I really did "care" about him. Afterwards he spoke much more easily of his "personal" problems.

Visiting a "paranoid" teen-ager in her home I discovered that her parents *were* constantly invading and intruding—on her room, her mail, her bureau drawers, her phone calls, even the pockets of her blue jeans. I obviously had to take her seriously when she told me that "they're as crazy as I am." She couldn't possibly become less "paranoid" until they changed.

Working with a "crisis intervention team" in the psychiatric emergency room of a municipal hospital, I discovered that the vast majority of those who would have otherwise been admitted could be helped to stay at home. With the intensive involvement of the crisis team (a psychologist, a nurse, and three paraprofessionals) a family could pull together to help one of its members during a psychotic episode or suicidal depression. While they assisted family members in dealing with external problems (welfare, job, housing, food), the team used the crisis as a lever to help them understand the particular dynamics that had precipitated it. Often, in a few weeks, without hospitalizing anyone, they were able to help a family resolve a situation that had seemed intolerable.

During the time that I was in charge of a hospital ward I discovered how much better off psychotic patients—and staff—could be if they were simply treated with the respect due other human beings. In the context of a community in which they were given power over their own lives, in which they took part in making rules and in working out cooperative living arrangements, a group of "mental patients" simply stopped being so disturbed. Given trust, or at least the possibility of it, by a staff that refused to disqualify their speech and behavior as symptomatology, the patients were often able to trust and get help from staff members; free to come and go, they tended to stay and try to work out their problems; allowed to regulate their own medication, they tended to use it occasionally, when necessary, and to avoid becoming dependent on it. "Everywhere else," one "chronic schizophrenic" young man told me, "I'm crazy; here I'm sane."

Still, I concluded that the reforms that could be made within the context of traditional mental health settings were severely limited by the structure of those settings and by the ideology of mental illness to which the professionals who dominate them subscribe. When I entered the U.S. Public Health Service, I decided to look for places in which troubled people could be helped—and could help themselves—without so many constraints.

Alternative Services

Six years ago I began to work—as consultant, researcher, and colleague—with "alternative human services." I wanted to see if the ideology of professionalism really did make it more difficult to meet the needs of some troubled people; if changing the setting in which help was given and the set of those who were giving it made a substantial difference in the people who received it; if some of the culturally alien but side-effect-free techniques they were using with their clients—meditation, massage, acupressure—might contribute to promoting their well-being; and if the skills I had developed in my psychiatric training could be shared effectively with and enlarged by groups of dedicated nonprofessionals. I am still working with alternative services. I do not think they have "the answer" to people's problems in living, but they are surely dealing with them in a way that is respectful, open-minded, and effective.

Alternative services are approximately 10 years old. Most of the early ones were founded by indigenous helpers, in direct response to the physical and emotional needs of the disaffected young people who in the mid- to late 1960s migrated to their communities—as alternatives to health, mental health, and social service facilities that the young found threatening, demeaning, or unresponsive.

The founders of the first alternative services resembled the earlier settlement house workers in their idealism and humanitarianism. They differed in their commitment to the kind of participatory democracy that animated the civil rights, antiwar, youth, and women's movements of the 1960s (Gordon, 1974). These activist workers believed that, given time and space to do it, ordinary people could help themselves and one another to deal with the vast majority of problems in living that confronted them. They questioned the appropriateness of professional services that labeled or stigmatized those who came for help, and, in their own work, blurred or obliterated boundaries between staff and clients: a teenager who was panicky one night might counsel another the next. Determined to remain responsive to their clients' needs, these early workers continually advocated the social changes that would make individual change more possible.

In 1967, a handful of switchboards, drop-in centers, free clinics, and runaway houses served marginal young people in the "hip" neighborhoods of a few large cities. Today there are approximately 2,000 hot lines, over 200 runaway houses, and 400 free clinics. They have been organized by people of all ages, classes, and ideologies in small towns, suburbs, and rural areas, as well as in the large cities. In Prince George's, a suburban and rural Maryland county, for example, one of three hot lines receives 1,400 calls a month, one of two runaway houses gives shelter and intensive counseling to over 350 young people each year, and a single one of the county's nine drop-in centers provides 600 hours of individual therapy each month (Gordon, 1978b).

In the early years, alternative services were preoccupied with responding to the immediate needs of their young clients—for emergency medical care, a safe place during a bad drug trip, or short-term housing. More recently, they have expanded and diversified. Drop-in centers work with the families and teachers of the teenagers who come to them as well as with the young people themselves. Runaway houses have opened long-term residences and foster care programs for those who cannot return home or would otherwise be institutionalized, and free clinics and hot lines have helped begin specialized counseling services for other and older groups—women, gays, the elderly, etc.

In the 1970s, the alternative service model has been adopted by people who have identified new community needs. They have created drug and alcohol counseling programs, rape crisis centers, shelters for battered women, peer counseling and street work projects, and programs designed specifically for old people and particular ethnic minorities.

During this same time, increasing numbers of people have realized that physicians are not providing substantial help to the 50–80% of their patients who complain of feeling poorly but lack demonstrable organic pathology. This failure has goaded both physicians and patients to question the definitions of physical and mental health and illness under which they operate and the kinds of treatment that these definitions dictate. The focus on pathology and disease, the too-rigid separation of physical and emotional problems, the destructiveness of so many pharmaceutical and surgical remedies, the assumption of an asymmetrical relationship between an all-powerful physician and a submissive patient, and the concommitant wrenching of the process of healing from a supportive social context have all prompted clinicians, researchers, and patients to look for therapeutic measures in other traditions and other techniques.

A new approach to healing—variously called "holistic," "integral," "humanistic"—is gradually emerging from this questioning. This approach conceives of and addresses itself to the "whole person in a total environment." Disease is seen as the result of an imbalance among a variety of social, personal, and economic, as well as biological influences, and healing as a method for restoring balance within the individual and between the individual and the environment. Instead of attacking the disease process with a technological armamentarian, physician and patient, healer and healee are learning techniques that permit them to make use of what Hippocrates called the *vis medicatrix naturae*, the healing force of nature.

There is a growing emphasis on diet, exercise, and life-style as the precursors of physical and emotional dysfunction and on the relationship between stress and physical and emotional illness. Attempts to restore physical and emotional balance are making use of the centuries-old preventive medical techniques of Chinese medicine, yoga, and herbalism, of homeopathy, massage, and chiropractic, and of such modern self-help techniques as biofeedback, guided imagery, and life-style counseling. All depend on a holistic or integrated view of mind and body, an attempt to rechannel energy and strengthen the whole person rather than to eradicate illness or erase a defect.

As many as 50 to 100 holistic health and "wellness" centers—and thousands of individual practitioners and numbers of alternative services for old and young people—have begun to incorporate these techniques, to use them to relieve stress and improve overall physical, mental, and emotional functioning. At the same time research in these areas is under way. Although the results are preliminary, they are nevertheless suggestive. Holistic practices and concepts or their modern modifications may, without destructive side effects, be able to alleviate such serious medical problems as hypertension (see, for example, Benson, 1977), chronic pain (Kroenig, Volen, & Bresler, in press), and cancer (see Simonton & Simonton, 1975), for which we have so far only fragmentary answers. Some of these disciplines can be learned and practiced by lay people. Increasingly, they are being regarded by workers in a variety of alternative services as a natural complement to a system of care that emphasizes the whole person in a supportive environment, the ability of people to help themselves and one another.

Characteristics of Alternative Services

Although alternative services are as diverse in their operation, staff, and structure as in their communities and clients, they share certain philosophical assumptions, attitudes, and practices that define their approach to mental health and illness as "alternative" and make them particularly useful and responsive to the people they serve. I have found the following to be among the most significant:

They respond to people's problems as those problems are experienced. A woman whose husband is beating her is regarded as a victim, not scrutinized as a masochist. A child who leaves his home is seen, housed, and fed as a runaway, not diagnosed as an "acting-out disorder" or judged as a "status offender." A man with chronic back pain and no demonstrable organic lesion is treated as a sufferer, not dismissed as a "psycho" or a "crock."

They provide services that are immediately accessible with a minimum of waiting and bureaucratic restriction. Hot lines, shelters for battered women, rape crisis centers, runaway houses, and many drop-in centers are open 24 hours a day, free, to anyone who calls or comes in off the street.

They tend to treat their clients' problems as signs of change and opportunities for growth rather than symptoms of an illness that must be suppressed. In drug-free alternatives to mental hospitalization like Diabasis and Soteria, even psychotic episodes are regarded as potentially transformative and illuminating experiences.

They treat those who come to them for help as members of families and social systems. This enables them to view their troubled clients' "symptoms" as reactions to and communications within their familial or social situation. It provides the underpinning for their treatment of pregnancy, childbirth, and dying primarily as shared family experiences and only secondarily, and occasionally, as medical conditions or emergencies. On a programmatic level this "systems" viewpoint encourages many alternative services to advocate and work with their clients in the arena—job, home, school, or court—in which their problems arise.

They make use of mental health professionals and the techniques they have developed but depend on nonprofessionals to deliver most of the primary care. In projects as diverse as runaway houses and home birth programs, free clinics and alternatives to mental hospitalization, professionals serve almost exclusively as consultants, trainers, and emergency backup. They are there to share their knowledge with staff and clients and not necessarily to run the service.

They regard active client participation as the cornerstone of their mental health service program and indeed of mental health. On an individual therapeutic level this means emphasizing the strength of those who seek help and their capacity for self-help: Teenage runaways are encouraged to see themselves as potential agents for a family's change rather than helpless victims of its oppression; battered wives to become strong enough to leave rather than endure their husbands' brutality. In dozens of "humanistic gerontology" programs and in hundreds of free clinics and holistic healing centers, clients are encouraged to use techniques like biofeedback, progressive relaxation, acupressure, and guided imagery, and disciplines like yoga and Tai Chi to experience, and then alter, physical and emotional states that they had always regarded as beyond their control.

On an organizational level, this emphasis on self-help leads most alternative services to include present and former clients in their decision-making structure. It means devoting time and energy to creating formal and informal ways for those who have been helped to use their personal experience as a basis for helping others.

They provide both clients and staff with a supportive and enduring community that transcends the delivery or receipt of a particular service. In a time when the extended family is losing its coherence, and ties to hometowns and neighborhoods are fraying, alternative services are providing a continuing focus for collective allegiance and an opportunity for long-term mutual support. For many who have long ago ceased to be official clients or workers they remain a retreat in times of trouble and a place to gather to celebrate joyous occasions.

They regard it as their responsibility to expand the work they do to meet the changing needs of their clients. It has become clear, for example, that no counseling—whether individual, family, or group—can adequately deal with the problems of a teenager who cannot read or find work. In a time of economic recession, workers in a variety of alternative services have begun to create meaningful vocational and educational programs for unskilled and previously unemployable clients.

They can provide care that is by any standards equal or superior to that offered by traditional mental health services. Many of the reports are anecdotal (i.e., the consistent finding that large numbers of young people with psychotic or borderline diagnoses are diverted from hospitalization by a variety of alternative services), but "harder" data are also beginning to accumulate: A 2-year follow up study of Soteria, a National Institute of Mental Health funded residential alternative to hospitalization, revealed that residents of the program "showed significantly better occupational levels and were more able to leave home to live independent of their families of origin" than a control group of people hospitalized on a crisis-oriented general hospital ward (Mosher & Menn, 1977); evaluation of the Senior Actualization and Growth Explorations (SAGE) project in Berkeley has revealed striking psychological, cognitive, and physical improvements in the older people who participated in the program of gentle physical exercise, meditation, and group discussion (personal communication from the evaluator, M. Lieberman, 1978); and a matched population study of 1,046 home births and 1,046 hospital births has revealed significantly more infections and birth injuries in the group of babies that was delivered in the hospital (Mehl, 1977).

They are in general more economical than the traditional services that their clients might otherwise use. Young people, many of whom come to runaway centers to avoid being hospitalized, provide an interesting example: In 1975, an NIMH study of 15 runaway centers around the country revealed that runaway centers spent from $32 to $50 a day for each young person housed; in contrast, the figures for acute care hospitalization ranged from $125 to $200 a day (Gordon, 1975). A more recent and sophisticated analysis of one runaway house, Someplace Else, in Tallahassee, Florida, revealed that this program was approximately three times as cost-effective as the services routinely offered by the county. Long-term residential alternatives to hospitalization for adults like Soteria and the Training in Community Living program of the Mendota Mental Health Institute tend to be

more expensive, but here, too, cost-benefit analysis seems to reveal significant advantages for the alternative services (Weisbrod, Test, & Stein,
1977).

They have financial problems. The desire to work with whoever comes
to them regardless of economic compensation; their attempts to provide
comprehensive and often unreimbursed services; their unwillingness to take
funds that restrict their work with clients; the complexity of federal, state,
and local funding procedures; and the general reluctance of many agencies
to fund service programs that are neither certified by a professional establishment nor proven in "scientific terms" all conspire to keep most alternative services chronically underfunded.

*They use their experience in trying to meet people's direct service needs
as a basis for advocacy efforts on their clients' behalf.* Hot lines that have
noted an increase in a particular kind of problem—battered women, child
abuse, etc.—have used their statistical information and their moral authority as service providers to prod local mental health and social service agencies to create programs to meet these needs. Groups that serve old people,
pregnant women, and runaways have organized on a state and national
level to advocate legislation and funding to further and protect their clients'
interests.

Recommendations for the Future

Many alternative services combine the skills and thoroughness of professionals with the commitment to service, the responsiveness, and the
organizational flexibility of nonprofessionals. They are already providing
effective low-cost mental health services to large numbers—probably several millions—of Americans of all ages, races, and classes (Gordon, 1978a).
Any attempt to make mental health services more responsive to people's felt
needs should take account of the kinds of programmatic innovations that
alternative services have been making, of the new techniques being developed in holistic health practice, and of the spirit that pervades the entire
alternative service movement. These objectives can be accomplished in two
ways: by encouraging the growth and development of those alternative
services that already exist, and by promoting the creation of a new kind of
smaller, more flexible, comprehensive human service facility.

Supporting Alternative Services

Some alternative services define themselves explicitly as part of an
emerging mental health movement, one that combines psychological attention with physical care and social activism to provide effective low-cost

mental health services. These programs—including approximately 50 residential alternatives to hospitalization, several thousand hot lines, and hundreds of crisis outreach programs and drop-in centers—already solicit and sometimes receive local, state, or federal mental health funding. They are eager to be funded as community mental health centers or to work out fee-for-service arrangements with third-party providers. Other services, including centers for runaway youth, battered women, and rape victims, and long-term residences for young people, receive local social service or Social Security Act (Title XX) money or obtain funding from the Administration for Children, Youth, and Families or the Law Enforcement Assistance Administration.

Although some of these programs are currently receiving attention and support from the mental health and social service establishment, many of them are still grossly underfunded, and many of those that are funded adequately are hobbled by restrictions on the kinds of clients they may serve or the way they deliver those services. To facilitate the current operation and continued evolution of these alternative services, funding agencies will themselves have to adopt some "alternative" attitudes and strategies. Among the changes that could be made in the way mental health and human service programs are legislated, organized, and funded are the following:

1. *Community groups that are already providing services—whether they be shelters for battered women, runaway centers, holistic health programs, or alternatives to mental hospitalization—should be involved in the legislative and funding process at each step.* They should be asked to testify and be included on agency review panels (from which, because of their lack of credentials or establishment connections, they are almost always excluded), and on the state or local boards that may ultimately decide where some of the monies go. When money comes directly from federal agencies, notice should be sent to alternative services that might be interested. (This recommendation has, incidentally, been accepted by the President's Commission on Mental Health, although no strategy for implementation is as yet under way.)

2. *Community groups that have already been providing services should be given first priority in receiving money for those services, in providing training for workers in them and in doing research on them.* The Family Violence Prevention and Treatment Act (HR 4948) introduced by Congresswoman Barbara Mikulski addresses some of these problems: "The most effective direct service programs for the victims of family violence have been developed in the private voluntary sector of dedicated volunteers, and the most effective approach to the delivery of social services to such victims has involved person to person support systems and an emphasis on self help." If experts—individuals, consulting firms, university professors—are

necessary for a particular research or training project, they should work as
subcontractors to the people who are providing the services, not vice versa.

3. *Legislation should always be designed for the broadest possible
group of people and that group should be defined in the least pejorative,
simplest way.* There is an enormous temptation in formulating legislation to
focus on problems. Perhaps it looks or feels good to be outraged by juvenile
crime, concerned about runaways, or troubled by the plight of the "mentally ill." As it happens, these attitudes often become part of the problem,
not their solution. Just as policemen cannot work without criminals, so
programs for runaways, juvenile delinquents, drug abusers, or the mentally
ill cannot survive without people to fit these categories. Programs are thus
induced to perpetuate the conditions and the labeling that they are supposed
to remedy. (The director of one drop-in center told me that to provide her
services it defined as a drug abuser a troubled young woman who smoked
two marijuana cigarettes a week, and that when funding switched from
"drug abuse" to "law enforcement money" he encouraged her parents to
declare her "in need of supervision," so the agency might continue its
services to her.)

Although categorical funding was useful in the creation of many alternative services, it is now often an impediment to their growth and development. A new mental health initiative could encourage rather than restrict
the natural evolution of these community-based alternatives by funding
them to provide a wider range of services to a broader population. Instead of
simply housing runaways or counseling drug abusers, runaway centers or
drop-in facilities could become comprehensive youth and family services;
experimental programs for "first-break schizophrenics" could become asylums for all community persons in need; and a house for battered women or
a rape crisis hot line could easily become the nucleus for a community
women's center.

4. *Legislation and regulations should help ensure the responsiveness of
all services (alternative and otherwise) to their clients by insisting that all
funded programs recruit clients and community people to work as volunteers and paid staff in their services, and to sit on their decision-making
boards.*

5. *Mental health agencies should promote effective and sensitive monitoring of grants and contracts by insisting that all project officers, and
indeed all program administrators, spend some part of their time involved in
direct service work in their local communities, preferably in projects similar
to the ones that they are charged with administering.*

6. *Mental health agencies should substitute a process of conscientious
and informed monitoring for some of the vast amounts of paper work normally required.* Lengthy client forms and reporting requirements prevent
many alternative services from applying for federal money and tend to

bureaucratize those that receive it and estrange them—or at least some workers in them—from their clients.

7. *Legislation should mandate a variety of mental health (as well as other federal and state agencies) to award small amounts of money with minimal application forms and reporting requirements to community service groups.* To a group of volunteers trying to rent a house for a shelter, or an office for a drop-in center, $5,000 can make the difference between survival and growth and organizational collapse. A similar bill for Youth Crisis Centers was introduced by Vice-President, then Senator, Walter Mondale several years ago.

8. *The executive should create an office within the federal government that would facilitate the exchange of information between alternative services and Congress and the federal agencies, and among alternative services.* This agency would also act as an "ombudsperson" for alternative services, continually raising federal consciousness about kinds of needs the community workers were discovering and what kinds of mental health services were being developed to meet them. This office could also provide community-based alternative services with technical assistance in preparing grant applications.

Learning from Alternative Services

If supporting alternative services is important, learning from them is crucial. The principles—and the spirit—that animate them are remarkably close to those with which the community mental health movement began. They could easily be the basis for creating new kinds of central places—or for reforming those that currently exist—where troubled and troubling people could be offered services. These new places could continue to be called community mental health centers, but they might better be called "human service centers" or "community centers" or simply "centers." The names, designed to indicate a responsiveness to people's needs, would avoid creating the feelings of deprecation inevitably associated with describing oneself as "mentally ill."

Instead of spending the majority of their time seeing patients in their offices, professionals in these centers would devote themselves largely to a much expanded version of the "consultation and education" that is now so often neglected. Their primary job would be to consult with community people about the services they have already begun, and to catalyze, but not dominate, efforts to create new residential, counseling, and community development programs.

Rather than define problems in mental health terminology, center staff would help people to define their own problems in their own terms. If a woman with five children were suicidally depressed because of the inadequacy of her welfare payments, the dreariness of her home, and the rats that threaten her family, the center's crisis team would work first of all on these realities: help her deal with the welfare department, assist her with child care, and bring in an exterminator. Instead of involving her in long-term psychotherapy or drug treatment, it might help her become part of a support group of parents in similar situations. In the context of this group she might at some point feel free to talk about the "personal problems" that so many mental health professionals would insist on "attacking" first.

For people who needed them, various kinds of residences would be available. Thus, someone experiencing the personality disintegration and overwhelming anxiety that often signal an acute psychotic episode would be able to go to a crisis house or to stay with a family where he could be guided and protected by a specially patient and skillful staff. There, symptoms would not be suppressed by drugs. Instead, the psychotic episode could become the kind of natural healing process that it is in some traditional societies and in such modern experimental communities as California's Soteria and Diabasis. Similarly, center workers might consult with or help start shelters for other groups—young people who could not live at home or "women in transition" or older individuals without social supports—where these people could gain perspective on their lives and share their problems without defining themselves as mentally ill.

Although a dangerous and uncontrollable few would continue to require institutionalization, the vast majority of those who need longer-term care could be kept in their own communities—in ordinary houses easily accessible to friends and relatives. Many of these people could—if staff workers provided organization and leadership—learn to take care of one another. Already some shelters for battered women and residences for older teenagers are run by clients; certainly old people who are healthy but homeless could supervise the care of young people who are chronically ill; and students at colleges or young workers could be subsidized—well below the cost of conventional foster care—to live with runaways who lack homes to return to.

The majority of people with problems do not, of course, need crisis intervention or residential services. Instead of assuming they needed "therapy," centers would offer them the resources—professional expertise, advocacy, and education—to help them deal with their own problems. People would be helped to understand themselves as participants in and, often enough, sufferers from the concrete situations of their life—a part of a family, an office, a work group, or a class. Techniques of family counseling, group therapy, and community organizing could be used to help make the family, the classroom, or the workplace more responsive to all its participants, to give them the tools to continue to work things out long after the center workers withdraw.

At the same time, some centers might begin to provide the kind of ongoing individualized health care that has been lacking in our society. Under the supervision of physicians who are developing a holistic perspective on health and mental health, physician's assistants, nurse practitioners, and neighborhood people trained by them could discuss and review each person's physical and emotional well-being, could investigate the economic, occupational, familial, and intrapsychic causes of stress in their lives. Together they could formulate a regime of diet, exercise, and relaxation, or help them to look for other employment, more education, or different housing.

Groups of people with special concerns or problems—women wanting to share with each other questions about their roles as women; parents of retarded or autistic children; old people wishing to improve their psychological and physical functioning—would be helped, if needed, to form groups with or without a leader in which they could discuss and deal with their common concerns.

Individual therapy would still be available, but there would be a shift in emphasis toward helping people to develop the capacity to analyze their social situations and physical and emotional needs and thus be able to use a network of helpers both within the center and outside. The biological aspect of their treatment would also change: Instead of relying on drugs to elevate mood or calm anxiety, to deaden headaches or stop gastric secretion, people would be taught to deal with these conditions through biofeedback, meditation, yoga, acupressure, Tai Chi, and massage. Learning to use these "self-help" techniques would enable people to avoid prolonged dependency on professional helpers, contribute to their sense of control over their own lives, and remove the possibility of dangerous side effects and diminished performance that always attend the use of psychotropic drugs.

This kind of center could be a continuing source of the kinds of "primary prevention" programs that the mental health establishment often talks of but rarely spends time and money to bring about. Together, staff and clients of the center could help other agencies develop education, recreation, and community action programs, and campaign for more responsive policies in the institutions that affect people's lives—from welfare offices to hospitals to factories. For the community as a whole, the center—which, like other federally funded programs, would have clients on its governing board—would be the kind of gathering place that alternative services already are, a place where people could come when they wanted to help as well as be helped, when they just felt like being with others, as well as when they were in trouble.

A mental health facility that regarded its mission as promoting health in a community rather than treating "sick" individuals, that reached out to people in flexible individualized ways rather than called them in for appointments, that saw itself as a center of community activity, not a "treatment facility" would probably be best funded under a system of block grants or as part of a National Health Service of the kind proposed by Representative Ron Dellums of Berkeley, California. A fee-for-service model—either as it exists now or as it might under a National Health Insurance —would inevitably be counterproductive, reintroducing the kind of labeling, strictures, and stigmatization that these centers would aim to eliminate.

Creating the kinds of programs I have described would, of course, have certain research implications. Among them are the following: (1) We will want to know what new community programs are most effective and why, and how working in this new kind of center changes the roles of mental health professionals and, indeed, our ideas about mental health and illness. (2) As a complement to programs that are seeking to promote health, we will want to know more about why our working and living conditions make us so tense and so prone to psychosomatic illness, hypertension, and alcoholism, and what we can, as individuals and as a community, do about these conditions. (3) We will also want to understand the basis for and potential of "alternative" therapies that turn out to be empirically useful. Their success may make us wonder why, for example, a neurochemical level of analysis should necessarily be more likely to lead us to the biological basis or correlates of schizophrenia than, say, an analysis undertaken at the level of energy balance in the acupuncture meridians.

Any attempt to make the kinds of changes in service and attitudes that I have described will also require a new kind of training, not only of the physicians, psychologists, and social workers who will help facilitate this change but of the paraprofessionals and the clients with whom they will work. Professionals need training that helps them to understand how their attitudes and convictions are formed by their own values and culture, and how these may at times prevent them from working effectively with people. They need to learn also that in addition to being bearers of knowledge and purveyors of new techniques, they are the servants of those for whom they work. At the same time, community people who crave a common purpose and some larger goal will have the opportunity to learn and use new skills.

In the context of a participatory healing community, the boundaries between helpers and helped will blur and the very nature of mental health work will be transformed. Even the most arduous tasks may well change their character: For most attendants the experience of working with mad people in a hospital setting is grim, demeaning, and uncomfortable; working with the same people in a place like Soteria or Diabasis or in one of the group foster homes that I have worked with is, though exhausting, enormously exciting and challenging.

The point of all this is not simply to produce another kind of treatment or another kind of professional, and certainly not to insist that all centers do all things in a particular way; but it is to change the structure of treatment and the delivery of services; to relate to troubled people on their terms; to insist that their needs—not the preconceptions or self-interest of any professional group—shape the kind of help they receive; to give them the opportunity to use their full potential and to heal themselves; and to support and enlarge—not usurp—the kinds of initiatives that alternative services have already taken. None of the reforms I have proposed is Utopian—and all of them together will not of course create a Utopia—but they are a start, a step toward relieving at least some of the human misery that we have too complacently and too long regarded as the symptoms of mental illness.

References

Benson, H. Systemic hypertension and the relaxation response. *New England Journal of Medicine*, 1977, *296*(20), 1152–1155.

Bryant, T. Preliminary report of the President's Commission on Mental Health, September 1, 1977.

Gordon, J. S. Coming together: Consultation with young people. *Social Policy*, 1974, *40*, 52.

Gordon, J. S. *Alternative services: A recommendation for public funding.* Unpublished, 1975.

Gordon, J. S. Final report of the Special Study on Alternative Services to the President's Commission on Mental Health, February 1978. (a)

Gordon, J. S. Statistics gathered by the Special Study on Alternative Services for the President's Commission on Mental Health, 1978. (b)

Kroenig, R., Volen, M., & Bresler, D. Acupuncture: Clinical applications and current status in America. In J. Gordon, D. Jaffe, & D. Bresler (Eds.), *Body, mind and health: Toward an integral medicine.* Washington, D.C.: National Institute of Mental Health, in press.

Mehl, L. E. Scientific research on alternatives in child birth: What can it tell us about hospital practice? In *Twenty-first century obstetrics* (Vol. 1). Marble Hill, Missouri: NAPSAC, 1977.

Mosher, L. R., & Menn, A. Z. *Community residential treatment for schizophrenia: Two year follow-up data.* Unpublished, 1977.

Simonton, O. C., & Simonton, S. S. Belief systems and management of the emotional aspects of malignancy. *Journal of Transpersonal Psychology*, 1975, *7*(1), 29–47.

Weisbrod, B. A., Test, M. A., & Stein, L. I. *An alternative to the mental hospital—Benefits and cost.* Unpublished, 1977.

21

International Health Planning: Psychosocial Issues and Implications for Development Assistance

Paul I. Ahmed and Renee White Fraser

International health planning has, for the last three decades, faced the challenge of providing effective health care for all the people of each nation. The donor nations have spent billions of dollars to improve the health status of people in the developing countries. The multilateral lending institutions, such as the World Bank, have made large health loans based on their perspective of what the countries needed. Technologies and advisors are pouring into developing countries to assist their bureaucracies in the management of their health systems, to train manpower, to supply drugs, and to clean water. Has this massive help been successful to date? Have the donor nations met the challenge of providing appropriate assistance to the developing countries? Are there new approaches to health planning that need to be considered?

Paul I. Ahmed • Office of International Health, U.S. Department of Health, Education and Welfare, Rockville, Maryland 20857. **Renee White Fraser** • University of Southern California, Los Angeles, California 90007. This chapter originally was a paper delivered to a session in International Health Planning, World Congress of Mental Health, Vancouver, B.C., Canada, August 21–28, 1977. A later version was presented at the International Congress of Anthropological and Ethnological Sciences, New Delhi, December 17, 1978. The views presented here are those of the authors, and no endorsement from HEW or USAID is assumed or implied.

This article tries to answer some of these fundamental questions, and offers an alternative approach to the challenge in a conceptual framework that includes sociocultural factors in international health planning. Many of the donor nation bureaucracies pay lip service to sociocultural factors as being good, helpful, and even important, but they have not found an operational method to include these elements in their project planning. It is our contention not only that sociocultural factors must be included systematically in international health planning but that the communities involved should participate in planning and providing services, no matter what the origin of money for the project. The work of one of the authors in mental health planning (Ahmed & Plog, 1976; Plog & Ahmed, 1977) has supported the thesis that roots of mental health lie very deep in the community, and that effective planning needs the participation of those affected by it. We suggest the same is true in health. This chapter will deal with a psychosocial framework for the conceptualization of health and health planning that will lead to community participation work. Community participation in itself is a subject for another time.

Where are we today in our efforts to help developing countries? The answer to this is given by the director-general of the World Health Organization, Dr. Hafsden Mahler, who stated that "the most signal failure of the World Health Organization, as well as of Member States, has undoubtedly been their inability to provide the development of basic health services" (Cahill, 1976).

Kurt Waldheim, as secretary general of the United Nations, reflecting on this remark, has supported the availability of basic health facilities for all. By "basic health services," it is meant: preventive health care for urban and rural populations, clean water, the provision of basic medicines, hygiene, decent standards of living, the disposal of sewage, balanced diets, and knowledge of birth control. Waldheim states that "it is our judgment that in the developing countries—where in some areas there is only one doctor to 40,000 people—it is *undoubtedly possible* to design a health-delivery system that has wide coverage, that people can afford, and that provides the primary essentials" (Waldheim, 1976).

Given the many, well-considered descriptions of what is needed to provide basic, effective health care and the equally well-considered evaluations that systems to provide such care *are possible* for the developing countries, we must ask ourselves what has gone wrong. Indeed, what attempts have been made; how may we profit from those experiences; and what do medical science and the social sciences have to offer the developing countries?

A review of comments from individuals who have been leaders in the field of providing for and studying health care in these countries leads to several mitigating and handicapping factors. However, one dramatic error stands out. According to Bryant (1969):

A root cause of these inadequacies in the less developed countries is that their patterns of medical care and education of health personnel are copied closely from the Western countries, particularly Britain, France, and the United States. There has been great reluctance to deviate from these patterns, even though they are often seriously irrelevant for the less developed countries.

What is known today as "Western" medicine is largely derived from European and American practices. It is only recently (the past 50 years) that this medicine has had a "scientific basis, has been able to systematically understand many diseases, and produce what Dubos calls "the magic bullets of medicine." Yet in a relatively short time, Western medicine has come to dominate most of the responses to health and illness throughout the world.

Along with this approach to health care, there has been a growing, if long overdue, appreciation that transferring Western medical technology, systems, and approaches to developing lands is often an absolute detriment to an effective and appropriate health delivery service (Cahill, 1976). It has become increasingly evident that many of the most intractable health problems are closely linked to factors of the environment, life-styles, social customs, and other crucial elements that are not part of the Western tradition.

The evidence abounds in developing countries of the problems associated with creating programs based on Western medical premises without consideration of the relevant cross-cultural variations. Benjamin Paul (1955) presents a series of case studies on this problem. One particularly devastating example comes from Somalia. When that East African nation attained independence, the European Economic Community (EEC) presented to that nation of nomads an ultramodern hospital—a building that belonged in Brussels. The structure almost reduced the nation's health budget to the breaking point while also centralizing almost all medical services in the capital city. The hospital served the wealthy few, but the great majority of the population, nomads, suffered even more neglect. Similar is the case in Liberia, where the budget of the JFK hospital is bigger than that of the Ministry of Health.

There are major deficiencies in our "scientific" curative approach to important diseases. The relative helplessness Western medicine has demonstrated in treating patients with schistosomiasis and liver-fluke diseases are well-known examples. McDermott has pointed out that Western medicine lacks truly decisive treatment or preventives for the leading causes of death and disability in young children: diarrhea and respiratory diseases. The malnutrition, he relates, is a consequence of the eating problems and cultural beliefs of these people. These observations lead to the important point that some of the leading causes of mortality and morbidity are not subject to the easily packaged cures of modern medicine but are tied up with culture, customs, and the ways in which people live their lives.

The Technology Transfer and Behavior Technology

For people in developing countries, part of the Western dream is the application of science and technology to health. To fulfill this dream, the West has exported its technology. With technology we implement the reduction and disposal of wastes; for populations we develop extensive drinking water and recreational water facilities. In part, because of the West's remarkable achievements, which have resulted in health improvements in this country, there exists a great desire to share this knowledge. However, neither the generic value of the technology nor the appropriateness of such technology to developing countries is clear. The introduction of technology brings inevitable problems. Chemical agents filtering water are now suspected to be cancer-provoking. Mosquitos have become resistant to DDT, allowing new outbreaks of malaria in Nepal and Pakistan. Many of the additives in bread and enriched flour may lead to cancer of the colon. Bacteria formerly treated with antibiotics are now immune to these same drugs. The limitations of Western technology are, however, rarely discussed fully in the developing countries. Complex technology, with its inherent risks for developing countries, is far from understood: even when understood, risk–benefit judgments are not always made. For example, drugs that are controlled in the West are distributed in the developing country openly, without prescription or warning. Chlormycitin is still being sent in loads without warning of its side effects to the dispensers or the users. The birth control pill is still distributed to women unaware of its side effects.

It seems clear now that the application of physical and biological sciences alone will not solve the problems; the solutions lie elsewhere. Only if people are willing to use birth control methods can better contraceptives control population. Clean drinking water is beneficial only if used consistently for all ingestion purposes and dishwashing, and only if it is accepted by the consumers as *better* water. Sanitation projects will work more effectively if they instigate the general practices of good hygiene among families. In short, physical and biological technology are less than fully effective without a supporting knowledge, some degree of understanding, and practice with behavior change.

In the developing countries there is a large gap between what medicine is capable of producing, what resources are available, and what is being produced. The possession of technology has not led to its effective application in the real local setting. For example, anemias, with nutritional origins, are common in the developing world. Young children, pregnant women, and nursing mothers frequently have a low level of hemoglobin and require more iron in their diet. Although iron is cheap and available to most who need it, we have not found a method of increasing the iron intake of vulnerable groups. Similarly, the same situation exists with vitamin A distribution, a deficiency of which leads to xerophthalmia and keratomalacia. Synthetic vitamin A is produced commercially at a relatively low price, yet the vitamin A problem is still with us. Thus, we have technology without the ability to translate it into local level action.

One reason offered for these problems is the developing nations' lack of motivation to apply therapeutic technology. It is argued that the expense is too great or that many donor technologies are unsuitable. While this may be true for some of the higher priced technologies, it is not a general rule, as illustrated by the problems with vitamin A and iron distribution. Probably the reason is somewhat deeper and understandable. The therapeutic technologies require health manpower resources, equipment, implementation techniques, and monies not at the disposal of a developing country. Most popular are those technologies that can be applied through the village. But application of even a preventive technology like inoculation requires social technology, for it involves significant modifications in the people's life-style and acceptance by them of Western concepts of medicine. No technology, whether therapeutic or preventive, can be transferred without changes in attitudes and behavior by the intended recipients. We must have social understanding along with technology.

The absence of social technology has made the donors of the Western world into the shippers of hardware technology. The donor agencies have become "shipping agents" instead of participants in a culture. The reasons for this concept of the aid function are found in the assumptions under which the donor programs operate (Foster, 1977). Some of the assumptions are:

1. Western clinical practices and institutional systems are universal in acceptance and application. The faulty expectation that accompanies this attitude is that other societies will naturally desire to emulate the West and will insist upon the adoption of modern medicine with its accompanying systems.

2. Problems encountered in developing a user population and in gaining acceptance are attributed almost exclusively to the locals. There is an implicit assumption that their attitudes and motivations must be changed rather than that examination of and/or change in the program or services be made. Reasons for lack of acceptance are most likely to be in both

camps. But the bureaucracies of donor nations must comprehend and acknowledge the incentives that history illustrates in order to make their programs effective.

3. The absence of the application of a careful social technology is also evident in the bureaucracies of some developing nations. The specialists and medical professionals who staff the bureaucracies in most receiving nations usually have been trained in the West. As such, they have grown to accept and appreciate the benefits of that system. Thus, the bureaucracies of developing nations accept the programs of donor nations due to familiarity and the recommendations of other bureaucrats, rather than because of the usefulness of the programs in meeting the needs and expectations of the local people.

4. Since the West has developed an effective health technology of infectious diseases, there exists an assumption that by the same means it can master all diseases. But this is not the case. In fact, the West has much to learn from the developing world. Healers in those countries have been able to identify and affect some of the psychosocial variables, impacting on heart disease, obesity, hypertension, etc. Many of those stress variables the West is just now discovering; it has now emerged in the United States that stress is a factor in eight out of ten leading causes of mortality.

The answer may be in a compromise between indigenous systems or traditional systems of medicine and the Western approach. Acute and infectious diseases yielding to treatment by antibiotics and vaccines should be treated by allopathic doctors. Disorders with major psychological components should remain the domain of the traditional healers, hakims, etc. Furthermore, both types of healers working together will create a more effective and more popular health system. So the developing countries, even if they are willing, should not abandon their own methods and only replicate the Western system.

The Patterning of Culture

A fundamental reason for the inadequacy in transferring Western medicine to developing countries is that each culture has its own way of organizing experience. In the area of health, communities vary in their manner of segmenting the gradient of health/illness and in the kinds of phenomena to which these states of health are assumed to be connected. The dividing line between normalcy and illness shifts from one group to another, and the categories of sickness are subject to cultural variation. Without awareness of these variations and sensitivity to the perceptions of health and illness in each culture, one cannot provide effective "health" care.

For example, the mestizo population of coastal Peru and Chile divide systems of medicine into two classes, scientific and popular, and diseases into five major categories: obstruction of the gastrointestinal tract, undue exposure to heat or cold, exposure to "bad" air, severe emotional upset, and contamination by ritually unclean persons. Household remedies are appropriate for all classes of sickness. "Scientific" doctors may be consulted, but only for illnesses assigned to the first two categories. For the other classes of sickness, only household remedies are deemed appropriate; if these fail, a folk specialist is called. Mestizos have patronized clinics and doctors for other matters but not for maladies popularly ascribed to air, emotional upset, or ritual uncleanliness. For those disorders, it has been thought that doctors' remedies from Western medicine are ineffectual or actually harmful because the Western-trained doctor does not "know" these illnesses and does not "believe" in them. Yet because of the similarities in symptomatology, tuberculosis sometimes masquerades as "fright" and so remains inaccessible to the doctor or the health center (Simmons, 1955).

The history of culture shows that communities and nations accept only *some* of the elements available for borrowing from another culture. Moreover, the borrowed idea or practice is usually *reinterpreted* and *modified* to fit the particular environmental and cultural framework (Paul, 1955).

Programs that seek to alter health practices and attitudes constitute efforts to change the local culture. These health innovations are subject to selective acceptance and modification. Indeed, acceptance or modification is not a random process but depends on (1) how the new idea is perceived by the potential recipients, (2) how it accords with their values and assumptions, (3) whether it is consistent with their system of social relationships, (4) the status of the innovation, and (5) the implications of that status for the various segments of the community.

Some resistances to change can be reduced by changing the presentation of the innovation to consider the particular culture. Certainly, any attempted change should not challenge established beliefs or practices that are fundamental to the stability of the particular social or cultural system. Any attempt to effect changes in health care must be considerate of these established beliefs and practices. In the past, the Western approach has been to provide needed changes in health facilities, treatment, and/or sanitation. But often these changes have not impacted the health situation because of a lack of foresight in considering the complete conception that a culture has of health.

The "Western" Approach

A basic proposition for providing effective health care in any non-Western culture has been to be aware of the basic beliefs and practices that are fundamental to a culture. It is clear that the imposition of the "Western" medical approach has proved ineffective. If we are to be sensitive to cultural variation and still attempt to provide the benefits of Western medicine to the developing world, how are we to accomplish it? Some translation must occur. Perhaps one should begin by understanding the "Western" approach.

The "Western" approach adheres to the medical model. Discussing both physical and mental illness, Ludwig (1975) posits that the medical model premises "that sufficient deviation from the normal represents *disease*, that disease is due to known or unknown natural causes, and that elimination of these causes will result in cure or improvement in individual patients." This reflects the dominant model of disease in Western culture, which is biomedical. Molecular biology is its basic scientific discipline. It assumes disease to be fully accounted for by deviations from the norm of measurable biological (somatic) variables. It leaves no room within its framework for the social, cultural, psychological, and behavioral dimensions that are so salient in the conceptions of illness held in developing countries.

Biomedicine constitutes the West's own culturally specific perspective about what disease is and how medical treatment should be pursued. Like other systems of belief, biomedicine is an interpretation that makes sense in light of Western cultural traditions and assumptions about reality (Fabrega, 1974).

The biomedical model was devised by medical scientists for the study of disease. Terms such as *diabetes, rheumatoid arthritis* or *multiple schlerosis* seem deceptively simple. A careful description will disclose that they represent a complex set of physiologic, chemical, and structural facts. Such diseases can implicate a host of social and phychological factors, but they are not seen as necessary features of the disease. As Fabrega (1974) points out, when examined logically, disease in biomedicine usually refers to undesirable deviations in a cluster of related physiological and chemical variables. An implicit assumption (and perhaps an erroneous one) is that many of the values of key variables that reflect physiological and chemical processes in man conform to narrow ranges that are common to the species as a whole. Verbal reports or behavioral changes, or both, constitute signals of biomedical disease. These behavioral changes have been abstracted out of Western custom and social behavior.

Engel (1977), in a recent article in *Science,* traces the historical origins of the reductionistic biomedical model. He examines the limitations of the biomedical model within Western medicine and particularly for psychological disorders. Engel suggests that concentration on the biomedical and exclusion of the psychosocial distorts perspectives and even interferes with patient care. The criticism Engel is making is even more important in the case of applying the methods, categories, and techniques of this system to developing countries.

Engel posits six hazards to the biomedical model in an application to the reality of diabetes and schizophrenia as human experiences as well as disease abstractions. The analogy that he draws between somatic and mental disorders provides an interesting characterization; however, the discussion has another useful purpose for this presentation. Engel has presented six liabilities of the model that account for many of the errors found in imposing Western medicine on the developing world.

The negative consequences for health that result from the application of this model are as follows:

1. The presence of the biochemical defect defines necessary, but not always *sufficient*, conditions for the occurrence of the human experience of disease. Attention to the variability in clinical expression and individual experience within a culture is necessary to accurately identify illness, but this is not promoted in the biomedical model. Instead, this leads to a false consensus between the doctor and the patient—a very crucial problem in creating health services in developing countries.

2. The biomedical model encourages bypassing patients' verbal accounts by placing greater reliance on technical measurements. At the same time, verbal expressions of sickness and symptoms are ambiguous and often a result of the specific socialization within a culture. At times the same words may serve to express primarily psychological as well as bodily disturbances, both of which may coexist and overlap in complex ways (for example, fright and tuberculosis among the mestizos; virtually each of the symptoms classically associated with diabetes may also be expressions of or reactions to psychological stress).

3. The role of psychosocial variables in disease causation is blurred with the use of this model. Cassel's (Waldheim, 1976) identification of higher rates of illness among populations exposed to incongruity between the demands of the social system in which they live and the culture they bring with them illustrates the importance of such factors. Certainly the adjective *developing,* applied to the third world countries, implies that the psychosocial factors would be critical in understanding sickness in these nations.

4. The biochemical defect may determine certain characteristics of the disease, but not necessarily the point at which the individual accepts the sick role or acknowledges the illness. In the case of providing a new health service to a people, this information would be critical for providing an effective health care system.

5. Treatment directed only at the biochemical abnormality does not necessarily restore the patient to health. Psychological and social variables

are often responsible for the discrepancy between correction of the biological abnormality and treatment outcome. Additionally, in developing countries, the shortsighted approach of the biomedical model leads to the identification of single causes for sickness, whereas attention to cultural and social factors is more likely to provide a multicausal perspective.

6. The behavior of the physician and the relationship between patient and physician powerfully influence treatment. Furthermore, the successful application of treatment is limited by the health practitioner's ability to influence and modify the patient's behavior. This is particularly true in developing countries where treatment techniques, and often the practitioners, are alien. The focus afforded by the biomedical model directs the practitioners away from the psychological, social, and cultural factors related to disease. Yet these are the aspects most immediate and important to the patients. Such a restricted viewpoint in a developing country enhances suspicion and decreases the credibility and trust people will place in health practitioners.

Engel has suggested that the biomedical model is disadvantageous for Western culture, and we have suggested that those disadvantages are even more critical in developing countries. In fact, it is the medical model itself that appears to be at fault in imposing Western medicine on the traditional cultures of developing countries.

Alternatives to the Biomedical Model

An alternative to the Western biomedical model is a biopsychosocial model suggested by Engel. This model would lead a physician to weigh the relative contributions of social and psychological as well as of biological factors implicated in the patient's case. Engel does not delineate how one goes about gaining this information. In particular, it is not clear how one deals with a variety of cultures. A reliance on cultural definitions of diseases would lead to a relativism that would defy utility.

Fabrega (1975) has postulated another approach, which he has labeled ethnomedical. He suggests that we find order and regularity in the forms of disease using a social frame of reference instead of the biomedical. This would include a set of more or less universal indicators of disease that are rooted in social categories. Thus, an illness could be diagnosed and labeled by the tasks and activities that *interfered* with daily lives and the degree of interference.

Ethnomedicine would require a model of illness behavior and perhaps several levels of behavioral analysis and diagnosis of disease. Such a model of illness behavior is an abstract and systematic statement of how treatment-related actions and causes unfold and how these actions and the causes might be explained. Such a model could be applied within any culture after information about the social categories, customs, and behavior had been obtained.

A more socially oriented illness paradigm would help doctor–patient exchanges and increase sensitivity to cross-cultural variations. Indeed, a social perspective toward disease and medical care that is grounded in ethnomedicine could dampen, if not eliminate, the hazards Engel has associated with the biomedical model.

In order to provide culture-specific information relevant to ethnomedicine, one would need a model for understanding how individuals process information about disease and make decisions on medical care. Fabrega (1974) has listed topics relevant to this concern. We have taken his topics and expanded them for utility in different cultures. The model we have developed is presented in Figure 1.

The model provides a framework for understanding how the individual processes information about disease and how he makes decisions regarding medical care. In order to effectively bring health care to other nations, we must understand their perspective of disease and medical care. This model suggests the components that feed into an individual's conception of disease in any culture.

The individual and his conception of sickness (biomedically known as disease) lies at the core of this formulation. The three-dimensional cube surrounding the person represents the different forces, concerns, and components that affect their conception of "being sick" and of requiring medical treatment. The individual surrounded by those immediate influences rests in a country or part of a country that is at a particular level of national development. That level can be raised or lowered and is important as it affects the availability and feasibility of certain types of medical care. At any given time, the individual is affected by his cultural heritage. It permeates his experience and is represented here as a bubble surrounding the individual.

Most salient to the individual are the factors depicted at the base of the cube. The individual's beliefs about how effective and useful certain systems of medicine are, his beliefs about what causes healing and sickness, his definition of being healthy, his beliefs about what is inside his body and how his body and mind function—all these must be considered in treating a health problem. Additionally, in order to affect health care, one must consider tendencies to rely on self-diagnosis and self-medication, the extent to which they are willing to cooperate with medical advice and treatment, the value and degree of importance they place on the sick role and on the suggestion of medical care, and the decision making they go through in order to recognize disease and healing.

This model presents portions of information that one must obtain to

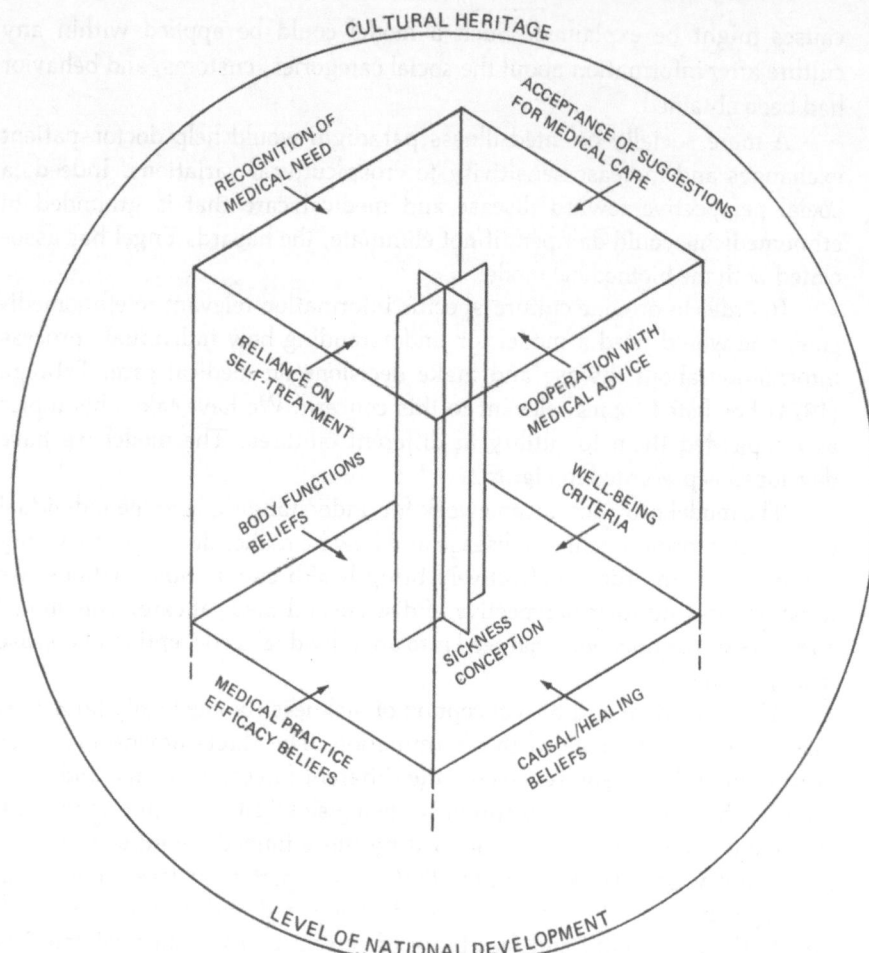

Figure 1. A framework for understanding how individuals process information about disease and make decisions on medical care.

design a culturally relevant health care system. The summation of this information should enable an outsider to comprehend the emic (i.e., from within) view of sickness and medical care.

Summary

This article presents where we stand in relation to the challenge of bringing health care to the developing countries of the world. It has become clear that imposing Western standards and medical technologies without consideration for specific cultural variation is ineffective and in some cases detrimental. Rather than stop at that point, this presentation has provided speculative reasons for the inefficacy of this approach. We have suggested that the biomedical model is at the heart of this approach and that it inherently predisposes this approach to be inadequate. We have also discussed some specific dangers it carries when applied within other cultures. This has led to the description of a new medical model, an ethnomedical model, and we suggest it would be more useful. The framework for understanding how an individual in any culture processes information about disease, presented here in Figure 1, is only one aspect of this new ethnomedical model. It provides a data-collection base that would be useful in understanding an individual's view of health within any culture. Indeed, its application will provide critical signs as to how we can better meet the challenges to provide effective health care for all the people of each nation.

In the end, we would like to raise some questions that still need answers: How can we, the rich, be sensitive to the needs of the poor and implement donor programs without creating massive resentment among those to be helped? How can we communicate our programs to the poor of the developing world with a philosophy of distributive justice and social equity?

The answers to these questions lie in many facets of donor programs such as program designs, and types of manpower used. The kind of personnel donor agencies use to direct and implement their programs is a crucial impacting variable.

If a physician or a social scientist with a biomedical orientation is at the helm of affairs, they will, in all sincerity, use the biomedical approach. Therefore, the need is for bureaucracies to be culturally sensitive, and to have a proper mix of health scientists, social scientists, and community participants like traditional healers. Another need is to train donor personnel in the country's culture. Western donor technocrats need to receive early education or training in a particular country. It may be that a 2-year assignment on an Indian Health Service reservation is needed; it is hard to learn of the health problems of those living in remote areas from an embassy compound with air conditioning, clubs, restaurants, etc.

An additional issue to consider is the motivation of the donor bureaucracies in implementing these programs. Is it self-interest or is it the spirit of mutual collaboration that has led to funding of the project by a donor nation? Are there legislatures and others giving humanitarian justifications while there are political reasons behind the funding? Answers to these questions are important to bring honesty into the process. Political motives are legitimate, provided we are honest about them. There may be multiple motives, but that, too, needs to be discussed openly. The motives will affect the effort, direction, manpower, and content of these programs. All these elements contribute to the effectiveness of a program and realistic planning to meet the goals of the donor and recipient nations.

Community participation is another step that we would like to see included in the agenda of donor projects. Most donor projects provide advisors to the ministers of health and do not advocate community participation. Direction and advice to the top personnel in the Ministry of Health are needed, but acceptance of such advice does not mean that a program will get implemented or that it will be successful. Needed is the emphasis that projects must be planned and managed to some degree by the local people. The donor bureaucracies could work directly with community boards and local healers, as we have started doing in the United States. The community participation approach is not simple, but it can be effective and it offers the greatest long-range benefits. Its bigger antagonists are donors and host country bureaucracies—not the people. International bureaucracies need more personnel oriented toward community work who are willing to take less influential positions very often in more remote places. This means less personnel to advise ministers and secretaries of health. More than that we need the determination of the leaders at the top that, God willing, they will help the poor of the world into managing their own affairs. This is as possible as is the approach to human rights.

References

Ahmed, P. I., & Plog, S. C. State mental hospitals: What happens when they close? New York: Plenum, 1976.

Bryant, J. Health and the developing world. Ithaca: Cornell University Press, 1969.

Cahill, K. M. Health and development. New York: Orbis, 1976.

Dubos, R. Mirage of health: Utopia's progress and biological change. New York: Harper & Row, 1959.

Engel, G. L. The need for a new medical model: A challenge for biomedicine. Science, 1977, 196, 129–136.

Fabrega, H., Jr. Disease and social behavior: An interdisciplinary perspective. Cambridge, Mass.: M.I.T. Press, 1974.

Fabrega, H., Jr. The need for an ethnomedical science. Science, 1975, 189, 969–975.

Foster, J. Medical anthropology and international health planning. Social Science and Medicine, 1977, 11, 527 534.

Ludwig, A. M. The psychiatrist as physician. Journal of the American Medical Association, 1975 235, 603–604.

Paul, B. D. Health culture and community. New York: Russell Sage Foundation, 1955.

Plog, S. C., & Ahmed, P. I. Principles and techniques of mental health consultation. New York: Plenum, 1977

Simmons, O. C. Popular and modern medicine in Mestizo communities of coastal Peru and Chile. Journal of American Folklore, 1955, 68, 57.

Waldheim, K. Health in a world perspective. In K. M. Cahill (Ed.), Health and development. New York: Orbis, 1976.

22

Health Care in the Year 2000

Peter G. Bourne

Introduction

In the last 25 years we have seen extraordinary and often unexpected advances in both scientific research and the quality of health care in America that have dramatically changed life expectancy and the quality of people's existence. It is reasonable to expect that we will see comparable or perhaps even greater developments between now and the end of the century. These new breakthroughs may be spectacular, unpredicted, and in some instances hard to conceive of at the present time. Until relatively recently, the major health problems that faced Americans were the same that had afflicted mankind from the dawn of history. Infectious diseases, malnutrition, and metabolic and genetic diseases for which there was little hope of cure or treatment took the lives of tens of thousands of Americans every year as they still do in the developing world. Those most likely to die were children, and their high mortality was an accepted part of the human condition. We have, however, made more progress in medicine and in the saving of human lives in the last 25 years than in the previous 2,500, and it is reasonable to believe that we are now in a phase of accelerated discovery and understanding that will yield similar changes in the quality of human life throughout the world by the end of this century.

Since 1940, we have seen the development of penicillin and other anti-

Peter G. Bourne • Coordinator, United Nations Development Program, International Drinking Water and Sanitation Decade, United Nations, New York, New York 10019. Former Special Assistant to the President for Health Issues.

biotics, the discovery of drugs that control mental illness and have made it possible for hundreds of thousands of people to leave mental hospitals and lead normal lives, and we have seen the most dramatic improvement in our ability to handle conditions that have become amenable to new surgical procedures.

In addition to the more spectacular surgical procedures such as heart transplant surgery, there have been innumerable, less publicized technical developments that have changed or saved the lives of hundreds of thousands of people. Even in the field of prevention we have seen dramatic breakthroughs. Poliomyelitis, once the scourge of childhood throughout America, has been essentially eliminated. As for other childhood diseases, if we merely were able to ensure that all young children were immunized, they would be largely eliminated. Our failure in this area has not been one of medical science but of managerial and administrative competence.

While there are still deficiencies in our health care delivery system, and we lag behind other industrialized nations in our ability to guarantee every American a basic minimum standard of health care, we have hospitals all over the country with highly trained staffs and the latest equipment unmatched anywhere in the world. Our problem is not one of lack of knowledge or technical ability, but rather one of equity of access, the result of geographic maldistribution of trained professionals and facilities, and continuing financial barriers to adequate care. These problems, too, are likely to be dramatically resolved in the next 25 years.

Health as a Global Issue

In considering what we can predict for the year 2000, we have to make a distinction between the United States and the rest of the world. While changes in our own country may be impressive, they will not compare with the progress we can anticipate in the developing world. It is in India, Upper Volta, Guatemala, Egypt, and the other nations of the third world that the greatest numbers of lives will be saved, and greatest human suffering alleviated.

In the 1840s, Britain, the first nation to industrialize, was in a comparable stage in its development to the developing world today. Health problems were rampant and largely tied to lack of adequate sanitation. The drains and sewers ran into rivers and into the wells from which people drew their drinking water. Cholera epidemics were recurrent, and life expectancy in the industrialized cities of Northern England was about 17 years because the majority of babies were dead of gastritis before the age of 5.

For 30 years, Edwin Chadwick, with a small group of supporters including novelist Charles Dickens, struggled against special interests, ignorance, and the conviction that "nothing can be done" to achieve one of the truly heroic engineering feats of the late Victorian period. Sewage was safely separated from drinking water, safe reservoirs were built with pumping and treatment stations. The result was an unprecedented reduction in infant mortality and a rapid elimination of cholera and other diseases that had always been taken for granted.

In many developing countries today, we stand on the threshold of making the same changes Chadwick made. For years there has been a sense of hopelessness. The diseases of squalor were accepted as part of the human condition. That is changing and in most developing countries there is a recognition that it can be different. The water can be cleaned up as it was in London 150 years ago. In particular, the success led by the World Health Organization in eradicating smallpox from the world has taught people that the traditional cripplers and killers of mankind are not as invulnerable as we once thought they were. It is possible to eliminate these diseases and to do it in a systematic and carefully planned way.

There is a long way to go. Malaria still afflicts 300–400 million people a year, killing a million children in Africa. Schistosomiasis affects 200 million and leprosy infects 15 million. Gastroenteritis kills tens of millions of children every year and countless others die from a wide range of diseases that are the inevitable accompaniment of absolute poverty, malnutrition, and poor sanitation.

The most dramatic change that will occur in the next 25 years will be the provision of sanitation and clean drinking water in the developing world and the control or elimination of most of these diseases. A vaccine for malaria will almost certainly come before the end of the century and the development of a heat-stable measles vaccine will save millions of children in Africa. The reduction in gastroenteritis that clean drinking water can provide will drop infant mortality and, in some countries, double the life expectancy.

Most developing countries lack not only adequate numbers of trained health professionals but also any semblance of a health care delivery infrastructure. It is to be hoped that in this they may benefit from the lessons learned in the United States, where our overfocus on tertiary care, and our highly trained physicians, has led us to develop a system that places its greatest emphasis on crisis care rather than prevention, and where access to care is tied not to need but to economic status. The Chinese and, to a lesser extent, the Cubans have taught us that you can provide basic health care for everyone without waiting to train a doctor for every village. Community health workers, or "barefoot doctors," clearly can offer the basic health care that is now lacking throughout most of the developing world. Within the next 25 years I believe we will see the development of an effective health care infrastructure in most developing countries that will follow the model of China much more closely than it will follow our own. There will be, however, an overall narrowing of the difference in the health problems of the developing and developed world. As infectious diseases and malnutrition are conquered, and as industrialization and affluence spread, the peoples of the developing world will be increasingly afflicted with the diseases of living well, which now afflict Americans and West Europeans. Traumatic injury from automobile accidents, alcoholism, obesity and heart disease, cancer, mental illness, and suicide all are likely to become the dominant concerns of the developing nations.

An uninformed and callous argument that is frequently made against improving health care in the developing world is that it will only lead to more mouths to feed in societies where food is already scarce. You will save them from disease to die of starvation, they say. Apart from the humanitarian arguments against such a position, it is clear that the number of children people have is directly tied to the infant mortality rate. Particularly in developing countries, people look upon children as a form of social security to take care of them in their old age. Once the quality of health care rises and infant mortality declines beyond certain levels, then the motivation to limit family size and accept birth control methods rises dramatically. It is also true that as people are afflicted less with debilitating diseases such as malaria, their work productivity increases correspondingly. This means not only greater agricultural production but also an increase in the overall gross national product for most developing countries.

By the year 2000, we can expect a population stabilization in the developing world with an age distribution that is shifting toward our own, in which 50% of the population is over 40 years instead of under 20 as is the case at present in many countries of the third world. Health problems will become more similar and homogeneous across the globe and the disparity in access to health care will be diminished markedly. The speed with which these goals are achieved depends largely upon the willingness of the developed nations to do their share in assisting less fortunate nations to make these changes.

Health in the United States

The population of the United States, and that of the rest of the world, is in transition and will be quite different in the year 2000 from what it is today. The birth rate in the United States has gone steadily down while life expectancy has been extended, a trend that is likely to continue. Not only are fewer children and young people dying from infectious diseases, but a higher percentage than ever before of those born today will live to be over 65. This means that quite apart from those diseases we are now able to treat that we could not 20 years ago, the types of illness will change anyway with the aging population. The bulk of the people in the United States already die from degenerative diseases that are an inherent part of aging, such as cardiovascular disease, cancer, or conditions that can be attributed to life-style, poor diet, alcoholism, drug abuse, automobile accidents, cigarette smoking, suicide, and homicide. In the year 2000, health care in America is likely to be even more concerned with these conditions, as the trends in Table I suggest.

The changing role of women in American society, which is likely to continue to progress during the next 25 years, will have a profound effect as yet not fully determined on the health and health care system of America. With the control of venereal disease, and a woman's ability to limit with considerable effectiveness the advent of pregnancy (an ability substantially enhanced by the ready availability of safe abortions since the Supreme Court decision in 1973), not merely women's sexual role but their total role in society has been affected. They are now free to compete in the market-place for jobs at all levels essentially on a par with men. Similarly, the health problems of women are likely to parallel increasingly those of men. Women smoke more and the incidence of heart disease and lung cancer is rising as a result. The traditional hazards of childbirth have been largely eliminated so that maternal mortality is now and is likely to remain negligi-ble in routine deliveries. A new problem has arisen, however, as a result of our increased knowledge and technology. As we have improved our skills in fetal monitoring, our concern with saving the lives of unborn children who in previous generations would have been lost has grown dramatically. The result has been a remarkable climb in the number of Caesarean sections performed, so that now more than 20% of all deliveries are Caesarean. The

Table I. Ten Leading Causes of Death, Precentage Distribution by Cause. Total Population 1+ Years of Age USA, 1976

Cause	No. of Deaths	Rate Per 100,000	Percentage of Total
Heart disease	723,049	341.7	38.9
Cancer	377,185	178.2	20.3
Cerebrovascular disease	188,473	89.1	10.1
Influenza and pneumonia	59,895	28.3	3.2
All other accidents	52,645	24.9	2.8
Motor vehicle accidents	46,778	22.1	2.5
Diabetes	34,492	16.3	1.9
Cirrhosis of liver	31,407	14.8	1.7
Arteriosclerosis	29,358	13.9	1.6
Suicide	26,828	12.7	1.4

result has been a resurgence in maternal mortality as we at the same time save the lives of more and more children. In addition, there has been a trend in recent years that will likely continue for women to have children at a later age. As women in the work force increase, so too will the number of first pregnancies over 30. This will heighten the risk of infant and maternal mortality and also of birth defects requiring long-term care or institutionalization.

More important, however, than the changing role and health of women will be the increasing shift of the population to the older age brackets. By the year 2000, 12.5% of the population, probably amounting to 31 million people in America, will be over 65 years of age. This means that in general, the level of demand on the health care system is likely to increase steadily, and the diseases of aging will assume even greater importance than they do now. Heart and vascular disease, lung disease and emphysema, arthritis and cancer are clearly the areas that will receive the most intense attention from the medical profession in the next 25 years. With the exception of cancer, it is unlikely that anything other than incremental improvement will be achieved in the treatment of these other conditions. With cancer, however, the situation may be different.

No single disease entity has ever received the intensity of research effort that we are currently focusing on cancer. More than a billion dollars of federal money alone is spent on cancer research each year. There has been for some time, and remains, considerable optimism that we are on the brink of discovering the causes and hence a cure for cancer. If this proves true, then the shape of our health programs in the year 2000 would be dramatically different. Roughly 300,000 lives a year would be saved and the reduction of the national health budget would be prodigious. Apart from the extraordinary alleviation of human suffering, not merely for those afflicted but also for their families, the elimination of cancer as a major health problem would radically alter the pattern of hospital bed utilization and particularly the practice of surgery. Unfortunately the prognostications about the future of cancer are mixed. Not all experts in this field are optimistic, and many point to the relative paucity of progress in the last 15 years, with the exception of childhood leukemia and lymphatic cancers, despite the intensity of intellectual talent and heavy investment of federal money. There is little reason, they argue, to believe that cancer will be any less of a problem 25 years from now than it is today.

The solution to the cancer problem, some claim, is to be sought not in the disease process within the human body but in the hazards of the environment in which we live. The influence of environmental factors ranging from cigarette smoke to commercial toxins to nuclear fallout in carcinogenesis seems overwhelming. It is clear that in coming years we will be forced to devote considerable attention to identifying and eliminating these factors if we are to control or eliminate cancer. However, because of the multiplicity of factors that seem to contribute to the conditions, our prospects of effectively cleansing our environment seem limited. The extent to which we succeed will significantly influence the pattern of health problems that we face by the end of the century.

Looking at the overall health trends in America in the last 10 years, what emerges is that the dominant factors affecting the health of our people are increasingly those related to life-style. First, as forcefully documented by the Lelond Report in Canada 5 years ago, it has become clear that cardiovascular disease aggravated by cigarette smoking, poor diet, lack of exercise, automobile accidents, drug and alcohol abuse, suicides, and homicides are preeminent causes of death and disability in Western industrialized societies. Particularly for those under 50, these factors combined far exceed all other causes of death. We will then be faced in the future with an entirely new set of concepts in our attempts to improve the quality of health in the country. Rather than dealing with external factors such as microorganisms, poor sanitation, crowded housing conditions, or malnutrition, we will in the future be trying to cope with what are exclusively behavioral, life-style problems that are determined by factors internal to the individuals we are trying to help. To alter for the better the health of Americans will require education to change life-styles and behavioral patterns, which past experience has shown it is extraordinarily hard to do.

The issue of cigarette smoking provides a clear example of the dilemmas we face. The tremendous detrimental health consequences resulting from chronic cigarette use are irrefutable and there must be very few smokers in America who are not aware of the health hazards they face. Yet, either because the consequences are so chronologically distanced from the act of smoking or because the addictive effects of nicotine and the immediately reinforcing effects of cigarettes are so strong, relatively few smokers heed the warning and give up smoking. It is clear that many smokers either have a fatalistic attitude toward the consequences of smoking or, while accepting the overall statistical risk, believe firmly that they will not individually be victims. At the same time, the evidence suggests that the majority of those who smoke would prefer to be nonsmokers but lack the will or ability to change. Even in the Soviet Union and China, where most other public health problems have been successfully dealt with by fiat, cigarette smoking continues unabated.

There have been in recent years intensive education programs aimed specifically at young people, who, it is argued, could be more susceptible to anticigarette warnings before they become habituated users. There is some evidence that this approach may be having some effect. However, the fact remains that we do not yet have the techniques necessary to change smoking behavior to a sufficient degree to significantly reduce the death rate and other health consequences. The same holds true for alcoholism and for acts of violence, whether perpetrated in automobiles or directly by one individual on another.

One area where we have achieved some success is in inducing people to exercise. Jogging is no longer an activity of eccentrics but has gained considerable social acceptance. However, even here the numbers involved are small. While still the most overweight nation in the world, we have been able also to achieve extraordinary public concern about dieting. This concern, however, seems to be tied more to vanity with regard to physical appearance than to concern over one's underlying health.

While we may be able to define people's behavior as unhealthy or even foolish, we cannot for the most part make them change. If we are then to reduce the adverse health statistics that these activities lead to, then the government must look for ways of minimizing the hazards involved. The government actively encourages the use of cigarettes with lower tar and nicotine; in some places this is encouraged by reducing the tax on those brands with less of these substances. We try to build cars that are safer, with air bags and seat belts, and we impose speed limits. We have seen, however, the strong public reaction to mandatory seat belts and the flagrant violation of the 55 mile-an-hour speed limit. There is clearly a point beyond which the public does not want to be pushed, even in the interest of saving lives.

It is clear that as we seek to come to grips in the next 20 years with these major causes of mortality and morbidity that are tied so significantly to life-style, we will have to grapple with some fundamental philosophical issues in society. The question of how far government can legitimately go in a free society to protect people from the adverse consequences of self-indulgent behavior is open to question. In totalitarian societies this issue does not arise, and government takes whatever steps are necessary to improve the health of society. However, the very essence of the democratic system is that it depends on allowing people to make informed decisions, with government's responsibility being to ensure that people have adequate information to make those decisions. If people elect them to satisfy short-term needs and seek immediate gratification at the expense of their own health in the long run, is it up to society to dispute their right to do so and dictate to them what is in their own best interests? Some would argue that it is.

I think that in the long run over the next 25 years the tendency will be for society to assume greater and greater responsibility for individual behavior. Not only will there be a greater attempt to change behavior through education but individual liberties are likely to be infringed upon in the interest of the larger society, with specific controls being imposed to prevent unhealthy behavior. As with the antihijacking procedure, the population is likely to accept that its own best interests are being served in the long run.

The Ethical Frontiers of Medicine

The scientific advances in the field of medicine in recent years have presented us with some extraordinary ethical dilemmas posing problems that have ramifications far beyond medicine to society as a whole.

Robin Cook[1] in his book and movie *Coma*, reveals a whole series of ethical dilemmas that will face us in the coming years as a result of the extraordinary advances we have achieved in medical science.

Genetic research, especially the problems raised in connection with recombinant DNA, and even the recently publicized prospect of cloning, all pose serious ethical dilemmas for society. How do we or should we decide the qualities of future generations? Should individuals be allowed to select their children's sex and other characteristics? If so, under what circumstances and with what restrictions? What should be the appropriate responsibility of government, the courts, the health profession, and the general public?

Our capacity not only to create but merely to prolong life with new technology produces serious social and ethical choices. Kidney dialysis is now taken for granted, but our resources reach only a fraction of those who need it, so that every day committees are making decisions about who will live and who will die. With the increasing success of organ transplants the problems are further compounded. Who is to decide whom to help? Do we help the 45-year-old bank executive with a family of four, the 60-year-old novelist, or the 17-year-old high school honor student? Should we commit the funds necessary to help a larger percentage of these people? If so, over what other kinds of health care does this take precedence?

What are the rights of organ donors? How shall we assure a proper balance between the need to prolong the life of the dying and the need to provide an organ for someone who can surely be saved?

Decisions as to what lengths we should go to keep a person alive also remain heated and unresolved. The controversy over the Karen Ann Quinlan case has shown the difficulty hospitals, courts, and families have in grappling with this issue; and the publicity surrounding the case indicates its importance to the public. In another, less well-known case, a Mongoloid infant had an intestinal obstruction. But the child's parents, feeling that having the child in the family would be unfair to their other children, refused to authorize the operation. The child starved to death within 2

[1]Robin Cook. *Coma*. Boston: Little, Brown, 1977.

weeks. What responsibility does society have to that child to intervene against the parents' wishes to save its life?

Of much longer standing and more familiar to the general public, but equally unresolved, are the problems associated with population control, contraception, abortion, and sterilization. You recall the case of the Relf children several years ago in Alabama. They were induced to undergo sterilization by a federally funded family planning agency. Although their mother signed a consent form, she was illiterate and likely did not understand the implications of her consent. Apparently, too, she thought she would lose her welfare benefits if she refused to consent.

If government, the courts, and the public were formerly content to leave health policy to the health professionals, they are not any longer. But at present all these groups exert their leverage only in a groping, piecemeal way, in the process generating much mistrust, misunderstanding, and outright warfare between themselves and the health profession.

Prompted by suits that have come before them, the courts have also made efforts to formulate health policy. The Supreme Court's decision on abortion, and the social and political controversy they have inspired, provide a major example of the thorny interrelationships among medicine, law, politics, religion, and ethics. Perhaps one of the best examples of a recent attempt by the judicial system to establish the court's role in health policy comes from the Massachusetts Supreme Judicial Court. Saikewica was a 67-year-old man with profound mental retardation, unable to talk, terminally ill with acute myeloblastic monocytic leukemia, but not in pain. The state school in which he had lived for most of his life was unsure whether or not it should prolong his life for several months by a long, painful process of chemotherapy in which the patient would not likely be able to cooperate, and which he certainly could not understand. No relatives wanted to have anything to do with the decision, so the school asked the probate court to appoint a guardian. The court did so, and the supreme judicial court subsequently affirmed the guardian's decision against treatment.

However, in its opinion, which was issued in November 1976, the court went on to address the broader question involved, and declared that only the courts ought to decide whether to continue or deny life-support treatment in such cases. To quote from Justice Paul Liacos's decision:[2]

> [W]e do not view the judicial resolution of this most difficult and awesome question—whether potentially life-prolonging treatment should be withheld from a person incapable of making his own decision—as constituting a gratuitous encroachment on the domain of medical expertise. Rather such questions of life and death seem to us to require the process of detached but passionate investigation and decision that forms the ideal on which the judicial branch of

[2]*Superintendent of Belcher Town v. Saikewica*, 1977. Mass Adv. Sh. 2461, 370, N. E. 2d, 417, 435.

> government was created. Achieving this ideal is our responsibility and that of
> the lower court, and is not to be entrusted to any other group.

The court went on to say that it would not, however, take upon itself the responsibility of formulating broad guidelines for use in emergency situations: these should be drawn up not by doctors, of course, but by the legislature.

The health professions are increasingly pushed aside in these important decisions, but no other responsible body has emerged with legitimacy to make these decisions. Various elements of the executive and legislative branches of the government in Washington have begun to address these issues.

The congressional Office of Technology Assessment and the General Accounting Office have conducted inquiries into the impact of different innovations in medical technology and services. Various Senate and House subcommittees and the Library of Congress have also begun to focus on the impacts of various scientific advances for our future. The Institute of Medicine of the National Academy of Sciences has also recently become heavily involved in several of these issues, particularly the controversy around DNA research.

The Bureau of Health Planning and Resources Development in HEW, the Office of Science and Technology Policy, and the National Advisory Councils of the National Institutes of Health have all been active. The PHS itself has been active in developing Patients' Bill of Rights, and since last year the Patients' Advisory Councils have provided consumer input.

One initiative that may be of particular significance, and in which Senator Kennedy and Vice-President Mondale have had special interest, is the Commission for the Protection of Human Subjects of Biomedical and Behavioral Research, which, as its name implies, has considered some of the issues of contemporary health policy during its 2-year life. It ended in October 1977, and the Congress is now considering the establishment of a similar commission on a permanent basis.

The commission in its permanent form would be composed of people from a wide variety of backgrounds, with expertise in the fields of medicine, law, theology, biological science, physical science, social science, philosophy, humanities, health administration, government, and public affairs. An important feature of such a commission, however, would be its independence from control by any of these groups. It would be an independent commission, able to reflect and study issues without the institutional and political constraints attendant upon attachment to a government agency or private institution. It would not be dominated by health professionals, for its chief purpose would be to foster widespread and broadly based debate, reaching out to all segments of society. For, on the broad ethical and policy issues it will condider, all people are equally affected and all views should be heard.

The commission would be able to clarify many issues for better understanding both by the public and by those more directly involved in decision making. Thus, although it would not itself decide issues, it would help society to decide who *should* decide them, and to explore what the implications of various decisions would be. The time has passed when we in the health profession can make all health decisions ourselves behind closed doors; the time has passed when we should want or try to do so.

The rest of the world looks to the United States for leadership on these difficult and ambiguous issues and the decisions we make here will affect health throughout the world. It represents truly the new frontier of medicine, and by the year 2000, if we cannot resolve these issues, our scientific discoveries in medicine may turn into a monster to destroy mankind rather than save it.

The Future of Health Care Delivery

Despite frequently expressed concern by opponents about the extent to which government seeks to alter the present nature of the health care delivery system, the impact of decisions in Washington has been remarkably little and certainly much less than many advocates would like. The pressures of the marketplace have in the past had much more influence on the manner health care is delivered in the country than have decisions by government health officials. The availability of a relatively restricted number of physicians in a sellers market has in the past allowed the fee-for-service system of delivery to continue to flourish. It is now predicted that we will have an adequate supply of physicians by 1980. After that, supply will at least equal, and perhaps in some areas exceed, the demand. This is already beginning to happen and it is beginning to change the nature of the physician's role. There is increasing willingness by the top young physicians to accept salaried positions to join group practices and to work for the government.

As the role of physicians changes, and particularly as the aura surrounding them has been reduced, there has been greater acceptance of broadened roles for nurses, physician's assistants, and other health personnel who were previously restricted to limited roles.

National Health Insurance has been discussed for a long time but it is probably a more viable possibility than at any time in the past. By the year 2000 there is every reason to believe we will have universal comprehensive coverage with the present financial barriers to full access to adequate health care removed. It will affect the nature of the health care delivery system in many ways, some of which may be inapparent for many years. Most important, however, it will put equal health purchasing power in the hands of people everywhere whether they live in rural areas, the inner city, or suburbia. It will tend to foster the development of health maintenance organizations and a greater emphasis on prevention and early detection.

It is not possible to predict all the changes that will occur in the health and health care systems in the world or even in the United States in the next 20 years. However, we do know that they will be profound and dramatic and that we will be living in a world that is very different from that of today.

Index